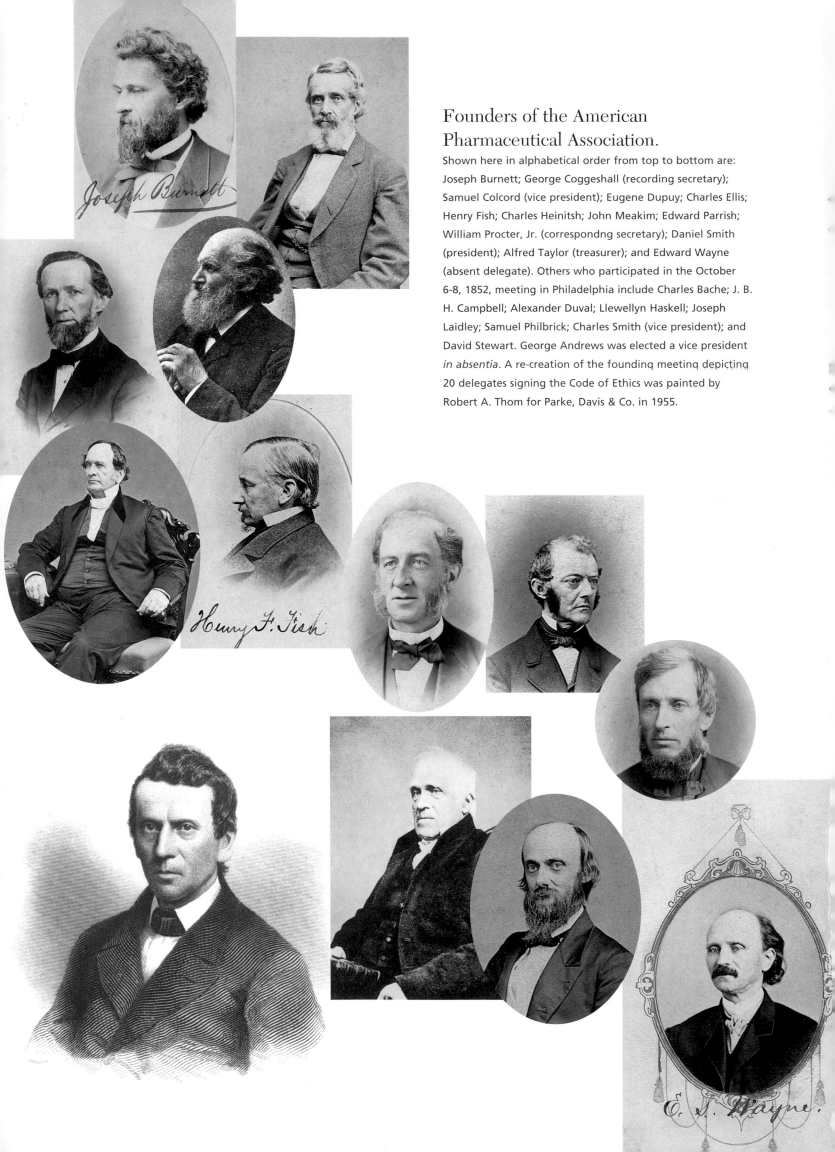

Founders of the American Pharmaceutical Association.

Shown here in alphabetical order from top to bottom are: Joseph Burnett; George Coggeshall (recording secretary); Samuel Colcord (vice president); Eugene Dupuy; Charles Ellis; Henry Fish; Charles Heinitsh; John Meakim; Edward Parrish; William Procter, Jr. (correspondng secretary); Daniel Smith (president); Alfred Taylor (treasurer); and Edward Wayne (absent delegate). Others who participated in the October 6-8, 1852, meeting in Philadelphia include Charles Bache; J. B. H. Campbell; Alexander Duval; Llewellyn Haskell; Joseph Laidley; Samuel Philbrick; Charles Smith (vice president); and David Stewart. George Andrews was elected a vice president *in absentia*. A re-creation of the founding meeting depicting 20 delegates signing the Code of Ethics was painted by Robert A. Thom for Parke, Davis & Co. in 1955.

150 Years of Caring

A Pictorial History of the
American Pharmaceutical Association

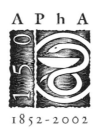

A P h A
1852-2002

By
George Griffenhagen

Collaborating Editors
Gregory Higby
Glenn Sonnedecker
John Swann

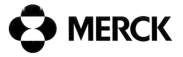 Editorial development and publication of *150 Years of Caring: A Pictorial History of the American Pharmaceutical Association* supported by a grant from Merck & Co., Inc.

Published by the
American Pharmaceutical Association,
2215 Constitution Avenue, N.W.,
Washington, D.C. 20037-2985
http://www.aphanet.org

Book Design by Mac Designs, Oak Hill, Virginia
Printing by Automated Graphic Systems, Macedonia, Ohio

        Library of Congress Cataloging-in-Publication Data
Griffenhagen, George B.
    150 years of caring: a pictorial history of the American Pharmaceutical Association /
  by George Griffenhagen ; collaborating editors, Gregory Higby, Glenn Sonnedecker,
John Swann
        p. cm.
    Includes index.
    ISBN 1-58212-040-4
      1. American Pharmaceutical Association--History. 2.Pharmacy--United
States--History. I. Title: One hundred fifty years of caring. II.Title.

  RS67.U6 G754 2002
615'.1'06073—dc21

                                                              2001053622

Printed in the United States of America

Table of Contents

Preface

This pictorial history of the American Pharmaceutical Association is much more than a narrative about bricks and mortar used to build an association headquarters and various memorials. The main focus of this book is neither the review of the periodicals and publications issued by the association, nor the description of the production, distribution, and proper use of home remedies and prescription drugs.

This book is primarily about the men and women who provided the leadership of the national professional society of pharmacists in the U.S.A. It describes the ways pharmacists have been transformed from compounders and dispensers of medication to professionals who are responsible for the appropriate use of medication to achieve optimal therapeutic outcomes. This volume is devoted to 150 Years of Caring by the men and women who chose pharmacy as their vocation.

Records, such as annual reports and membership promotional brochures, of any association can lead one to believe that an inanimate organization was responsible for various achievements and services the association offers to its members. This is equally true for the records produced by the American Pharmaceutical Association over the past 150 years.

Evander Francis Kelly, APhA's chief executive officer from 1926 to 1944, recognized this when he observed that, "No organization can function by itself, and no organization can operate without direction which must be supplied by its members."

In recognizing APhA's leaders, Henry Armitt Brown Dunning counseled: "It is fitting that in honoring our leaders, we recognize our own obligation to give something of ourselves to the service of our calling." In looking to the future, Hugh Cornelius Muldoon predicted, "APhA will continue to be strong because of the character and motivation of its leaders, and the deep concern of its members."

As you review the more than 300 illustrations in this book, you will see that with few exceptions they depict the leaders and the members of the American Pharmaceutical Association. "It is these men and women who give the color of history," according to Simon Strunsky.

Since this is a story about "members in association," rather than an "association of members," the chapters in this book have been organized by areas of endeavor of the people who provided APhA guidance and support. Chapters 6 through Chapter 16 relate to the practitioners of pharmacy. This is followed by chapters on pharmaceutical scientists, pharmaceutical educators, law enforcement officials, drug manufacturers, and pharmaceutical distributors. There are also chapters on women, minorities, students, and the military.

For the first time all the men and women who served as officials of the American

Pharmaceutical Association and all of its sub-divisions from 1852 to 2002 are identified in Appendix D. Since "history is the essence of innumerable biographies," according to Thomas Carlyle, each APhA president from 1852 to 2002 is further recognized with a portrait and biographical sketch in Appendix C. An Index makes it possible for the user of this book to learn some of the ways that each of the more than 1,500 men and women played a role in 150 Years of Caring.

Oliver Wendell Holmes wrote that, "A word is not a crystal, transparent and unchanged; it is the skin of a living thought and may vary greatly in color and content according to the circumstances and the time in which it is used." Therefore, the terminology found in this book (such as "druggist" vs. "pharmacist" or "drugstore" vs. "pharmacy") is consistent with the circumstances and the time in which each term was used. Since acceptable nomenclature has undergone considerable transformation, the evolution of pharmacy's terminology is described in Chapter 42.

Many of the national and state pharmaceutical associations mentioned in this book have changed their names, some as many as three times since their formation. In keeping with the concept of the "time in which it was used," association names are provided in this book as they existed at the time being discussed. Readers who desire to learn more about the numerous organizations associated over the years with the American Pharmaceutical Association will find helpful guidance in the "Sources of Information" appearing as Appendix E.

An inscription on the U.S. National Archives building in Washington, D.C., reads, "What Is Past Is Prologue." Not only is this message an appropriate epitaph for this pictorial history, but there is another meaningful relationship. John

Russell Pope was the architect for both the U.S. National Archives building and the American Institute of Pharmacy, APhA's Washington headquarters.

As you will read in "Chapter I. Recording the APhA History," Ivor Griffith's 1944 presidential address noted, "I have been surprised, in searching the annals of the Association to find so little continuity in its recorded history. We cannot look forward to our tomorrow with hope of accomplishment unless we know our yesterdays with love and with understanding."

We hope this volume will achieve the desire envisioned by Ivor Griffith, and realize the full importance of the U.S. National Archives epitaph, "What Is Past Is Prologue."

If this is attained, it will be due to a number of people who have provided indispensable assistance in the development and production of this pictorial history. We are especially indebted to our collaborating editors Gregory Higby, Glenn Sonnedecker, and John Swann for their careful review of the historical accuracy.

APhA staff members who have been especially supportive in the development of this book include John Gans, Sam Kalman, and Lucinda Maine; the latter has been so helpful that she should really be listed as a collaborating editor. Special thanks goes to Dorothy Smith for copy-editing, and to Jim McGinnis who is responsible for the layout, design, and production of this book. Even with the invaluable assistance of many people, the publication of this book may not have become a reality were it not for the generous financial support provided by Merck & Co., which we acknowledge with appreciation.

George Griffenhagen

CHAPTER 1

Recording the APhA History

A number of 19th-century APhA presidents devoted a portion of their presidential addresses describing briefly the history of the American Pharmaceutical Association. The first concise histories of APhA were presented by Conrad Lewis Diehl in 1896, and Frederick Hoffmann who wrote the keynote address at the 1902 APhA semi-centennial meeting in Philadelphia.

To preserve the history of APhA, a committee was appointed at the 1868 APhA annual meeting to solicit photographs from members "to be kept in an album [and] to be on exhibition at each meeting." By 1871, photos had been received from 125 members. Ten years later, the photograph album was exhibited at the annual meeting, and all members were invited to insert their portrait photograph in the album. It was then suggested that the effort be discontinued, but this gave rise to a resolution in 1883 that "the photograph album and the collection of pictures of members should not be abandoned." In 1990, the portraits of all APhA past presidents, many coming from this early effort to preserve the APhA history, were installed in the Board Room at the American Institute of Pharmacy in Washington, D.C.

Pharmaceutical journalist of *Druggists Circular*, Clyde L. Eddy, in his capacity as chairman of the Historical Pharmacy Section in 1922 called for "a complete down-to-the-minute history of American pharmacy." He proposed the following chapters: Pharmaceutical Education; Pharmacy Laws in America; Pharmaceutical Associations; Practice of Pharmacy; Commercial Pharmacy; *U. S. Pharmacopeia* and *National Formulary*; Biographical Sketches; Manufacturing Pharmacy; Wholesale Distribution; and Pharmaceutical Journalism.

Eddy thought that such a work could be ready for presentation at the 1923 meeting, and APhA granted $100 to the Section to carry out this bold project. But by 1924, Eddy had to admit that he had been over-optimistic. "While it is my hope," he said, "that the history will be completed in 1927, the 75th anniversary of APhA, it may require ten years for completion." Disturbed by the mounting criticism and the obvious lack of progress, in 1926 the Council appointed a "Commission on the History of the Association," charged with the investigation of the prospects of the project. The report of the Committee, read before the House of Delegates on August 24, 1928, recommended "that the subject be dropped for the present, and the committee be dismissed. We feel," the report said, "that if such a work is to have a popular appeal, it should be an individual effort, written in a uniform easy flowing style, free

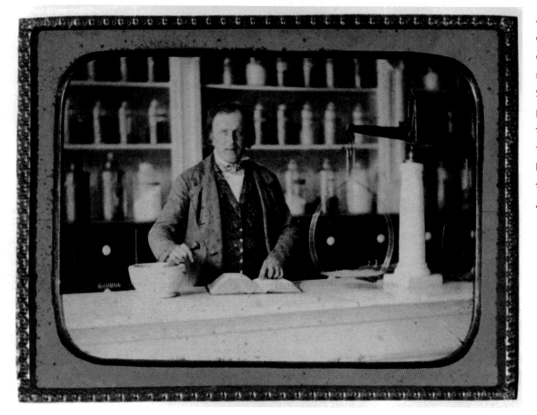

An unknown pharmaceutist checks his pharmacy dispensatory while using a mortar and pestle. This Smithsonian Institution photograph, taken about the year that APhA was founded, is the earliest known daguerreotype of the interior of an American pharmacy.

from dryness or ponderosity. Such a book could not be written to advantage by a committee, even if the subsequent manuscript were carefully written."

In the August 16, 1937, issue of *Drug Topics*, distributed at the 85th annual meeting held August 16-22, in New York City, a dozen photographs of various annual meetings from 1890 to 1916 were featured. *Drug Topics* then offered "two orchestra tickets for the best show in New York to the man or woman attending the [1937] APhA convention who is able to supply us with the names of the largest number of association members found in the photographs of old convention pictures." There is no record of who won these theater tickets, or the number of persons who were correctly identified.

In 1944, President Ivor Griffith recommended, and the APhA House of Delegates approved, a resolution that "the Committee on Publications be directed to proceed to assemble and print an authen-

tic history of this Association from its inception to its 100th birthday, the work to be undertaken by one or more persons competent to interpret this history in painstaking details, blessed with readability." The resolution was referred by the Council to the Committee on Publications for study.

Ivor Griffith's 1944 presidential address adds, "I have been surprised, in searching the annals of the Association to find so little continuity in its recorded history. We cannot look forward to our tomorrow with hope of accomplishment unless we know our yesterdays with love and with understanding."

Beginning in 2000 (volume 40), the *Journal of the American Pharmaceutical Association* has published a series of articles commemorating the APhA Sesquicentennial. They include:

■ "American Pharmacy's Great Transformation: Practice 1852-1902," by Gregory J. Higby, vol. 40, pp. 9-10, 2000.

- "Pharmacy Organizations 1852-1902," by George Griffenhagen, vol. 40, pp. 139-140, 2000.
- "Governance of Pharmacy 1852-1902," by David B. Brushwood, vol. 40, pp. 347-348, 2000.
- "American Pharmaceutical Education 1852-1902," by Robert A. Buerki, vol. 40, pp. 458-460, 2000.
- "The Pharmaceutical Industry 1852-1902," by Dennis B. Worthen, vol. 40, pp. 589-591, 2000.
- "The Pharmaceutical Sciences in America, 1852-1902," by John Parascandola, vol. 40, pp. 733-735, 2000.
- "The American Practice of Pharmacy 1902-1952,"by Glenn Sonnedecker, vol. 41, pp. 21-23, 2001.
- "Pharmacy Organizations 1902-1952," by George Griffenhagen, vol. 41, pp. 166-170, 2001.
- "Governance of Pharmacy, 1902-52," by David B. Brushwood. vol. 41, pp. 376-377, 2001.
- "American Pharmaceutical Education, 1902-1952," by Robert A. Buerki, vol. 41, pp. 519-521, 2001.
- "The Pharmaceutical Industry 1902-1952," by Dennis B. Worthen, vol. 41, pp. 656-659, 2001.

This series is expected to be completed in the *Journal of the American Pharmaceutical Association* by the end of 2002.

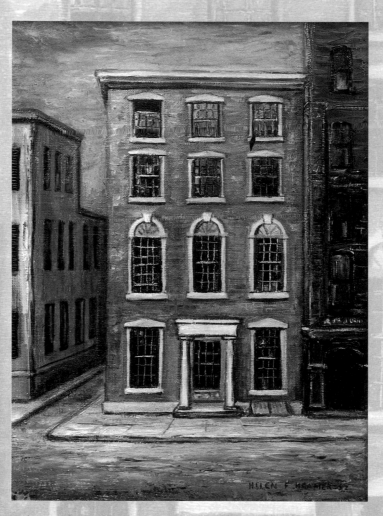

APhA was founded in 1852 at the Philadelphia College of Pharmacy on Zane Street in Philadelphia. This painting by Mrs. John Kramer, wife of PCP's registrar, was presented to APhA during the 1952 Centennial meeting and is on exhibit at the American Institute of Pharmacy.

CHAPTER 2

Founding of APhA

Until 1852, the concept of a national professional society was only the dream of a few local pharmacy societies. The immediate incentive for the founding of APhA was the dangerous condition of the drug market. In New York, Ewen McIntyre had discovered that a portion of supposed calcium carbonate imported from England was actually calcium sulfate. McIntyre's employer, John Milhau, brought the matter before the New York College of Pharmacy. Other preparations were examined and proved to be substitutions, adulterations, or deficient in strength. A petition to Congress, signed by pharmacists as well as physicians, led to the subsequent enactment of the Drug Importation Act of 1848. Another factor in the passage of this law was the use of adulterated drugs by American troops during the Mexican-American War; this led a misinformed Congress to claim that drugs were chiefly responsible for wartime casualties. The corrupt system of appointing port inspectors based on political spoils rather than qualifications, and the lack of established standards prevented the law from achieving its objectives.

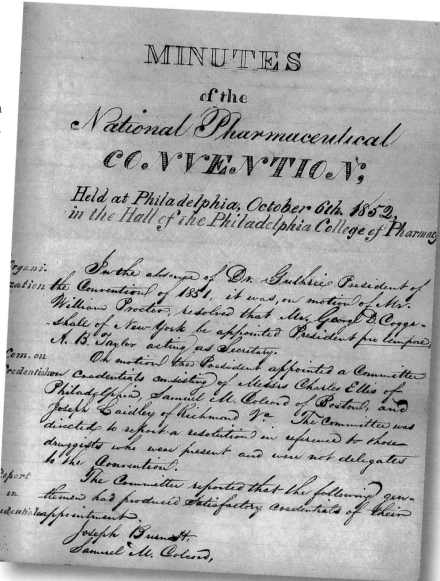

Handwritten minutes of the National Pharmaceutical Convention held at Philadelphia, October 6-8, 1852, in the Hall of the Philadelphia College of Pharmacy. The original is in the APhA Foundation Archives.

In an effort to remedy the latter problem, the New York College of Pharmacy convened a group from several colleges of pharmacy in New York City on October 15, 1851, "for the purpose of

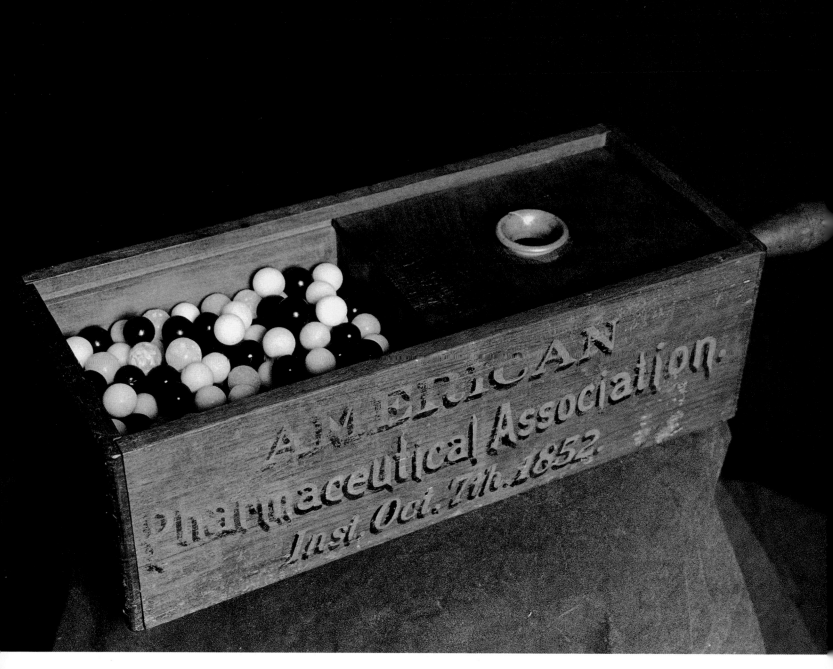

This ballot box was used in the 1870s to elect new APhA members. More black marbles than white marbles placed in the ballot box meant that the new member was "black-balled."

considering the propriety and practicality of fixing a set of standard strengths and qualities for drugs and chemicals for the United States inspectors."

Subsequently, William Procter, Jr., wrote, "when the invitation...was received, several of the members expressed the opinion that although the call was for a special object, the convention might take a wide range in its influence." It was agreed that a convention of "pharmaceutists" be held in Philadelphia the following year.

The Philadelphia convention convened at 4:00 p.m., October 6, 1852, in the Hall of the Philadelphia College of Pharmacy located on Zane Street, with a total of twenty in attendance. The first order of business was the nomination and election of officers, followed by the presentation of nine objectives for the consideration of the convention.

- To create a national association with a constitution and code of ethics;
- To support schools of pharmacy;
- To improve the selection and training of pharmacy apprentices;

- To investigate secret medicines and quackery;
- To urge enactment of laws for the inspection of imported drugs;
- To adopt our National Pharmacopeia as a guide in preparing medicines;
- To curb indiscriminate sale of poisons;
- To separate pharmacy from the practice of medicine;
- To encourage presentation of original papers on pharmacy and science.

The second day saw the convention delegates adopt a Constitution and a Code of Ethics to which members were willing to subscribe. The final day, delegates drafted and approved a preamble to the Constitution and then gathered around a table to affix their signatures to the new association's Constitution and Code of Ethics.

When Did APhA Hold Its First Meeting?

The founders of APhA recognized October 6, 1852, as the date of its first "organizational meeting" in Philadelphia. However, a number of the founders (including Edward Parrish and George D. Coggeshall) believed that the APhA "initial meeting" was held in New York City on October 15, 1851. So important was the role of the 1851 convention in the evolution of APhA that in 1865 the Association reprinted the proceedings of the 1851 convention for the benefit of all APhA members.

When APhA was officially incorporated on February 21, 1888, the incorporators chose to include in the official seal the words "Initial Meeting at New York 1851 / Organized at Philadelphia 1852." On December 12, 1887, ten APhA presidents and five other APhA officials [1] affixed their signatures to the Certificate of Incorporation. Thus the 1888 official APhA "family" acknowledged that an "initial meeting" was held on October 15, 1851, even though the Association was not organized until October 1852.

[1] Signatories to the 1888 APhA Certificate of Incorporation included APhA presidents Maurice Alexander, Conrad Lewis Diehl, Albert Ebert, Alexander Finlay, James Good, Lewis Hopp, John Uri Lloyd, William Saunders, William Scott Thompson, and Karl Simmon. Other signatories included APhA general secretary John Maisch, APhA treasurer Samuel Sheppard, and three APhA first vice presidents: Philip Candidus, Albert Hollister, James Vernor, and the 1887-1888 members of the APhA Council.

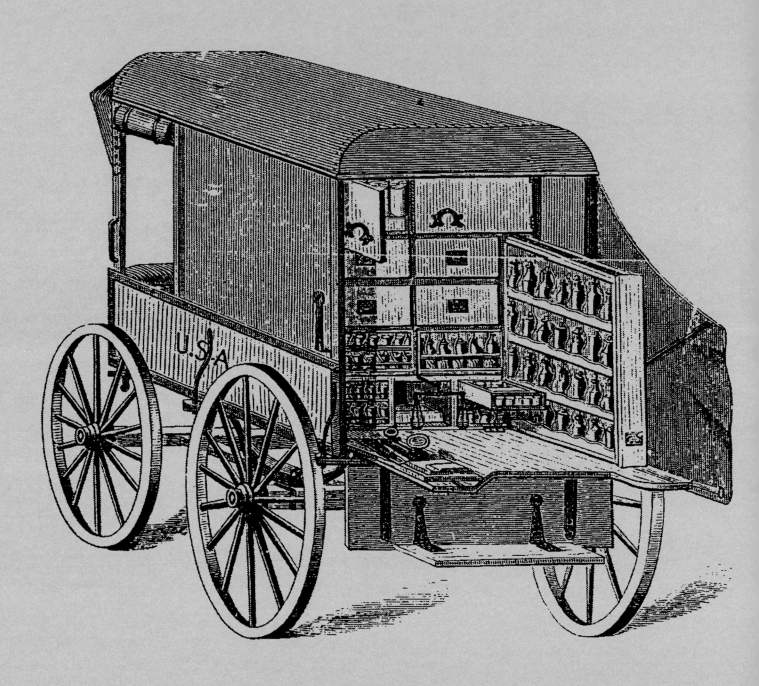

One of several types of wagons used during the Civil War. When the back of the wagon was opened, shelves filled with bottles of medicine and a work counter for compounding prescriptions were pulled out to create a pharmacy on wheels. From *The Medical and Surgical History of the War of the Rebellion*, Government Printing Office, Washington, DC, 1883.

CHAPTER 3.

Sharing in National Crises

A variety of events during the years touched everyone in the country, including the American Pharmaceutical Association and its members. The following represents specific examples that are recorded in the APhA proceedings.

An early trauma to pharmacy and the country was the American Civil War. In 1860, president Henry Taylor Kiersted was gratified to report that, "at a time when sectional strife and jealousy has sown the seeds of discord, it has been eminently gratifying in such times to witness the dignified indifference with which this scientific body has pursued the even tenor of its way. No clamor of demagogues has found an echo here. With true patriotism you have met year after year, from North and South, to discuss like brothers questions involving the common good of all." But this soon changed.

The 1861 annual meeting was to have been held in St. Louis, Missouri, but was cancelled because of "the pending political upheaval." The Civil War began on April 15, 1861.

The 1862 annual meeting was held in Philadelphia in spite of the gloom that surrounded the sessions. The 24 pharmacists who attended the meeting learned that APhA 1854-1855 vice president Joseph Laidley had died from a detonation while developing explosives for the Confederate Army. APhA member Charles Junghanns had died from wounds suffered at the battle of Shiloh. Most of the local pharmacy associations had disbanded, and there was fear that the meeting might be the last one for APhA.

At the 1864 annual meeting held in Cincinnati, Ohio, Jacob Ferris Moore sadly reported that, "the continuance of the war materially affects the usefulness as well as the prosperity of the Association by calling many of our associates in other pursuits and cutting us off from many of our brethren."

Among APhA presidents who served in the Union Army were William Baker Chapman, Conrad Lewis Diehl, Joseph L. Lemberger, Albert Prescott, and Enno Sander, while those who served in the Confederate Army include Philip C. Candidus, Gustavus Luhn, and William Simpson. APhA 1866-1893 secretary John M. Maisch served as chief chemist at the U.S. Army Medical Laboratory in Philadelphia producing drugs for the Union Army.

The 1865 annual convention met in Boston, September 5-8, five months after Robert E. Lee had surrendered to Ulysses S. Grant. "A livelier and more animated spirit prevailed," president William J. M. Gordon rejoiced over the end of the war; he noted

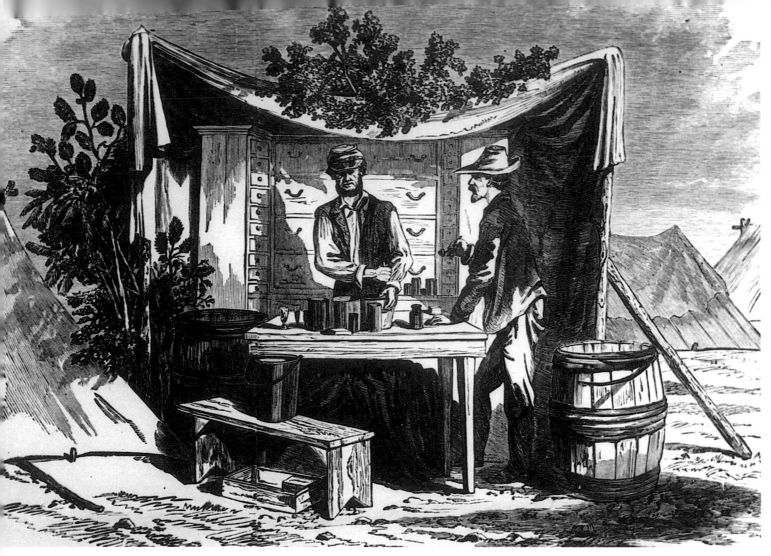

A hospital steward fills a surgeon's order at a Union Army drugstore during the Civil War. This engraving originally appeared in *Frank Leslie's Illustrated Newspaper*.

that "many of our members, particularly in the Southern States, have been practically cut off from connection with our association during the last four years." A moment of silence was observed for those who did not return, such as member John Dodge who fell mortally wounded while leading his company in the attack on Fredericksburg.

It was mainly through the efforts of William Procter, Jr., that APhA held its annual meeting in Richmond, Virginia, September 16-19, 1873. This act of unity helped bring together a war-torn association.

The APhA annual meeting held in Kansas City, Missouri, August 23-25, 1881, was also caught up in an event that jarred the nation. The opening address of the meeting reported that "the President's life is in balance," referring to U.S. President James Garfield who was shot at the Washington, D.C., railroad station on July 2, 1881. He died four days prior to the APhA annual meeting, but the news had not yet reached Kansas City.

Yet another assassination coincided with an APhA annual meeting.

Two days before the 1901 annual meeting in St. Louis, Missouri, President William McKinley died of gunshot wounds received in Buffalo at the Pan American Exposition. APhA's convention proceedings were suspended "until after the conclusion of this day of grief" [McKinley's funeral]. The attempted assassination of President Ronald Reagan took place during the 1981 annual meeting in St. Louis. This time, television broadcasts in the exposition hall virtually closed the exhibits for the remainder of the day.

Members were involved in other conflicts than the Civil War. At the annual meeting in Baltimore, Maryland, in 1898, president Henry Martin Whitney told attendees that, "we honor our Naval Apothecaries who have been working in iron clad ships with the temperature ranging from 130 degrees to 160 degrees F." He was speaking of the Spanish-American War, and took special note of member Walter A. Sellers "who was killed in the *Maine* catastrophe in the harbor of Havana, Cuba, on the night of February 15, 1898." APhA 1929-1930

president Henry Armitt Brown Dunning also served during the Spanish American War.

At the 1906 annual meeting, president Joseph Lemberger described the "great calamity, an earthquake followed by fire which devastated San Francisco [April 18-19]." He went on to report that, "a large proportion of the population was involved in unspeakable sorrow and loss of property, including many pharmacists who are members of the Association. William Martin Searby [who was to become 1907-1908 APhA president] lost his library, but the California College of Pharmacy will carry on."

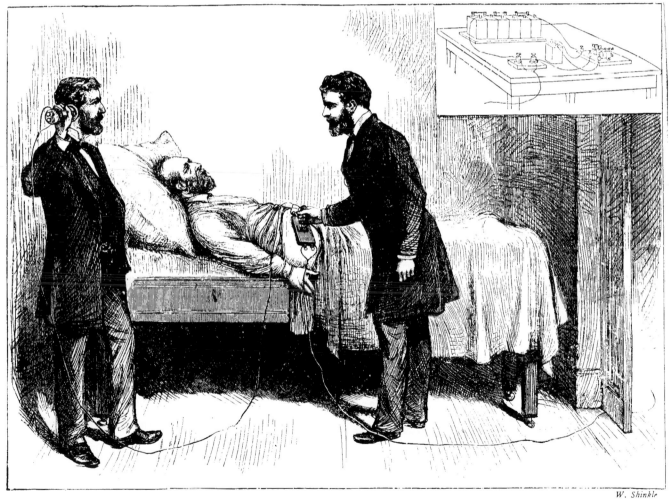

W. Shinkle

U.S. president James Garfield was shot on July 2, 1881, and died four days before the 1881 APhA annual meeting leaving delegates in a state of shock. This engraving from *Harper's Weekly* depicts how Alexander Graham Bell used his newly invented electrical detector to locate the bullet.

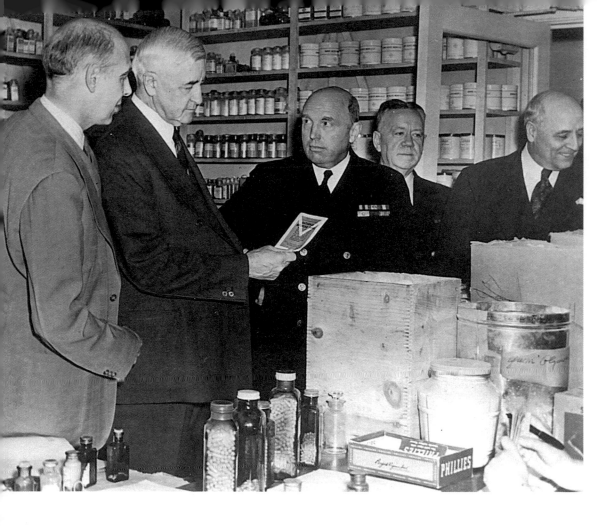

The basement of APhA headquarters was turned into a warehouse to receive contributions of desperately needed quinine during World War II. APhA assistant secretary Charles Bohrer (left) escorts U.S. Secretary of Commerce Jesse H. Jones through the stockpile. Looking on (left to right) are U.S. Navy Surgeon General Ross McIntire; Medical Corp Captain J. J. Kaveney; and member of Congress Andrew T. May, chairman of the House Military Affairs Committee.

President Frederick Wulling dispatched a telegram to President Woodrow Wilson from the 1917 APhA annual meeting in Indianapolis, pledging "the support of the Association in the present crisis of the country [World War I]." At the next annual meeting, president Charles LaWall told attendees, "as the great war continues, we grow increasingly conscious of the enormous task before us. There is a great need for qualified pharmaceutical service for the American soldiers in the U.S. Army." He noted that one of the first "sacrifices" was the death of Kenneth B. Hay who had been a student at the Philadelphia College of Pharmacy before enlisting with the Pennsylvania Hospital Unit and sailing to France on May 18, 1917. APhA presidents who served in the military during World War I include Joseph B. Burt, Patrick Costello, Sylvester Dretzka, Henry Gregg, Earl Roy Serles, and Newell W. Stewart. Following the end of World War I, APhA established a World War Veterans Section that continued for several years.

The December 1941 issue of the *Journal of the American Pharmaceutical Association, Practical Pharmacy Edition*, editorialized: "On December 7th the enemies of freedom, democracy, and our 'way of life' declared war on this country and attacked our Pacific possessions." The following month, APhA published a *Manual for Pharmacists in Civilian Defense*, and provided instructions for the blackout of pharmacies. It was also reported in 1941 that pharmacist's mate Edgar McLaughlin Dodd received "meritorious conduct in action" for the rescue of survivors after the *USS Reuben James* was sunk in the North Atlantic.

In March 1942, the *Journal of the American Pharmaceutical Association, Practical Pharmacy Edition*, reported that seizure of the Dutch East Indies by the Japanese early in 1942 had cut off more than 90 percent of the world's supply of cinchona from which quinine is derived, and announced that any pharmacy having more than 50 ounces of quinine, needed for the treatment of malaria, should report the extent of their inventory to the War Production Board.

On January 11, 1943, at the request of the War Production Board, U.S. Secretary of Commerce Jesse H. Jones, appointed APhA as the agent of the government to receive all stocks of quinine donated for use by the armed forces. This led APhA to set up a National Quinine Pool and the basement of the American Institute of Pharmacy was cleared and allocated to store the incoming quinine. Funds were provided for the employment of six clerks to receive, check, and repack the donated products. Soon the

clerks assigned to this work were unable to cope with the tremendous influx of quinine, and APhA invited the Army and Navy to lend pharmacists to assist. Twelve Navy pharmacists and pharmacist's mates, plus six Army pharmacists from the Walter Reed Hospital, worked around the clock at APhA headquarters. The operation was coordinated by APhA secretary Evander F. Kelly aided by assistant secretary Charles Bohrer and *Journal* editor Robert W. Rodman.

Within the first two months, 63,542 ounces of cinchona derivatives were received from 7,868 pharmacists. Over 16,000 packages containing

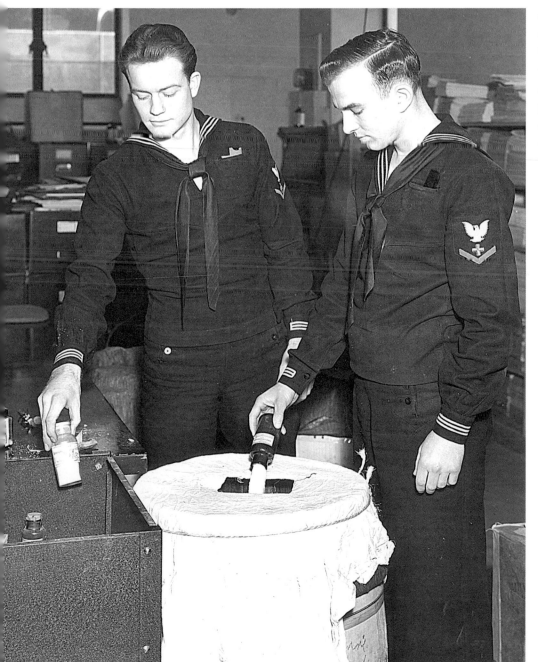

APhA invited the Army and Navy to assist in receiving and repacking the influx of quinine that was arriving at the National Quinine Pool located at APhA headquarters. Twelve Navy pharmacists and six Army pharmacists worked around the clock during the first few months of 1943.

By May 1943, over 16,000 packages containing 150,000 ounces of quinine had been processed by APhA, and each contributor received a *Quinine V-Card* as official recognition for their role in the World War II effort.

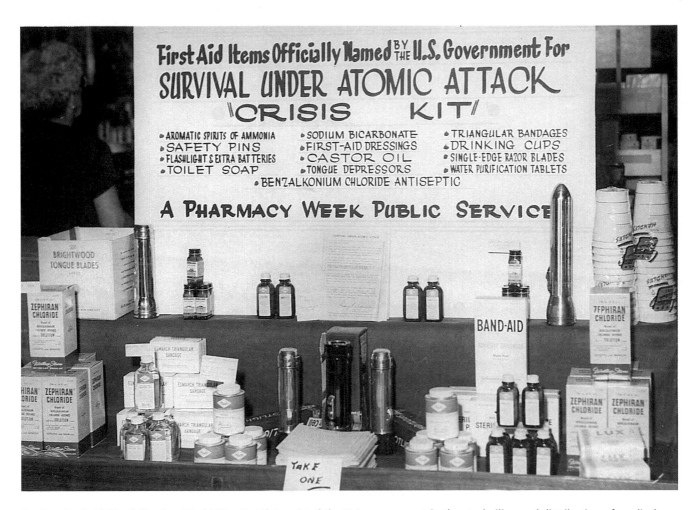

During the Cold War following World War II, APhA assisted the U.S. government in the stockpiling and distribution of medical supplies for use in case of a nuclear attack. This 1960 pharmacy window display advises the public on first-aid measures.

150,000 ounces of quinine and other cinchona salts had been processed by APhA for the National Quinine Pool by May 1943, and were turned over to the military for the troops in North Africa and the Pacific. [See illustration of the *Quinine V-Card* as official recognition for this important war effort.]

Annual meetings continued throughout World War II until APhA announced an "indefinite postponement of the 1945 meeting" as "authorized by the [APhA] Council." The action was taken "since war conditions offered little hope that the Office of Defense Mobilization ban on conventions would be lifted in time to make the necessary arrangements this year [1945]."

Following World War II, and during the Cold War with the Soviet Union, APhA offered assistance to the U.S. Office of Civil and Defense Mobilization created in 1958. APhA inaugurated a program to assist the government's plans for stockpiling, distribution, and utilization of medical supplies in case of a nuclear attack.

After the Bay of Pigs disaster in Cuba, APhA came to the aid of the International Red Cross to fulfill the exchange of pharmaceuticals for the release of

1,113 Cuban prisoners captured in 1961, which had been initiated by President John F. Kennedy. Staff members James and Linda Hawkins spent a month in Havana to aid in evaluating the pharmaceutical needs for completing the prisoner exchange agreement.

Many pharmacists were involved in the conflicts of Korea and Vietnam. More recently, Operation Desert Storm (1990-1991) included the U.S. Army's 47th field hospital in Bahrain, and pharmacists served aboard several hospital ships. [See Chapter 45. *Awards and Memorials*.]

CHAPTER 4

APhA Organizational Structure

APhA was organized as a federation rather than as an association of individual members. The 1852 Constitution stated that "the members shall consist of delegates from regularly constituted Colleges of Pharmacy and Pharmaceutical Societies," and added that "every local pharmaceutical association shall be entitled to five delegates." The local associations seated as delegations at the 1852 founding meeting included pharmacy societies in Baltimore, Boston, Cincinnati, Hartford, New York City, Philadelphia, and Richmond. All but two of these were designated as "Colleges," a term based on English custom. The two 1852 local societies not designated as a "College" were the Connecticut group described by APhA as an "imperfect association;" and the Richmond Pharmaceutical Association whose membership was restricted to "pharmacy proprietors."

Three years later, the APhA Constitution was amended to read: "Every apothecary and druggist of good moral and professional standing, whether in business on his own account, retired from business, or employed by another...is eligible to membership." To gain membership status, each applicant had to be "elected by two-thirds of the members present on

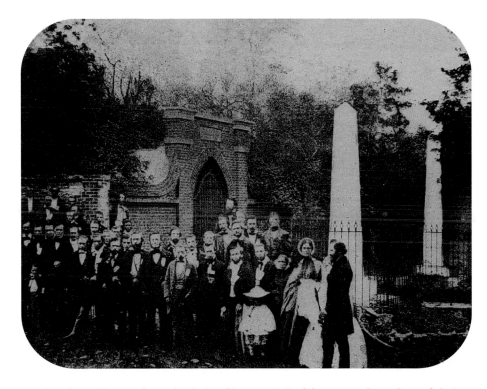

During the 1858 annual meeting in Washington, D.C., delegates and members of their families sailed down the Potomac River to Mount Vernon on the steamer *Thomas Colyer*. This earliest known photograph of an APhA gathering shows the group at George Washington's tomb. Identified on the original photograph are Samuel Colcord; Eugene Dupuy; Samuel Garrigues; Edward Parrish; William Procter, Jr.; and Frederick Stearns.

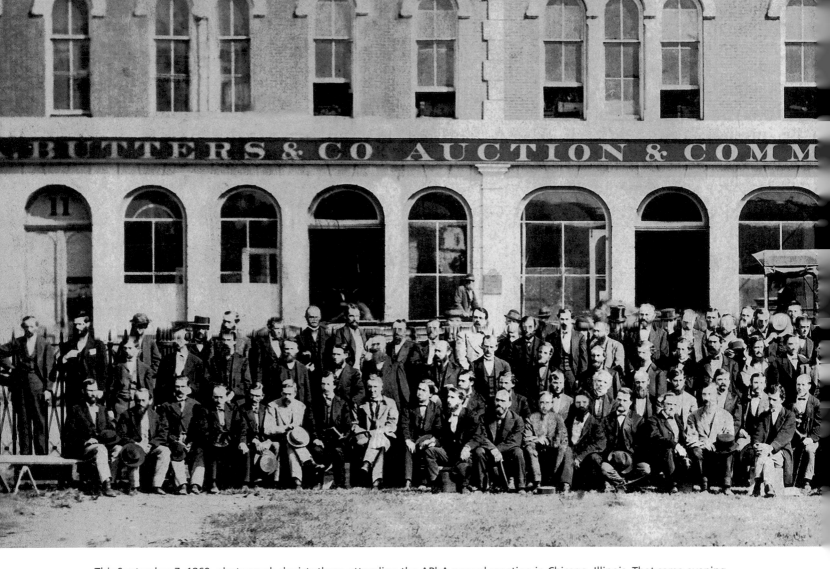

This September 7, 1869, photograph depicts those attending the APhA annual meeting in Chicago, Illinois. That same evening, APhA members and their wives attended a reception in the dining hall of the Tremont House. The program cover for the 17th APhA annual meeting is shown in the inset on the far right.

ballot." However, to be designated as a voting delegate, applicants were "required to present a certificate signed by a majority of the delegates from the place whence they come" or by "obtaining the certificates of any three members of the Association."

By 1858, corresponding secretary Edward Parrish urged pharmacists to organize a local association "in all towns which contain over eight or ten reputable pharmaceutists," stimulating the formation of other societies including Memphis, Tennessee; St. Louis, Missouri; and Washington, D.C.

Two new types of pharmacy societies appeared at APhA annual conventions after the Civil War. The first was a delegation from the Alumni Association of the Philadelphia College of Pharmacy in 1865 which sought to be recognized as a local society. APhA member Edward Squibb objected, pointing out that it could not be a local association because its "members were scattered all over the U.S." However the alumni group was accepted by a vote of those in attendance at the meeting. Two years later, the annual meeting received word of the founding of the Maine Pharmaceutical Association; it was initially considered to be another local association, but in time, it was recognized as something quite new — the first state pharmaceutical association.

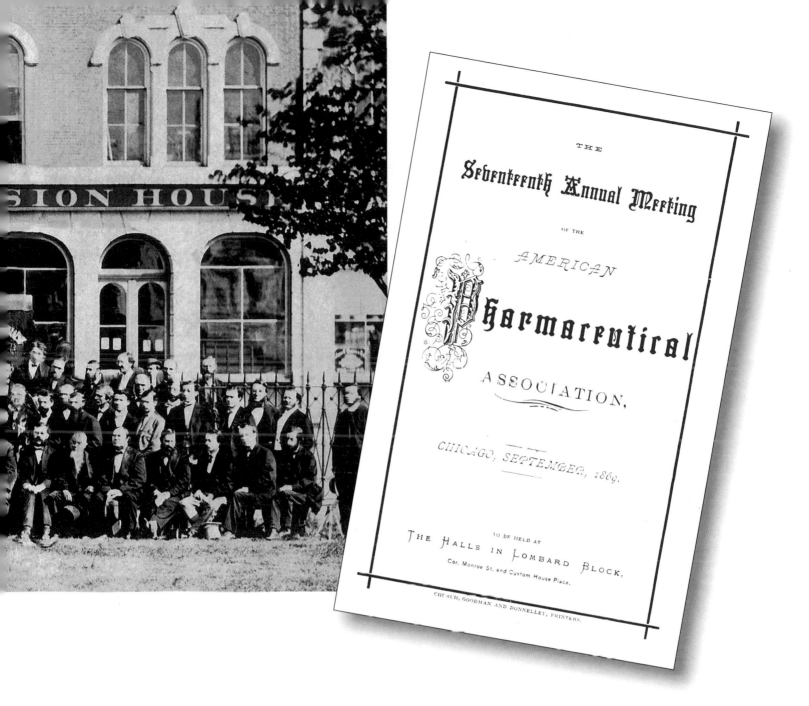

Within 15 years, between 1871 and 1887, a total of 36 state pharmaceutical associations were organized. Representatives of eight state pharmaceutical associations sent delegates to the 1876 annual convention; by 1880, 14 state pharmaceutical associations were represented. This caused concern over the inequality of voting; some associations had up to five voting delegates while other associations had only one or two voting delegates. This led some to urge that there should be one vote for each organization.

Membership in the Association was restricted exclusively to pharmacists from 1852 to 1867 when membership qualifications were extended to include "teachers of pharmacy, chemistry, and botany." In 1863, Edward Squibb proposed life membership, but his suggestion was not accepted. The following year, APhA decided to grant life membership to those who remained a member for at least ten years. Free life membership was abolished in 1867 because of the loss of revenue, although 112 members declined to relinquish their title. A debate ensued in 1866 on establishing an associate member class for "druggists" as proposed by Edward Parrish, but Edward Squibb, Frederick Stearns, Samuel Colcord, and others objected. The creation of a class

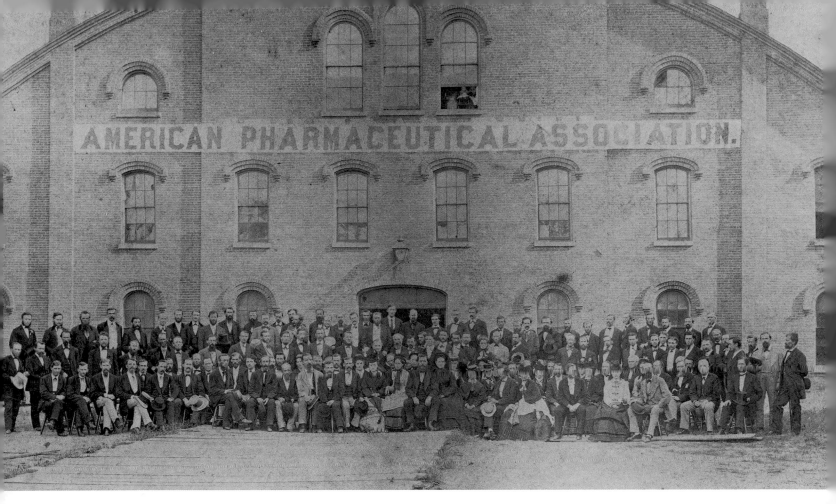

On September 4, 1872, during the 20th APhA annual meeting, 136 members and their ladies posed for this photograph in Cleveland. The building in the background, decorated with a large banner welcoming APhA, was known as the "Rink," and was the site later the same day of a "promenade concert" staged for members and guests.

for foreign members was discussed in 1868, but it was decided not to accept foreign members except as honorary members.

In 1905, "editors and publishers of pharmaceutical journals" were officially added to those qualified for membership. By 1920, the list of persons qualified for APhA membership had become so cumbersome that the Constitution was revised by deleting all references to specific persons other than "pharmacists and other persons interested in the progress of the science and art of pharmacy."

This provision remained in effect until 1945 when the APhA Bylaws were modified to include active members, associate members, student members, life members, and honorary members. This did not satisfy those who wanted to change the definition of "active members" which included "nonpharma-

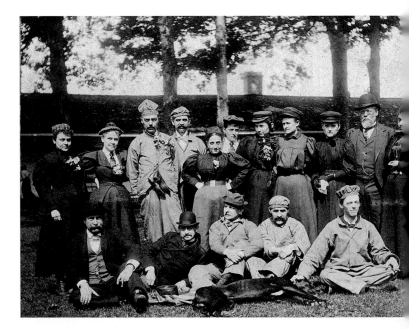

Sixty APhA members and their ladies spent ten hours touring the subterranean wonders of Mammoth Caves at the conclusion of the 1874 APhA annual meeting in Louisville, Kentucky. Those identified in this photo at Mammoth Caves are (standing) Mrs. Henry Whelpley, Mr. and Mrs. James Lilly, and on the far right Mr. and Mrs. Conrad Lewis Diehl.

cists who are desirous of advancing the profession of pharmacy." In 1957, the APhA House of Delegates recommended that active membership be limited to pharmacists; in 1961, APhA amended the Bylaws limiting "active membership" to pharmacists, later defined as "individuals licensed to practice pharmacy in the United States or holding an earned degree in pharmacy which qualifies the individual to obtain such a license."

APhA's total membership had reached 700 in 1866, and broke the 1,000 mark in 1874. It was not until 1913 that membership reached the 2,000 mark from a total of 20,000 pharmacists in the U.S. The 3,000 mark was exceeded in 1920; 4,000 in 1923. By 1943, membership exceeded 5,000, one-quarter of which were student members. In 1947, membership stood at 15,707 (including 5,433 student members); 24,458 (with 9,850 student members) in 1952; 30,000 (including 12,256 student members) in 1958; and a high of 53,460 (with 13,901 student members) in 1980. The total membership has ranged from 39,000 to 47,200 from 1990 to 2000, including an average of 14,000 student members.

In 1852, the officers of the Association included "a President, three Vice Presidents, a Recording Secretary, a Corresponding Secretary, a Treasurer, and an Executive Committee of three." The recording secretary kept the Association's minutes, while the corresponding secretary "attended to the official correspondence of the Association." In 1865, the two secretaries were merged into a single office called "permanent secretary," and then commencing in 1895 the office was called "general secretary." The title of APhA's chief executive officer changed to "executive director" in 1959, and then to "executive vice president" in 1989. From 1866 to

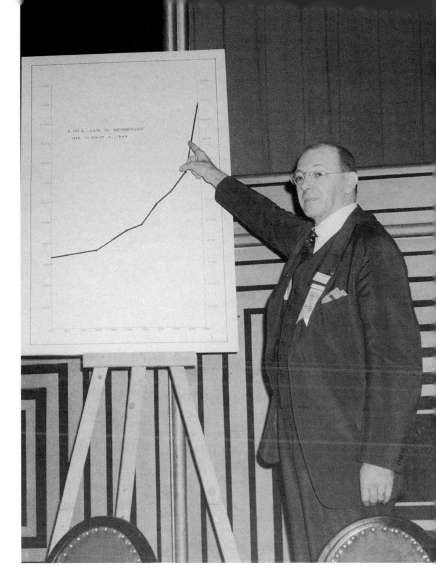

APhA secretary Robert Fischelis reports on the membership of APhA at the 1946 annual meeting in Pittsburgh, Pennsylvania. The membership stood at 15,707, including 5,433 student members in 1947, a three-fold increase from four years earlier.

1925, there was also a "local secretary" who was responsible for annual meeting arrangements.

The office of third vice president was eliminated in 1924; the office of second vice president was dropped in 1969; and the office of first vice president was eliminated in 1980. For a period from 1981 to 1988, the title of the chief executive officer was "president" while the title of the Association's elected president was "chairman of the board." To avoid confusion, the temporary use of different titles is ignored in these pages. (See a listing of all APhA officers in Appendix D.)

For the first time, three candidates were nominated for president in 1864 (William Gordon,

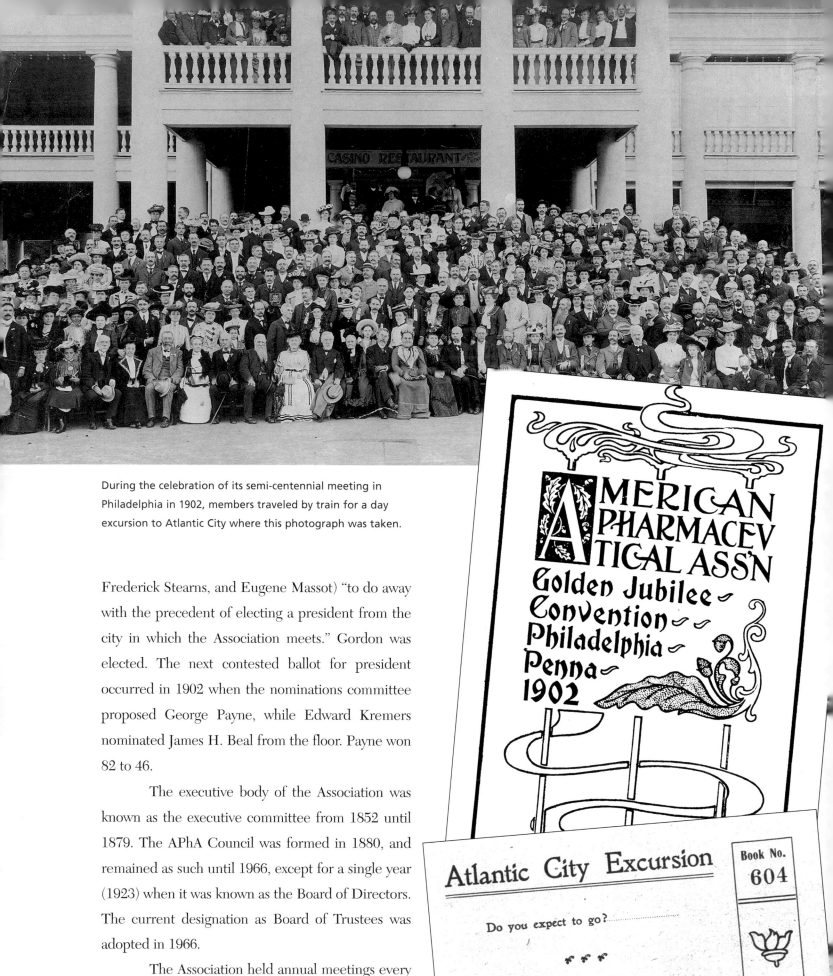

During the celebration of its semi-centennial meeting in Philadelphia in 1902, members traveled by train for a day excursion to Atlantic City where this photograph was taken.

Frederick Stearns, and Eugene Massot) "to do away with the precedent of electing a president from the city in which the Association meets." Gordon was elected. The next contested ballot for president occurred in 1902 when the nominations committee proposed George Payne, while Edward Kremers nominated James H. Beal from the floor. Payne won 82 to 46.

The executive body of the Association was known as the executive committee from 1852 until 1879. The APhA Council was formed in 1880, and remained as such until 1966, except for a single year (1923) when it was known as the Board of Directors. The current designation as Board of Trustees was adopted in 1966.

The Association held annual meetings every year from 1852 to the present, except for 1861, cancelled because of the Civil War, and 1945, cancelled because of World War II. In the early years, most annual meetings (90) were held in August or September; during the last 60 years, most (54) have been held in March, April, or May. The earliest time of the year for an APhA annual meeting was February 16-21, 1985; the latest was November 26-29, 1878, postponed from the first week of September because of a yellow fever epidemic. Cities where APhA has most often held its annual meetings include Philadelphia, New York City, and Washington, DC (8 each); Boston (7); Chicago, Detroit, and San Francisco (6 each); Baltimore and New Orleans (5 each). States in which the annual meeting was held in various cities include California and New York (each 12 times); Ohio (9); and Florida (6), plus five annual meetings in Canada. (See a complete listing of APhA annual meetings in Appendix A.)

Members stop at the Yosemite big trees on their way to the 1909 Los Angeles, California, annual meeting. This was the second time that APhA met in California, the first time being in 1889 in San Francisco.

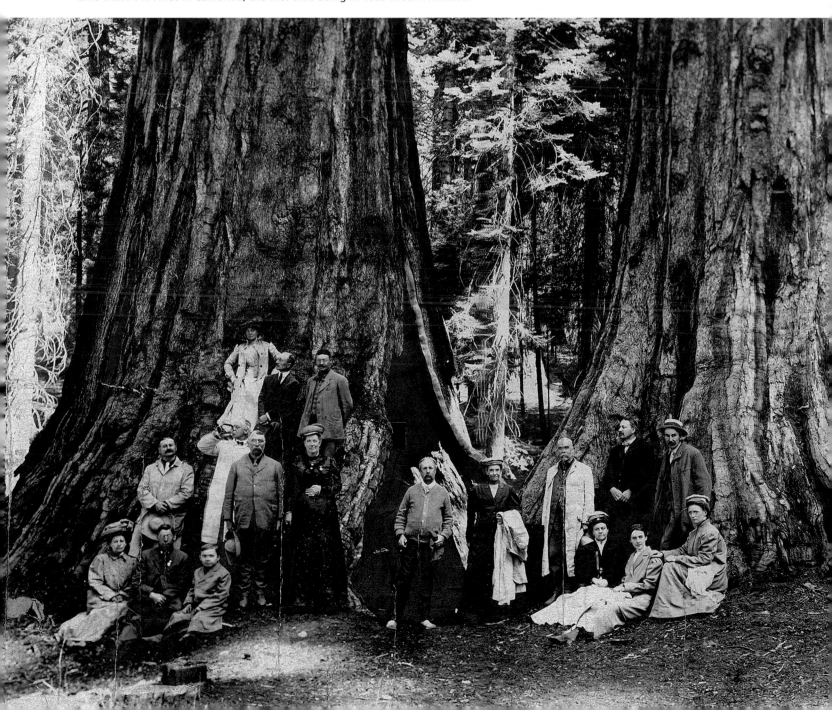

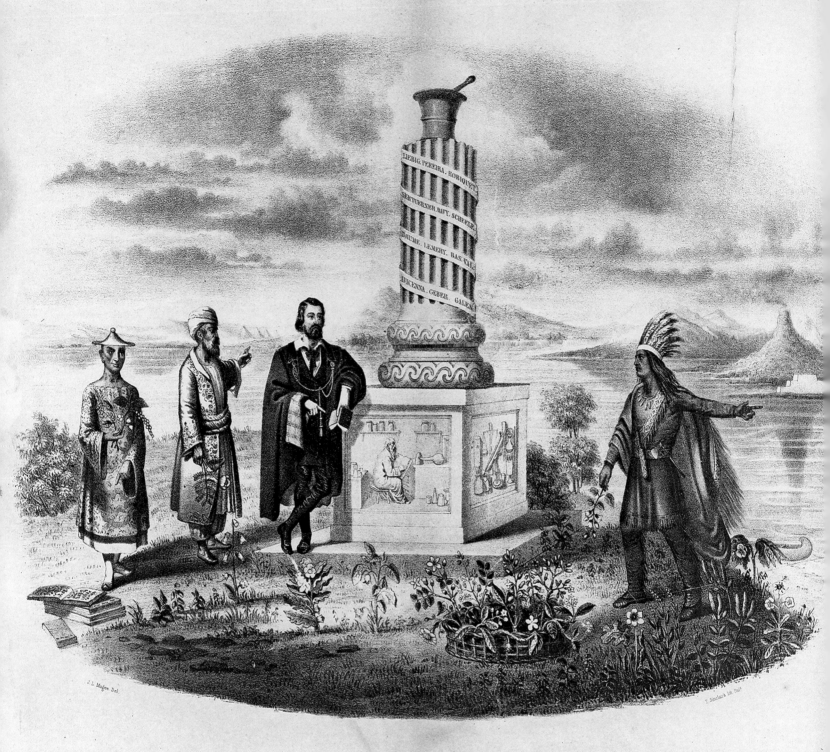

AMERICAN PHARMACEUTICAL ASSOCIATION.

FOUNDED A.D. 1852.

This is to Certify that *John F. Hancock* has been elected a Contributing Member of the American Pharmaceutical Association

ATTESTED this *Ninth* day of *September 1863.*

In Testimony whereof are hereunto affixed the names of the proper officers.

William Evans Jr. SECRETARY.

J Faris Moore PRESIDENT.

J. M. Maisch V. PRESIDENT.

CHAPTER 5.

Membership Certificate

A suitable certificate of membership was considered by the APhA founders as one of the their first obligations. A committee was created in 1853 to develop a membership certificate, but a design was not approved until 1856. The ornate format was laden with symbolism depicting a classic column with a curling scroll listing some of the great names in the history of pharmacy. Four figures represented the Far East (signifying Oriental pharmacy); the Middle East (symbolizing pharmacy of the Arabs); Europe (representing the development of scientific pharmacy without making any reference to nationality); and the Americas (exemplifying the variety of medicinal plants discovered in North and South America).

Objections were soon voiced by members because the design was based on the certificate employed by the Pharmaceutical Society of Great Britain. Members felt that the design should include only "American ideas." But it was probably the pretentiousness of the certificate that shortened its life. Pharmaceutical manufacturer Frederick Stearns was the most severe critic of the certificate, calling it

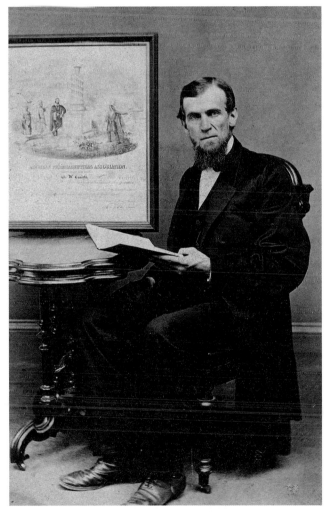

1865-1866 president Henry Lincoln sits beside his framed membership certificate which some members felt was too imposing and ostentatious.

Opposite Page: The first membership certificate was proposed in 1853, but was not adopted until 1856. The certificate shown was awarded to John Hancock who subsequently became APhA president in 1873-1874. The symbol-laden certificate had a short life, and was replaced in 1865 by a new membership certificate without illustrations.

"unfitting evidence of membership in such an important scientific body." In 1860 Stearns introduced a resolution providing for the development of a new design, but it was tabled. The ornate design quietly died when the Executive Committee reported in 1863 that there were only 22 copies remaining, and noting that nearly 50 certificates had been "wasted by mistakes." The last six copies were distributed in 1865, and the following year a new membership certificate was introduced without illustrations. The original APhA membership certificate made its last appearance in 1902 in historical usage on the printed program of the 50th anniversary meeting of the Association.

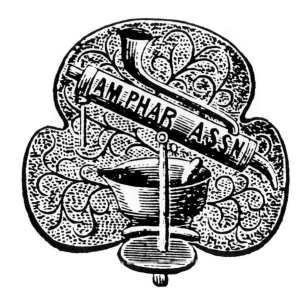

The first membership pin created by APhA was authorized by the executive committee in 1876; they described it as "a leaf with mortar and pestle and condenser representing materia medica, pharmacy and chemistry."

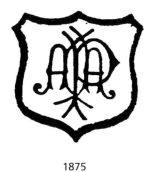
1875

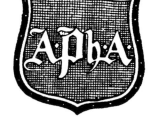
1912

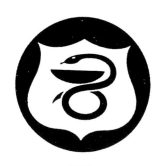
1964

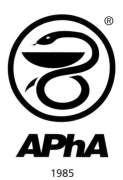
1985

The logo was first introduced in 1875 (using the letters "APA"), and was revised in 1912 (using "APhA"). The Bowl of Hygeia was introduced into APhA's logo in 1964, and was modernized in 1985.

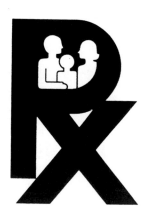

In 1995, APhA introduced the "One Symbol for Pharmacy" to unite the profession and to assist the public in identifying pharmacies and pharmacists.

CHAPTER 6.

Protecting the Druggist

One of the first four sections created by APhA in 1887 was the Section on Commercial Interests which was charged with finding a way to "protect the business interests of its members." Competition in the sale of proprietary medicines for less than the usual resale price established by the manufacturers, called "price-cutting," was demoralizing and resulted in the failure of many drugstores. Significantly, many of the most successful cut-rate drugstores were operated by enterprising non-pharmacist businessmen rather than by pharmacists.

By the early 1880s, there was a growing feeling that the business interests of practicing pharmacists ("druggists") could not be adequately taken care of within APhA. There had been an organization created in 1883 by a group of "retail and wholesale druggists" called the National Retail Druggists Association (NRDA). It soon became obvious, however, that "the wholesale druggist and the retail druggist did not have identical interests, and that no quick results could be expected, especially with regards to price cutting," so the NRDA was dissolved. It was in this atmosphere that the Section on Commercial Interests was asked to support the business interests of drugstore owners. Some described this as a merger between APhA and the National Retail Druggists Association since "it was found that the membership of the two organizations was almost identical," and the last president of NRDA, Albert H. Hollister, was elected the first chairman of the APhA Commercial Section.

During the year following its establishment, "the new Section was unable to agree on a resolution on price cutters." In 1891, the Section chairman reported, "the cut-rate problem is still agitating and disturbing the mind of the drug fraternity. Numerous plans have been proposed, but as yet none seem to be practical." William Alpers, later to become APhA president, didn't help when he told the group, "I believe it will be better for us to devote our time to scientific research and such things as are strictly professional than to spend a whole day in discussing how we shall manage to get ten cents more on an article in which we have no interest, either scientific or professional."

Hoping to understand the workings of the price-cutter, the Commercial Section elected Joseph Jacobs of Atlanta, Georgia, as the 1897-1898 chairman who told the group in his chairman's address, "I have been at variance with what I understand to be the object of the Commercial Section. I think you have made a mistake! You have made an arch cutter chairman of the Commercial Section, and a fellow who is proud to be a cutter." Another Section member promptly responded, "we thought this would settle the cut-rate question," to which Jacobs answered, "it will not settle the cut-rate question. If you intend to kill the Section, you are going at it in the proper manner, but I think it would be better to vote to disband the Section and be done with it."

A growing number of "druggists" felt that APhA could no longer protect their business interests. The establishment of the Section on Commercial Interests failed to allay this concern, and APhA president Henry Whitney admitted in 1898 that, "there is no national body of pharmacists that represents the commercial side of pharmacy."

This led Joseph Price Remington to tell the Section members that, "there is a need for the retail druggists to get together and form an organization in which they will not admit the wholesaler, the professor in the college of pharmacy, or the proprietor of a remedy; but a retail druggists association pure and simple which shall be controlled by the retail druggists of this country."

On the initiative of the Chicago Retail Druggists Association, the National Association of Retail Druggists (NARD), now known as the National Community Pharmacists Association, was founded in 1898. The same year, the Commercial Section moved to endorse the effort being made to

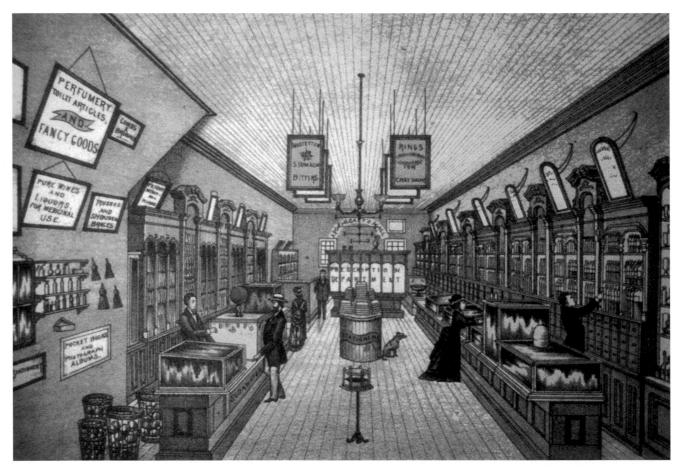

By the 1870s, many pharmacies featured marble counters, costly mirrors, and artistic show globes as seen in this 1876 print of the Elmore Drugstore in Batavia, New York. It was during this period that concern grew that APhA could not adequately take care of the business interests of these pharmacies.

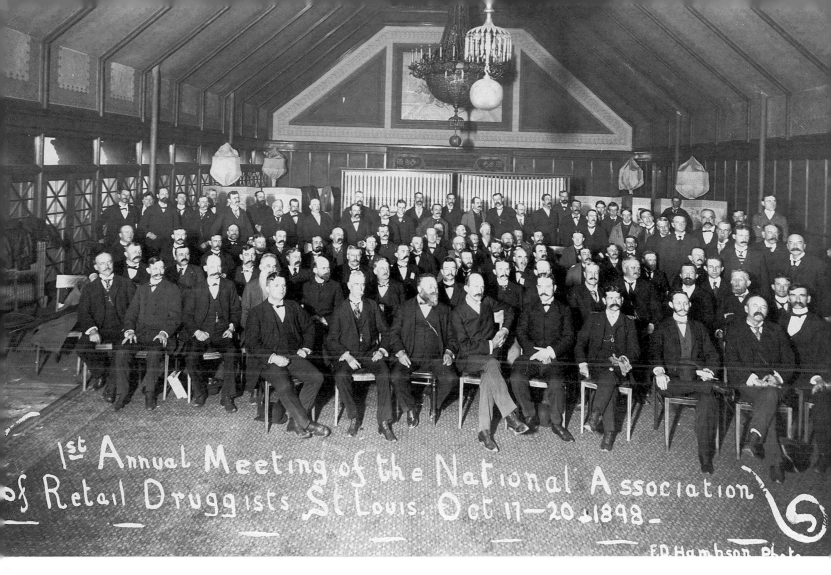

1st Annual Meeting of the National Association of Retail Druggists St. Louis. Oct 17—20 1898. F.R.Hambson Photo

With the support of the Section on Commercial Interests, the National Association of Retail Druggists was founded in October 1898. This photograph from the APhA Foundation Archives captures the organizers in St. Louis, Missouri.

form a permanent national organization of retail druggists in St. Louis, but the motion was tabled. A similar motion was adopted the following year after APhA president Charles Emile Dohme announced that "the National Association of Retail Druggists has sprung into existence since our last meeting and is actively engaged in the very laudable attempt to eliminate the much dreaded and despised cut-rate evil. I sincerely hope the NARD will succeed in its efforts."

To establish closer ties, NARD president Henry P. Hynson was elected chairman *pro tem* of the 1899 APhA Commercial Section. Then in 1901, NARD president William C. Anderson addressed the Commercial Section, anticipating the day when

"these two organizations, standing shoulder to shoulder, shall form the firm foundation on which is built the magnificent structure, American pharmacy." In 1902, NARD executive secretary Thomas Wooten was elected chairman of the Commercial Section, telling the group, "You are charged — unjustly I know — with being out of touch with the man behind the prescription counter. If pharmacy is to continue to be a remunerative calling, the commercial side of pharmacy always must have a champion."

APhA proposed in 1902 that the National Association of Retail Druggists and APhA hold a joint convention, but no mutually acceptable location and date could be found. So in 1905, APhA president Joseph Lemberger suggested that the Commercial

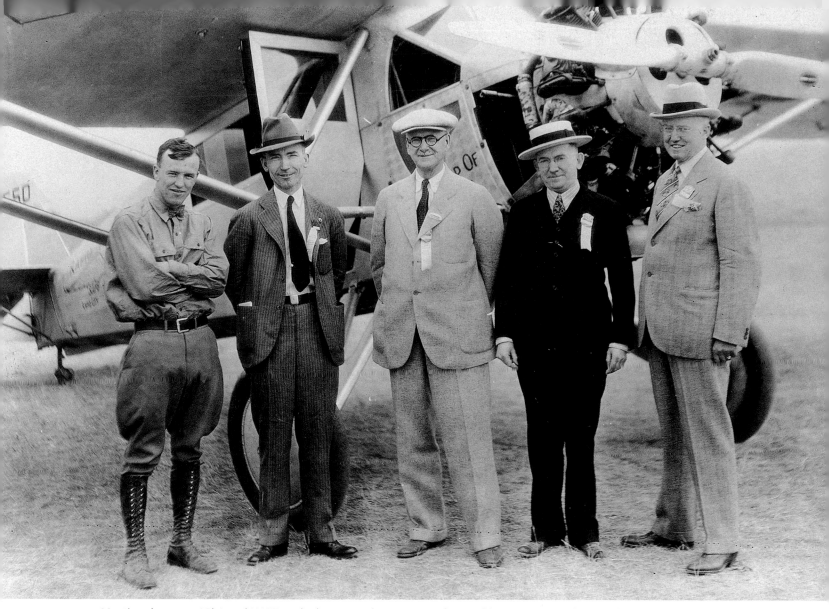

Meetings between APhA and NARD took place to explore matters of mutual interest. One such example occured during the 1929 APhA annual meeting in Rapid City, South Dakota. The photograph shows a group of officers after a flight over the Black Hills. They include (left to right) pilot Ed Hefley; APhA secretary Evander Kelly; APhA president David Jones; NARD president Denny Brown; and APhA local secretary Floyd Brown.

Section be disbanded. But in 1909, Commercial Section chairman Harry Mason reaffirmed the importance of the Commercial Section when he argued that its "paternity has often been regretted, [and] it has usually been treated as an illegitimate son, [yet] I hope that all efforts to kill or stupefy the Commercial Section will cease." The Commercial Section remained active until 1937 when the name was changed to the Section on Pharmaceutical Economics.

It was some years before meaningful areas of cooperation between APhA and the National Association of Retail Druggists materialized. One

such joint effort took place when NARD and APhA established the National Retail Drug Code Authority in December 1933, under authority of the National Recovery Act (NRA). However this effort of President Franklin D. Roosevelt to offset the depression was short-lived. The Supreme Court invalidated NRA, and the National Code Authority ceased to exist on June 8, 1935.

A more lasting cooperative venture involved in NARD's efforts to obtain retail price maintenance for products sold in the pharmacy. As early as 1928, APhA "heartily and unreservedly" endorsed efforts to obtain "fair trade" legislation that would require a retailer to sell at or above the retail price set by the manufacturer. Then in 1935, APhA extended congratulations to eight state pharmaceutical associations "for having secured the enactment of fair trade legislation patterned after the California Fair Trade Act" which was enacted in 1931. In 1936, APhA supported NARD's lead in obtaining the enactment of the Miller-Tydings Federal Enabling Act (1937 amendment to the Sherman Anti-trust Act). Then when the U.S. Supreme Court handed down their 1951 decision that the "non-signer clause" (requiring compliance by all distributors even if they had not signed a "fair trade" contract) could not be enforced in interstate commerce, APhA urged "any movement to restore fair trade to its former effectiveness." Until 1958, APhA repeatedly promised to "cooperate fully toward the passage of a national Fair Trade Act," after which the "fair trade" concept came under increasing

attack by both consumer groups and the Federal Trade Commission. The end came in 1976 when Federal legislation made it illegal for manufacturers and distributors to agree on minimum resale prices.

World War II led APhA and NARD to hold joint sessions of their respective executive bodies to coordinate war efforts. The third APhA-NARD joint meeting was held at APhA headquarters November 9, 1945, at which time they jointly agreed that state associations should form special committees "to act in an advisory capacity to the Veterans Administration [as a way] to encourage the 10,000 pharmacist-veterans to return to the profession." At the same joint meeting, they agreed that "pharmacists should be urged to identify themselves with community health, educational, cultural, and other civic activities as a contribution of pharmacy to community betterment."

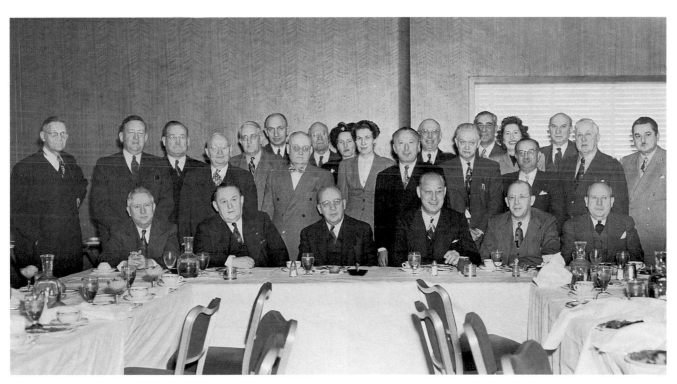

During World War II, the executive bodies of APhA and NARD held joint meetings to coordinate the war efforts. Those seated in this photograph include (left to right) Roy Sanford (APhA), John Dargavel (NARD), George Beal (APhA); Frank Moudry (NARD), Robert Fischelis (APhA), and John Tripeny (NARD).

In 1971, a meeting of five national pharmacy associations was held to consider the creation of a task force to study the organizational needs of the profession of pharmacy. A subsequent meeting between APhA, the American Society of Hospital Pharmacists, and the National Association of Retail Druggists was set for January 28, 1972 in Washington, DC. Representatives of NARD failed to attend, claiming that they had not agreed on a Task Force, and they could not enter into any meeting where a resolution might be proposed.

Two years later (1973), APhA and NARD joined forces to form the Committee on Pharmacy Economic Security (COPES) "to identify courses of action to help pharmacists gain a reasonable return on their educational, professional, and capital investments." The first success of COPES was the *amicus curiae* ("friend of the court") brief supporting the North Dakota Board of Pharmacy which resulted in the U.S. Supreme Court holding the pharmacy ownership law as constitutional. However, aside from its symbolic importance, this Supreme Court decision did little to change pharmacy ownership laws in the various states.

CHAPTER 7

Section for Practicing Pharmacists

When APhA was founded, there were two distinct types of pharmacists. One was called the "druggist" which the founders described as those who were selling drugs at both "retail and wholesale." The other type consisted of pharmacists, variously described as "apothecary" or "pharmaceutist," who mainly "dealt in prescriptions." During the ensuing 50 years, this dichotomy led to the distinction between those mainly interested in commercial activities and those who favored a professional pharmacy.

So while the APhA Commercial Interests Section devoted its attention to the commercial aspects of pharmacy, a new Section was established in 1900 for those pharmacists who desired to improve their professional practice. It was called the Section on Practical Pharmacy and Dispensing, which APhA president John Patton described as "one of the most important moves this Association has made in recent years."

In 1904, the chairman of the Section on Practical Pharmacy and Dispensing announced that, "the Commercial Section has lost a great deal of its attraction for our members," and recommended that "these two sections should be combined." But in 1909, Harry Mason countered that "such a combination would cripple both sections."

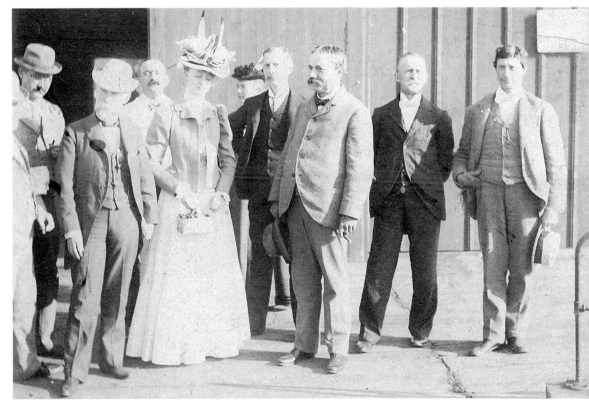

During the 1899 APhA annual meeting in Put-in-Bay, Ohio, members gathered to discuss the need for the formation of a Section on Practical Pharmacy and Dispensing.

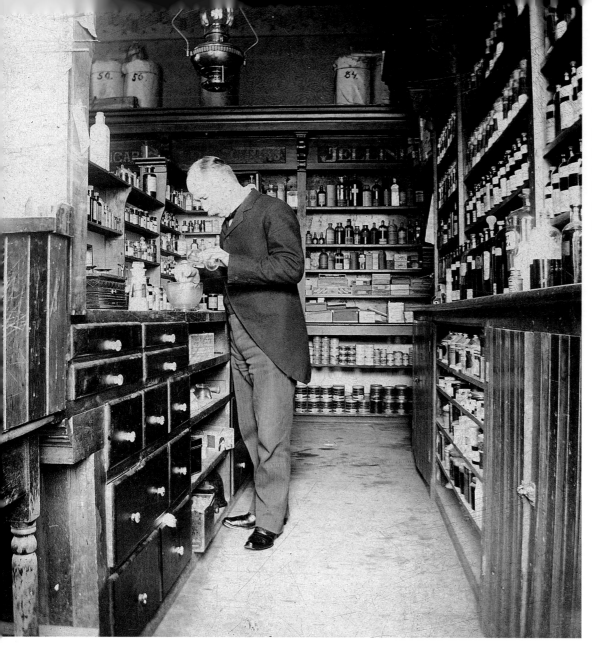

This 1900 photograph shows a pharmacist compounding prescription medication. The APhA Section on Practical Pharmacy and Dispensing was established to assist pharmacists like this one.

During the first four years of its formation, members of the Section on Practical Pharmacy and Dispensing heard lectures on such subjects as prescription incompatibilities, a review of available suppository molds, an apparatus for making a solution of iodine, and prescription surveys. Ampules and sterile solutions were discussed at the Section for the first time in 1909, and the birth of the APhA *Recipe Book* took place in the section in 1910. The Section name was changed in 1914 to Section on Practical Pharmacy with the term "Dispensing" being dropped as redundant. In 1924, Robert Ruth introduced the concept of National Pharmacy Week, and in 1930 incompatibilities in prescriptions were given more attention. In 1932, William J. Husa introduced

methods for producing enteric coating of capsules using salol. The name of the Practical Pharmacy Section was changed in 1966 to Section of Pharmaceutical Technology. (See subsequent chapters for the evolution of this Section.)

In 1966, APhA introduced a model agreement for pharmacists and pharmacy owners as recommended by the House of Delegates which included hospitalization and retirement benefits, plus disability and professional liability insurance. In 1977, APhA introduced a package of insurance and retirement options for members, including liability, fire and casualty insurance for owners of community pharmacies, and a pharmacy employer plan to enable pharmacy owners to insure their employees.

CHAPTER 8

Prescription Pharmacists

In 1914, Henry Vincome Arny (who was to become president in 1923) presented a paper before the APhA Section on Practical Pharmacy and Dispensing in which he stated: "Let us imagine the practicing prescriptionists of this association — not the manufacturers, not the professor, nor the frankly commercial retail druggists — forming an organization called the American Institute of Prescriptionists."

But it was not until 1939 that this was realized with the establishment of the "Conference of Professional Pharmacists," which became the American College of Apothecaries in 1940. The two primary organizers were Charles V. Selby and Robert A. Abrams.

Eugene V. White of Berryville, Virginia, introduced on April 9, 1960, a Patient Record System to strengthen the pharmacist-patient relationship,

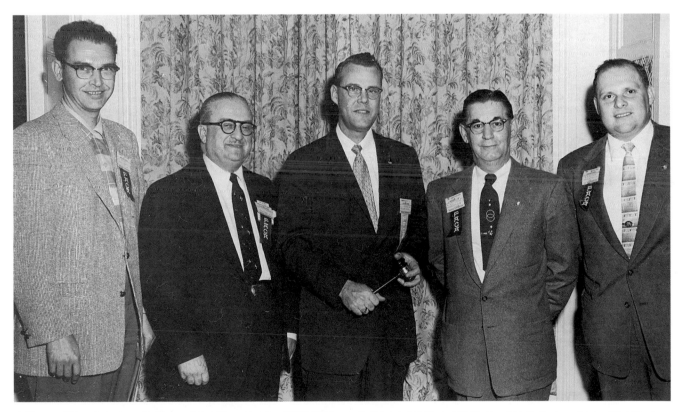

Officers of the American College of Apothecaries for 1956-1957 are (left to right) Kenneth Heinz; Calvin Berger; Leroy Weidle, Jr.; Gerald Nutter; and Robert Abrams. Berger subsequently served as vice speaker of the APhA House of Delegates (1958-1959), and Abrams subsequently served as secretary of the APhA Economics and Administrative Science Section (1966-1969).

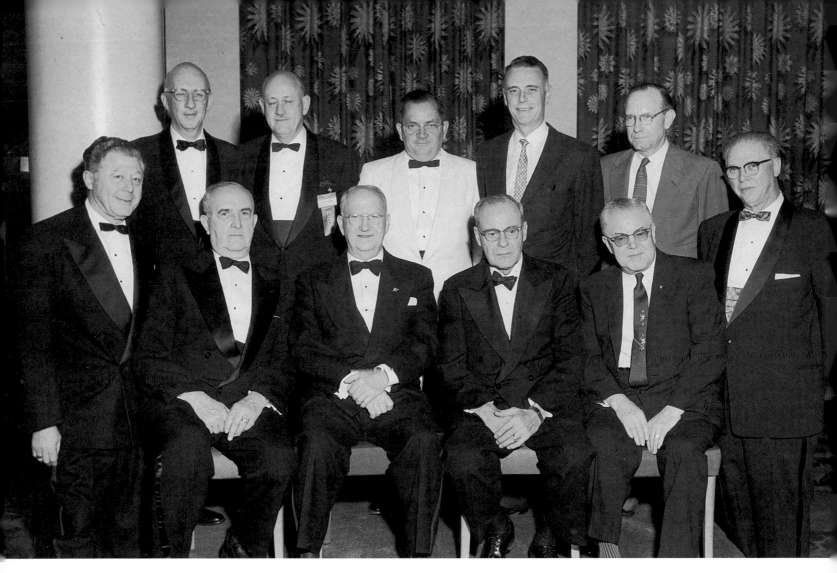

The American College of Apothecaries in 1957 included four APhA presidents, and two first vice presidents, whose names appear in bold face. They are (seated left to right) Louis Longaker, **J. K. Attwood**, Leroy A. Weidle, Max N. Lemberger; (standing left to right) **Louis Fischl**, **Frederick Lascoff**, **Mearl Pritchard**, C. J. Masterson, **Ronald Robertson**, James Hill, and **John Heinz.**

even though Jack W. Dorsey had been keeping "a personalized prescription record card system" since January 1, 1947. As one of the first state requirements for maintaining a Patient Record System, the New Jersey State Board of Pharmacy regulation in 1972 required the pharmacist to examine the patient profile before dispensing any medication to determine the possibility of a harmful drug interaction or reaction.

APhA unveiled the "Pharmaceutical Center" at its 1965 annual meeting which, according to William S. Apple, was based on a concept developed by Eugene V. White. Pharmacist White had purchased a traditional drugstore in 1960 and converted it into an "office practice of pharmacy." Gone were the soda fountain, greeting card racks, and gondolas of proprietary medicines. In came a waiting room, modern furniture, and background music. With the cooperation of McKesson & Robbins, Vice President (and pharmacist) Hubert H. Humphrey cut the ribbon on the new Pharmaceutical Center, proclaiming that this is "the opening of a new professional life for thousands of pharmacists in the years to come."

A "Concept Pharmacy" premiered at the 1996 annual meeting in Nashville, Tennessee. This learning center, developed by APhA and the National Wholesale Druggists Association, was designed to demonstrate pharmaceutical care in action. (See Chapter 22. *APhA Foundation* for additional information on pharmaceutical care projects.)

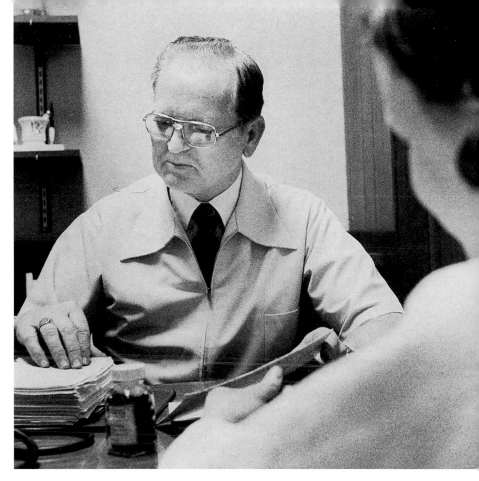

Eugene White of Berryville, Virginia, introduced a new concept in community pharmacy. In 1960, he purchased a traditional drugstore and converted it into an "office practice of pharmacy." He is shown in this photograph taken in 1984.

U.S. Vice President Hubert Humphrey and McKesson & Robbins chairman of the board Herman Nolan cut the ribbon to premier the Pharmaceutical Center during the 1965 annual meeting in Detroit. The sign over the pharmacy entrance refers to APhA's first president, Daniel B. Smith.

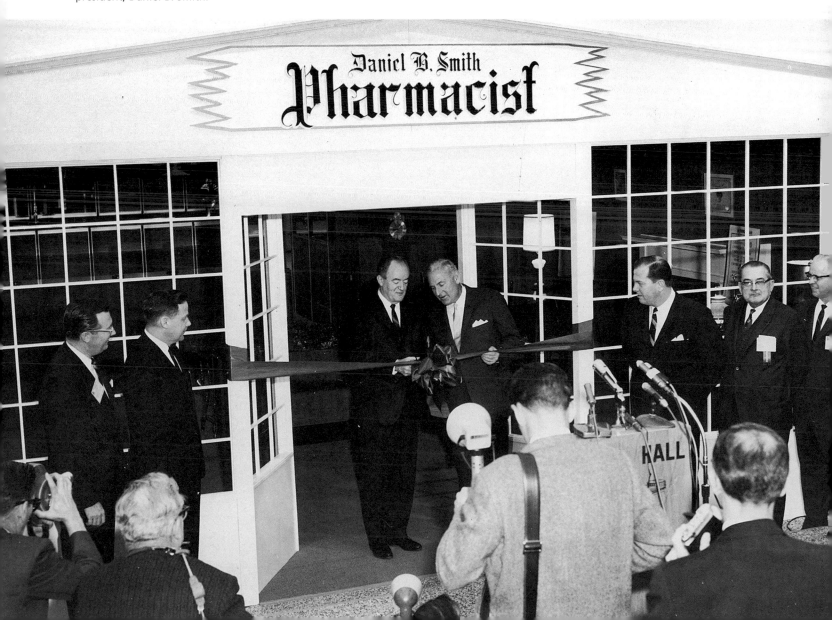

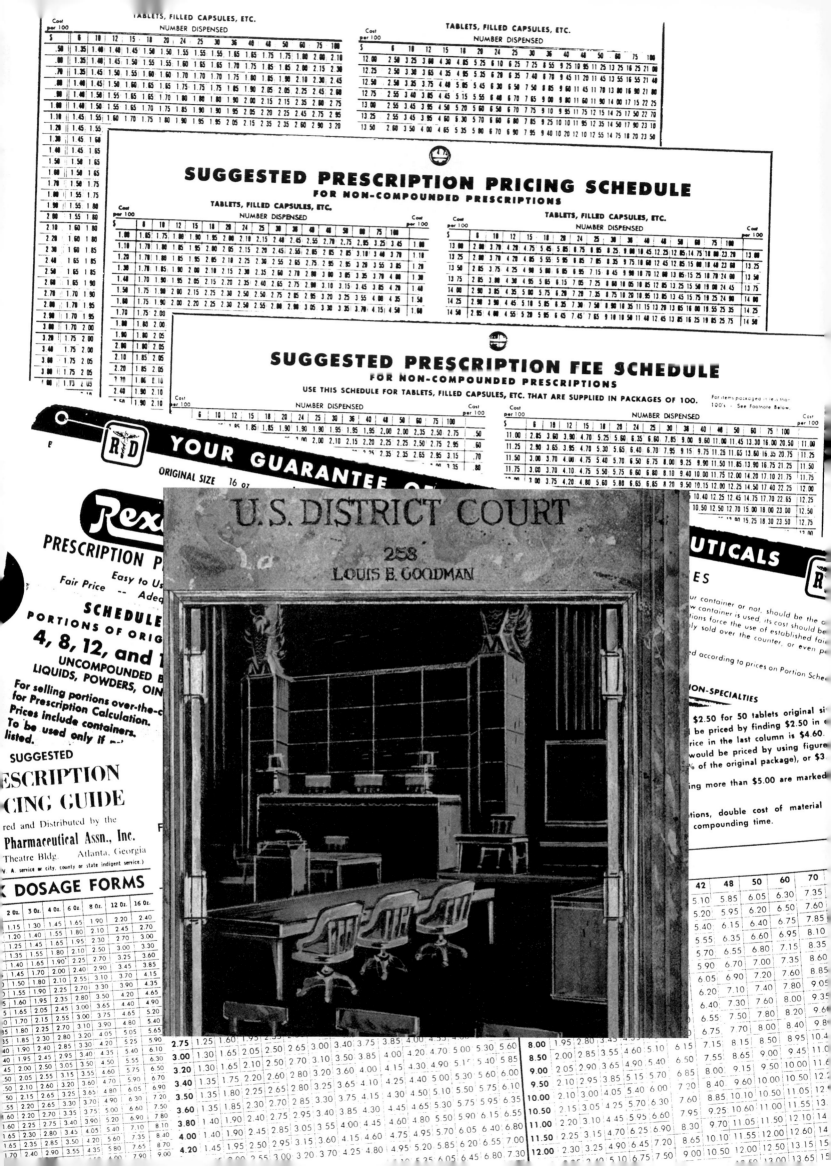

SUGGESTED PRESCRIPTION PRICING SCHEDULE
FOR NON-COMPOUNDED PRESCRIPTIONS

SUGGESTED PRESCRIPTION FEE SCHEDULE
FOR NON-COMPOUNDED PRESCRIPTIONS
USE THIS SCHEDULE FOR TABLETS, FILLED CAPSULES, ETC. THAT ARE SUPPLIED IN PACKAGES OF 100.

U.S. DISTRICT COURT
258
LOUIS E. GOODMAN

CHAPTER 9

Prescription Pricing

Shortly after 1900, practicing pharmacists began looking for a more equitable manner of charging for their services. In 1908, NARD published a "Prescription Pricing Schedule" which called for a charge for the ingredients plus a compounding charge; this worked when ingredients were inexpensive. But after World War II with the introduction of the newer chemotherapeutic agents, the cost of the ingredients increased sharply, and a pricing method again had to be reviewed.

In 1924, the *APhA Journal* published the first of many "Price Schedules" which would eventually come back to haunt APhA. A 1930 APhA report on "Prescription Pricing" still recommended that the charge for prescription medication should be determined by whether they were "hand made pills, suppositories, or liquids," without regard to the ingredients. In 1936, the South Dakota Pharmaceutical Association adopted a new uniform schedule for pre-scription pricing which included compounding fee, minimum fee for various types of preparations, and, most important of all, "the pricing of ready-made items which are too expensive for pricing under type of preparation." The following year, Joseph Goodness told members that there were three ways to price prescriptions: (1) Cost of materials doubled plus labor charge; (2) Materials at selling price plus a compounding fee; or (3) Minimum price list for prescriptions having inexpensive materials.

As early as 1940, Evander F. Kelly editorialized in the *APhA Journal* that health professions are subject to the Sherman Anti-Trust act. It was another twenty years before APhA had to face the consequences of prescription pricing schedules. On June 21, 1960, the U.S. Justice Department filed an antitrust complaint against the Arizona Pharmaceutical Association and the American Pharmaceutical Association maintaining that the defendants established and maintained uniform consumer prices for prescription drugs. Similar complaints were filed against the Northern California Pharmaceutical Association, the Idaho Pharmaceutical Association, and the Utah Pharmaceutical Association. To subsidize the defense of these charges, APhA promptly launched a "Defend the Profession" campaign that raised $68,600 from 4,000 members.

Opposite Page: From the 1930s through the 1950s many "Prescription Pricing Schedules" were produced which in 1960 led to a series of anti-trust complaints by the U.S. Justice Department. Here are three editions of the Northern California "Prescription Pricing Schedule" and the San Francisco courtroom where the association was found guilty of "fixing prices."

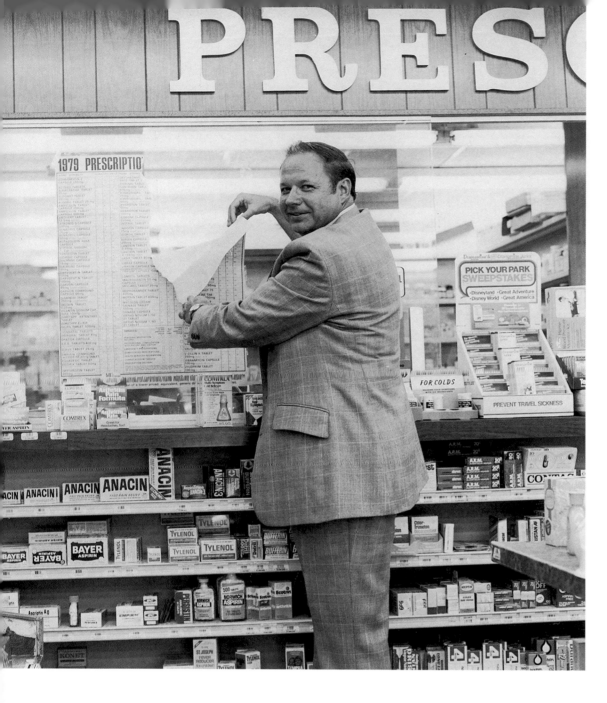

1974-1975 APhA president Robert Johnson removes a prescription pricing poster from a California pharmacy after mandatory price posting was repealed in 1979. The California experience proved that prescription price posting confused consumers rather than helped them.

At the anti-trust trial in San Francisco, the government charged that the Northern California Pharmaceutical Association had approved in 1955 a prescription pricing schedule that had been developed by Donald K. Hedgpath, an officer of the state association. During the 1960 trial, George Griffenhagen was set to testify that prescription pricing schedules had been employed for more than a century, but Federal judge Louis E. Goodman forbade such testimony ruling that "the historical background would only muddy the waters. This case only involves what the parties to this case agreed to do with a particular document [the Hedgpath

Prescription Pricing Schedule]." The jury took 5-1/2 hours to bring back a guilty verdict on June 16, 1960, and the Association was fined $40,000, while Hedgpath was fined $1,000.

The anti-trust trial against the Utah Pharmaceutical Association was held November 21-22, 1962, and on January 31, 1962, Judge A. Sherman Christenson handed down a verdict in favor of the government, concluding that the officers of the Utah Pharmaceutical Association used a "prescription pricing schedule" to "restrain trade and commerce in the sale of prescription drugs."

The anti-trust trials provided new incentive

for APhA to seek a better method for pricing prescriptions. As early as 1940, W. Paul Briggs had expressed the hope that "the day will come when pharmacists receive a definite professional fee for services rendered," even though he knew that the traditional method of applying a percentage mark-up to the cost of medicaments was the most widely employed. APhA appointed a special committee in 1955 "to study and analyze the economic and social ramifications of prescription pricing concepts." Horace A. Fuller was among the first to advocate in 1957 a "professional fee schedule." In 1963, Joseph D. McEvilla explained that the professional fee must be sufficient to cover all costs of compounding and expenses such as rent, light, heat, etc., which should be added to the cost of the ingredients. With this explanation, APhA began promoting the use of the professional fee. Executive director William S. Apple observed in 1960 that "unless pharmacy adopts a pricing method which clearly delineates to the public the difference between the value of professional services and the value of the physical commodity, the profession forfeits its best opportunity for public appreciation and recognition." The following year, APhA endorsed the "the use of professional fees." APhA launched the Uniform Cost Accounting System (UCAS) in 1977, described as "the key to the economic survival of our profession."

In 1938, APhA expressed its "profound interest in all plans prepared for extending medical care," but strongly urged, "the retention of free choice of physician, dentist, pharmacist, and nurse by the patient as an essential feature in whatever system may be adopted." In 1949, APhA affirmed its stand "opposing compulsory national health insurance," providing a detailed statement the following year on APhA's position, which was re-affirmed annually through 1958. Blue Cross and Blue Shield were urged by APhA in 1950 to revise their policy coverage "so as to provide a place for pharmacists which will assure professional supervision of the dispensing of drugs."

But until the 1960s, it was difficult to get pharmacists seriously interested in prepaid pharmaceutical services, and few prepayment plans existed. So in 1969, APhA created the National Pharmacy Insurance Council, representing various pharmacy organizations, to assist pharmacists faced with difficulties in obtaining adequate reimbursement from the rapidly increasing number of prepaid prescription plans. The project was short-lived, however, because on June 5, 1973, the APhA Board of Trustees voted to terminate its membership for "the failure of NPIC to resolve any significant third-party payment problem confronting the nation's pharmacists."

Commencing in the 1990s, APhA worked closely with the National Council on Prescription Drug Programs to build standards and reimbursement systems for both pharmaceutical products and professional services in third-party prescription plans.

In 1999, APhA, the National Association of Chain Drug Stores, and the National Community Pharmacists Association jointly released a "white paper," seeking to improve administrative systems and payment strategies to allow community pharmacists more opportunities to deliver quality patient care.

Enter Mail Order Prescriptions

On December 7, 1959, the Sub-committee on Antitrust and Monopoly of the Senate Judiciary Committee chaired by Senator Estes Kefauver launched Congressional hearings into the pharmaceutical industry. One conclusion reached was to recommend requiring generic prescribing.

Among the disclosures at the hearings was testimony by Ethel Percy Andrus, president of the American Association of Retired Persons, who explained how this organization had instituted a prescription mail-order service. To further explore these "Mail-Order Prescription Schemes," APhA convened a meeting on January 6, 1960, in cooperation

Presidents of various organizations met at the 1960 APhA annual meeting to discuss the impact of mail-order prescription schemes. They include (left to right) Ralph Ware (National Association of Boards of Pharmacy); Cecil Stewart (National Conference of State Pharmaceutical Association Secretaries); Ronald Robertson (APhA); Henry Gregg (American College of Apothecaries); and Clifton Latiolais (American Society of Hospital Pharmacists).

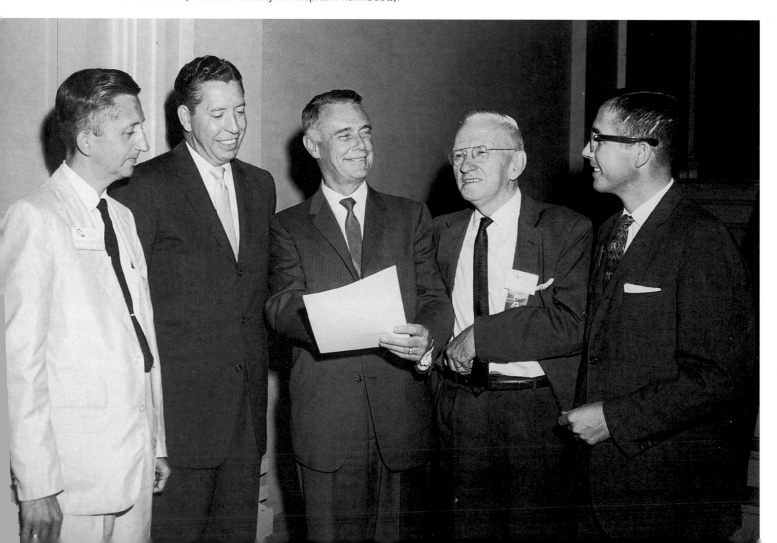

with the National Association of Boards of Pharmacy and the National Conference of State Pharmaceutical Associations. The conclusion reached was that "this new mechanism is enveloping and imposing a threat to pharmaceutical service."

In 1977, Federal Prescription Service, Inc. of Madrid, Iowa, a mail order firm, instituted litigation alleging an antitrust conspiracy against a number of pharmacy organizations; later all defendants were dismissed except APhA and William S. Apple. The case went to trial on October 29, 1979, with the plaintiffs claiming $2,300,000 in damages which would be automatically tripled to $6,900,000. On February 14, 1980, the U.S. District Court found APhA to be legally responsible for certain actions in violation of the Sherman Antitrust Act and awarded damages of $34,000, which were automatically tripled to $102,000.

APhA appealed the decision, and on August 12, 1981, the U.S. Court of Appeals ruled that APhA did not engage in any "actionable conspiracy under the antitrust law in its two decades of efforts to secure legislative and legal controls on mail order prescription services."

There were enough prescription mail order firms in existence by 1975 that they formed the National Association of Mail Order Pharmacists; the group has since changed its name to the Pharmaceutical Care Management Association.

Following the adoption of model mail order regulations approved by the National Association of Boards of Pharmacy, APhA began to accept and publish classified ads for "mail order pharmacists." Then, in 1993, there was a surprising purchase by Merck & Co., one of the largest U.S. pharmaceutical manufacturers, of Medco Containment Services, a holding company that owns one of the nation's largest mail order pharmacy services. Similar purchases the following year were made by SmithKline Beecham who bought United Health Care's subsidiary Diversified Pharmaceutical Services; and by Eli Lilly and Company who bought McKesson's PCS Health Systems.

By the year 2000, the only one of these purchases to sustain its original manufacturer/mail service/pharmaceutical benefits management model was Merck-Medco. The other two manufacturers divested their acquisitions.

the Department of Health, Education and Welfare jointly released a "Model Drug Product Selection Act," that was endorsed by APhA. By 1982, drug product selection laws had been enacted in 49 states. The following year, the APhA House of Delegates supported the "pharmacists' role in the selection of pharmaceutical alternates," and in 1987, the House encouraged "continuing dialogue with other health care organizations on the role of the pharmacist in therapeutic interchange."

In 1889, the House of Delegates supported "a uniform procedure for designating the source of the drug product selection decision on a prescription claim." In 1997, APhA supported "informed decision-making based upon the professional judgement of pharmacists" in drug product selection; and promised to "assist pharmacists and pharmacy students in becoming knowledgeable about complementary and alternate medications to facilitate the counseling of patients regarding effectiveness, proper use, indications, safety, and possible interactions."

CHAPTER 13.

Pharmacy Specialization

With the creation of a Section on Practical Pharmacy and Dispensing in 1900, APhA president Albert Prescott announced that, "we should now be ready to welcome the service of specialists in the field of pharmacy." Prescott's idea would be implemented decades later as organization developed ways of maintaining competency assurances

One cornerstone was the founding of the American Council on Pharmaceutical Education in 1932. Through ACPE, APhA, the American Association of Colleges of Pharmacy, and the National Association of Boards of Pharmacy have been partners in drafting standards and sending inspection teams periodically to evaluate compliance with published accreditation standards for each school of pharmacy.

In 1973, APhA and the American Association of Colleges of Pharmacy established a joint task force to evaluate the continuing competence of the practicing pharmacist. This was partly a result of various states (California, Florida, Kansas, New Jersey, and Ohio) establishing regulations requiring mandatory continuing education to maintain competence.

The American Council on Pharmaceutical Education then assumed the responsibility of approving continuing education providers, but not continuing education programs. Completion of continuing education credits became mandatory for pharmacists who wanted to continue to practice their profession.

In 1978, Samuel H. Kalman (APhA) and John F. Schlegel (AACP) developed a new set of Standards of Practice that described the general management and administration of the pharmacy; activities related to processing the prescription order, patient care functions; and education of health care professionals and patients.

Perhaps the first specialty in pharmacy practice to emerge was "clinical pharmacy." As early as 1922, John C. Krantz, Jr., defined "clinical service as anything done to expedite the recovery of the sick, whether at the bedside of the patient or at the laboratory. The pharmacist renders a valuable clinical service, but his role is not large enough." As Krantz urged, "clinical services must be a phase of pharmaceutical service."

The mature concept of clinical pharmacy was first put forward in 1945 by L. Wait Rising. In 1965 Glenn Sperandio observed that clinical pharmacy includes both community and hospital pharmacy. And in 1968 both ASHP and APhA arrived at a definition of clinical pharmacy that included the key phrase, "patient-oriented practice."

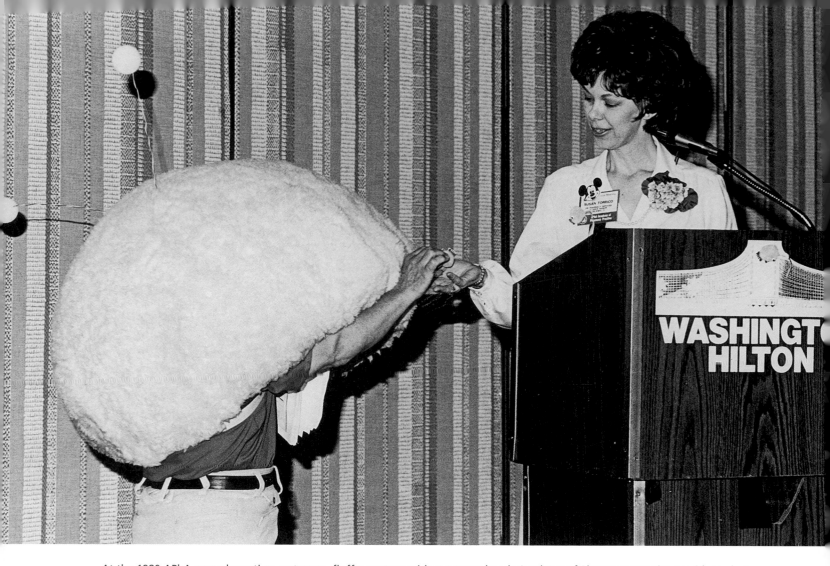

At the 1980 APhA annual meeting, a strange, fluffy creature with antennae hands Academy of Pharmacy Practice president-elect Susan Torrico a mysterious-looking pad of multicolored paper, called a PANG, on which was printed proposed Standards of Practice. The workshop, "Putting the Standards of Practice to Work for You," was developed jointly by the American Association of Colleges of Pharmacy and APhA, sponsored by Lederle Laboratories.

In 1971, the APhA House of Delegates urged the creation of "an organizational mechanism within the structure of APhA for recognition of specialties and certification of specialists." A task force was created in January 1973, and among their 1974 recommendations was the establishment of a Board of Pharmaceutical Specialties.

The Board of Pharmaceutical Specialties (BPS) came into existence on January 5, 1976, and promptly established criteria for the recognition of certain specialties. On June 19, 1978, BPS declared that Nuclear Pharmacy be recognized as a specialty.

William Jay Schieffelin had presented a paper in 1914 at the APhA Scientific Section dis-cussing the importance of radium emanation as a therapeutic agent. He pointed out that pharmacists should be prepared to meet the demand for radium as required by physicians.

The first radionuclides became available for civilian medical use following World War II; and in 1945, Abbott Laboratories launched the first commercial program to harness the atom for use in medicine. APhA advised members in 1947 that the production of radioisotopes in quantity brings medical and pharmaceutical science to full-scale development of a new frontier. In 1954, APhA observed that pharmacists were not active in handling radioisotopes in hospitals and proposed that a four week

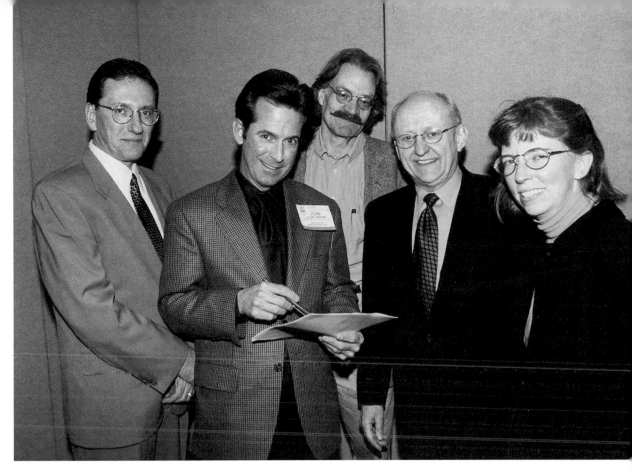

A panel reviews the first decade of pharmaceutical care at the 2001 annual meeting. Participants include (left to right) APhA past president Calvin Knowlton; AIHP president John Swann; University of Minnesota College of Pharmacy professor Peter Morley; ASHP staff member William Zellmer; and University of Wisconsin School of Pharmacy professor Jeanine Mount, moderator.

course be established at the Oak Ridge (Tennessee) Institute of Nuclear Studies. By 1957, pharmacists at the University of Chicago Clinics were involved in the preparation of radioactive medications. Among the pioneers were John F. Christian in 1950, G. B. Hutchison in 1954, and William H. Briner in 1968.

The Academy of General Practice sponsored a symposium on Nuclear Pharmacy in 1974, and the following year the APhA Section on Nuclear Pharmacy was officially formed. The Food and Drug Administration published guidelines for the clinical evaluation of radiopharmaceuticals in 1975, and the Nuclear Pharmacy Section encouraged state boards of pharmacy to adopt regulations covering the practice of nuclear pharmacy.

In 1986, the Board of Pharmaceutical Specialties received a petition requesting that clinical pharmacy become a specialty, but the following year, BPS rejected the petition, considering "clinical pharmacy practice as too broad and too general to be recognized as a specialty." The sponsoring group, the American College of Clinical Pharmacy which was established in 1979, crafted a new petition, defining more narrowly the tasks and skills described in the clinical pharmacy petition and gave the new specialty the name "pharmacotherapy." Eventually in 1988, BPS approved both Pharmacotherapy and Nutritional Support Pharmacy as recognized specialties.

In 1991, BPS received a petition to recognize Psychiatric Pharmacy Practice as a specialty, which was accepted in 1992, and Oncology Pharmacy was accepted in 1996. In January 2001, over 3,000 pharmacists held BPS certification distributed across the five specialties. Pharmacists who wish to retain BPS certification must be recertified every seven years. On its 25th anniversary (2001), BPS took note of the fact that it has worked with several organizations, including APhA, the American College of Clinical Pharmacy, the American Society of Health-System Pharmacists, and the American

Society of Parenteral and Enteral Nutrition in developing these specialties.

Prior to 1980, APhA endorsed the term "pharmacy aide" to designate supportive personnel utilized in pharmacy practice, and advocated the training of these pharmacy aides "via in-service or on-the-job training programs." Then in 1988, APhA officially changed the terminology to "pharmacy technician," and the Michigan Pharmacists Association began to administer voluntary certification examinations for these pharmacy technicians. The Illinois Council of Hospital Pharmacists introduced a certification program the following year, and both Michigan and Illinois collaborated with other state associations to administer technology certification. In 1993, APhA, ASHP, the Michigan Pharmacists Association, and the Illinois Council of Hospital Pharmacists commenced discussions to develop a national voluntary certification program for pharmacy technicians. In January 1995 the Pharmacy Technician Certification Board (PTCB) was formed. The following year, APhA and ASHP published the "White Paper on Pharmacy Technicians," and estimated that 150,000 pharmacy technicians were being employed nationwide.

The Pharmacy Technician Certification Board administers a voluntary test three times a year at more than 120 sites across the country. A technician who passes the examination is designated as a Certified Pharmacy Technician, and by the end of 2001, more than 100,000 pharmacy technicians had been certified.

In 1997, the American Society of Consultant Pharmacists, founded in 1970, created the Commission for Certification of Geriatric Pharmacy. The following year, the National Institute for Standards in Pharmacist Credentializing was founded by the National Association of Boards of Pharmacy, the National Association of Chain Drug Stores, and the National Community Pharmacists Association to offer certification in the management of diabetes, asthma, dyslipidemia, and anticoagulation therapy.

The Council of Credentializing in Pharmacy was created in 1999 by a coalition of eleven national pharmacy organizations to provide leadership, standards, public information, and coordination for all professional voluntary credentializing programs in pharmacy. A "white paper" published in the January-February 2001 issue of the *APhA Journal* included a comprehensive glossary of key terms relating to pharmacist credentialing.

CHAPTER 14.

Hospital Pharmacists

Another lasting contribution of the Section on Practical Pharmacy was the creation in 1936 of the APhA Sub-Section of Hospital Pharmacists. In 1908 J. T. Harbold, pharmacist at the Pennsylvania Hospital, offered one of the first presentations on hospital pharmacy at the Section on Practical Pharmacy.

As early as 1921, APhA president Charles H. Packard pointed out that "there are in the whole country over 6,000 hospitals; probably over 500 of these employ pharmacists." He therefore recommended that a hospital pharmacists committee be created and given a part in the annual program of the Section on Practical Pharmacy and Dispensing. In 1922, all officers of the Section were hospital pharmacists which led to a proposal that a section for hospital pharmacists be organized. Edward Swallow, pharmacist at the outpatient department of Bellevue Hospital in New York City, writing in the *APhA Journal* supported "the proposed movement for organizing hospital pharmacists," and presented a plea for the formation

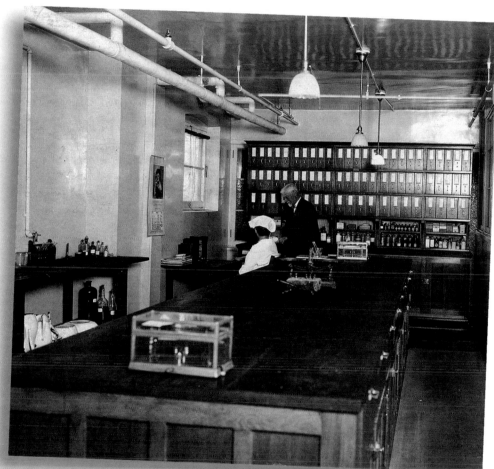

In the 1920s, there were less than 500 pharmacists employed by the 6,000 hospitals in the U.S. One of these hospital pharmacists can be seen in this photograph at Muhlenberg Hospital in Plainfield, New Jersey.

of a special group of hospital pharmacists within APhA.

For the remainder of the 1920s, there was a leveling off in hospital pharmacy organizational efforts, but in almost every issue of the *APhA Journal* from 1926 to 1935 there were articles on hospital pharmacy. By 1935, a nucleus of proponents had

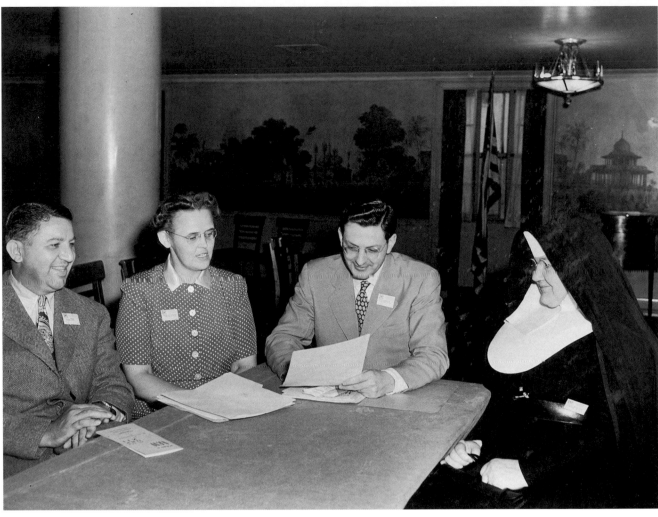

The American Society of Hospital Pharmacists was established on August 21, 1942, at the APhA annual meeting, electing Harvey Whitney as its first chairman. The newly elected officers at the 1944 meeting (shown here) included (left to right) secretary Thomas Reamer, vice chairman Hazel Landeen, chairman Don E. Francke, and treasurer Sister Mary John.

developed, and both the American Hospital Association and the Catholic Hospital Association had recognized hospital pharmacists as either a section or a committee.

A group of hospital pharmacists at the APhA annual meeting in 1936 persuaded APhA officials to establish a sub-section on hospital pharmacy within the Section on Practical Pharmacy and Dispensing. J. Solon Modell, one of the early leaders of the hospital pharmacy movement, described it as "a turning point and milestone in the development of hospital pharmacy practice." Louis C. Zopf was elected as the chairman of the sub-section, and Harvey A. K.

Whitney was appointed to serve as secretary.

As early as 1925, the Hospital Pharmacy Association of Southern California was established. Then in February 1936, the Minnesota Hospital Pharmacists Association was created; and in May 1937, the Nebraska Hospital Pharmacy Association was founded. By 1939, there were hospital pharmacists associations established in California, Illinois, Indiana, Iowa, Minnesota, Nebraska, New York, Ohio, Pennsylvania, and Wisconsin.

In 1940, the APhA House of Delegates expressed "a real need for a unified organization of hospital pharmacists," and approved a resolution that

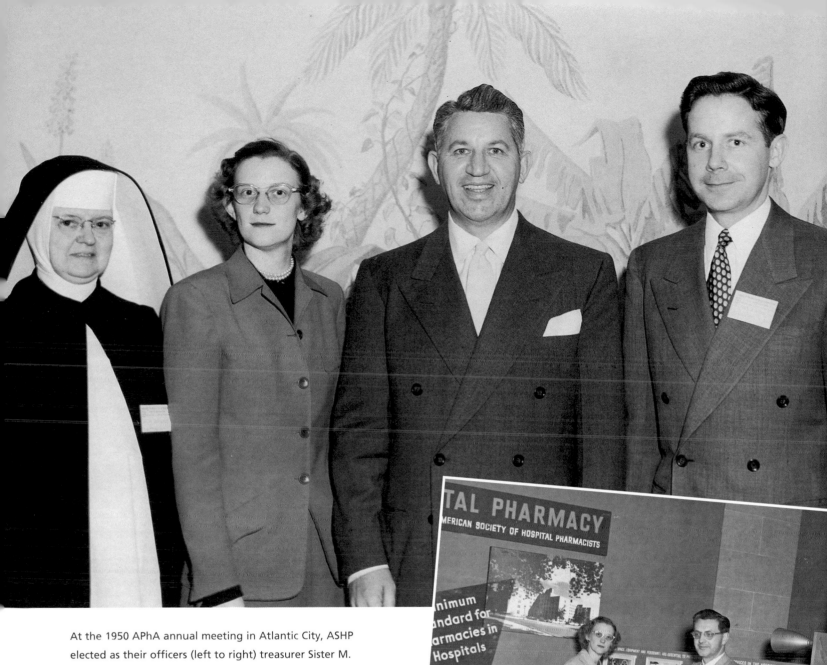

At the 1950 APhA annual meeting in Atlantic City, ASHP elected as their officers (left to right) treasurer Sister M. Jeanette, secretary Gloria Niemeyer, chairman Thomas Reamer, and vice chairman Grover Bowles. The titles of chairman and vice chairman were changed in 1947 to president and vice president.

At the 1951 APhA annual meeting in Buffalo, New York, Gloria Niemeyer and Don Francke are shown staffing the exhibit of the American Society of Hospital Pharmacists.

the APhA sub-section on hospital pharmacy should be abolished, and a new group should be formed. Then on August 21, 1942, the new organization, American Society of Hospital Pharmacists, was approved by the APhA Council as an affiliate. The sub-section was dissolved, and the inaugural meeting of ASHP was held at the 1943 APhA annual meeting with Harvey A. K. Whitney as the first president.

In 1947, the APhA Council, with the concurrence of the ASHP executive committee, established

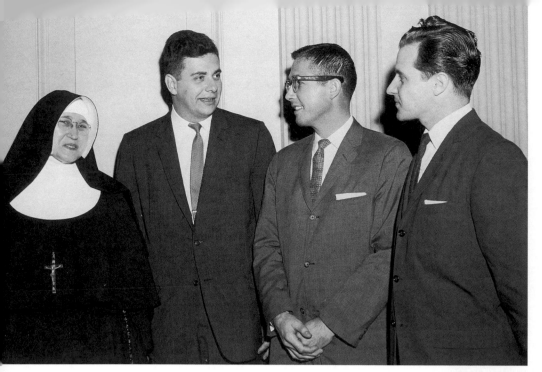

Joseph A. Oddis (far right) was selected ASHP executive secretary in 1960. Other ASHP officers at the 1960 APhA annual meeting in Washington, D.C., include (left to right) Sister Mary Berenice, treasurer; Peter Solyom, vice president; and Clifton Latiolais, president.

a division of hospital pharmacy with Robert P. Fischelis as director and Gloria Niemeyer as secretary. The following year, Niemeyer was elevated to assistant director of the APhA division of hospital pharmacy, as well as ASHP secretary, and associate editor of the ASHP *Bulletin* which was first published in June 1943 by Leo W. Mossman. Don E. Francke assumed editorship in 1944. ASHP was incorporated in 1955, and launched the *American Hospital Formulary Service* in 1959.

Joseph A. Oddis was employed in 1960 as director of APhA's division of hospital pharmacy, and as executive secretary of ASHP. When APhA dissolved the division in 1962, Oddis was named ASHP's full-time executive secretary. ASHP moved from APhA headquarters to its own office in Bethesda in 1966, and the name was changed in 1994 to the American Society of Health-System Pharmacists. ASHP held its annual meetings with APhA from its inception until 1979.

The only other new APhA section created during the first half of the 20th century was the Section on Historical Pharmacy, established in 1902. This Section subsequently merged in 1967 with the

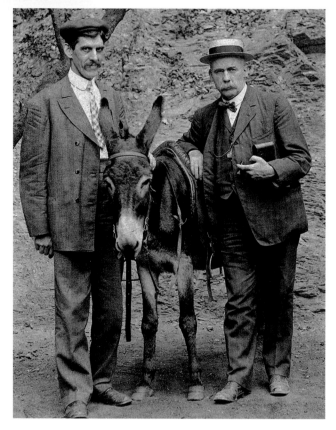

1903-1904 Historical Pharmacy Section secretary Ezra Kennedy (right) and 1909-1910 Scientific Section chairman Martin Wilbert find a long lost friend during the 1908 APhA annual meeting in Hot Springs, Arkansas.

American Institute of the History of Pharmacy which was founded in 1941 by Edward Kremers and George Urdang, both noted pharmaceutical historians. Since its first organizational meeting in 1941, AIHP has met jointly with APhA.

CHAPTER 15.

Chain Pharmacies

Prior to 1890, there were few instances where an individual operated two or more pharmacies under the same management. By 1900, there were no more than 25 pharmacies in the country that were combined into chains. There were in the U.S. 315 individuals and corporations operating three or more drugstores by 1920. These chains represented a total of 1,565 chain pharmacies or 3.12 percent of all pharmacies in the country. The largest included: The Louis K. Liggett Company of New York City with 211 pharmacies; the Owl Drug Company of San Francisco with 32 pharmacies; and the Walgreen Drug Company of Chicago with 21 pharmacies.

Louis K. Liggett commenced buying out most major competition, expanding from 229 pharmacies in 1921 to 627 in 1930. Concerned over this type of operation, New York enacted a law requiring that all pharmacies opened after passage of the law should be owned by registered pharmacists. Other states followed, and in 1927, Pennsylvania enacted an even stronger law. Louis Liggett purchased two new pharmacies in Pennsylvania after the ownership law was enacted, and the Pennsylvania Board of Pharmacy refused to grant Liggett pharmacy permits. Liggett in turn sued claiming that the law was unconstitutional. The lower court ruled in support of the State, so Liggett appealed to the U.S. Supreme Court who ruled on November 19, 1928, that a state cannot "under the guise of protecting the public, arbitrarily interfere with private business." The profession of pharmacy was stunned, but took heart in the dissent of Justices Holmes and Brandeis who questioned whether it is appropriate for a "business to be owned by people who do not know anything about it."

The 1928 decision was reversed in 1973 when the U.S. Supreme Court held constitutional a North Dakota statute requiring that majority ownership must be in the hands of North Dakota pharmacists in good standing, and described "the Liggett case a derelict in the stream of law [which is] hereby overruled." (See Chapter 6. *Protecting the Druggist*.)

Independent of APhA, the National Association of Chain Drug Stores was organized in 1933 by Wallace J. Smith of Read Drug and Chemical Company (now Rite Aid) to establish "a unified voice" to represent chains to accommodate the requirements of the 1933 Retail Drug Code Authority. When NRA was eliminated, including the Retail Drug Code Authority, NACDS directors decided to continue the organization composed of owners of pharmacy chains.

As early as 1930, the APhA House of

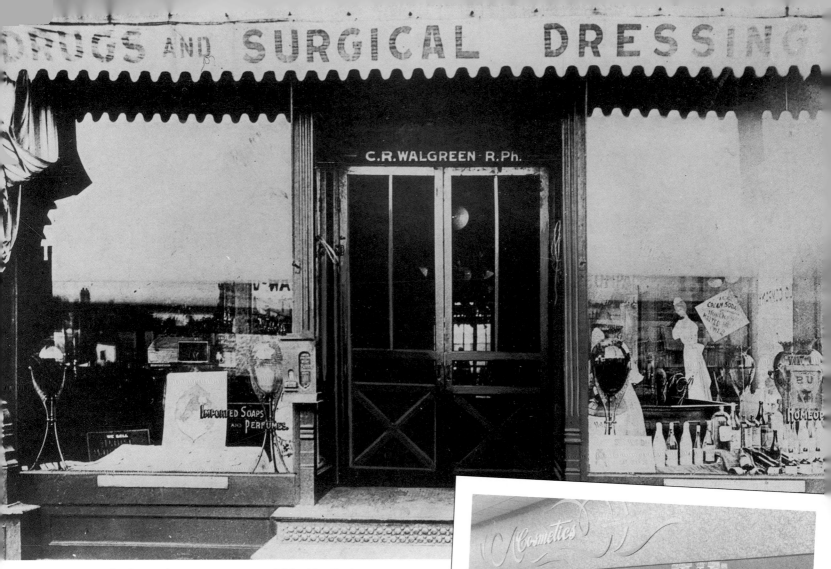

The first Walgreen Drugstore, established by Charles Walgreen, Sr., was opened in June 1901 at 4134 Cottage Grove Avenue, in Chicago, Illinois. By 1920, there were 1,565 chain pharmacies, or 3.12 percent of all pharmacies in the U.S.

Delegates adopted a resolution urging "the curtailment of merchandise unrelated to the usual departments of pharmacy," and the following year, the House expressed "vigorous disapproval of the establishment of pharmacies or drug departments in supermarkets or other retail establishments unrelated to pharmacy." Then in 1950, APhA voiced "vigorous disapproval" against any form of self-service (including vending machines) for the sale of drugs.

A cooperative venture was implemented in 1984 with the National Association of Chain Drug Stores to educate the public on proposed legislation to counter crimes against pharmacist (i.e. narcotic thefts).

Charles Walgreen introduced self-service pharmacy in 1942. The public awareness of the pharmacists' presence was lost in a maze of merchandising until chain owners recognized that the public wanted to interact with their pharmacist.

CHAPTER 16

Employee Pharmacists

A trend with great repercussions in pharmacy resulted when state pharmaceutical associations limited their membership to pharmacy owners. For a time, such a restriction was of little concern to employee pharmacists because most could eventually realize their ambition of becoming the owner of a pharmacy. By the end of the 1870s, it was becoming a goal more difficult to achieve, and this resulted in separating pharmacists into two distinct groups. The pharmacy owners called themselves "druggists" or "apothecaries," while employee pharmacists were designated by the pharmacy owners as "drug clerks." By the 1870s, these employee pharmacists began to organize in an effort to obtain better working conditions.

In 1874, APhA studied the salary of drug clerks, which they called "assistant pharmacists." While the druggist associations feared that these drug clerk societies could lead to unionization, APhA welcomed with open arms the representatives of the local associations of drug clerks from Chicago, St. Louis, and Washington, D.C.

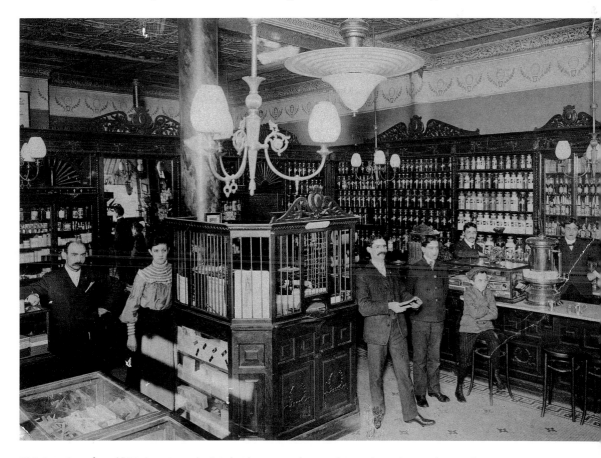

This interior of an 1897 drugstore depicts both owner pharmacists and employee pharmacists who were still called "drug clerks." As late as 1903, president George Frederick Payne told APhA members that "the art of cleaning bottles, pasting labels, and selling goods are the chief part of a week's work" for drug clerks.

As late as 1903, APhA president George Payne told APhA members that "a college graduate may be well versed in pharmacy, chemistry, and botany...yet he may make a failure as a drug clerk. Scientific pharmacy, chemistry, and botany are only needed a comparatively small portion of the time, but the art of cleaning bottles, pasting labels, and selling goods successfully are the chief part of the week's work."

The first national organization for employee pharmacists was established in 1893 under the name, Drug Clerks' Mutual Benefit Association. Additional organizations of employee pharmacists created in the early 20th century included the American Registered Pharmacists Association founded in 1900, and the Drug Clerks' Brotherhood founded in 1908. The National Drug Clerks Association operated a home for "aged and infirm drug clerks" from 1924 until the group was dissolved in 1934.

Commencing in the late 19th century, drugstore owners were concerned that these local as well as national organizations were leaning toward unionization of employee pharmacists. The House of Delegates debated the issue of unionization for decades, and unionization was officially opposed in principle by APhA as a possible infringement on the professional responsibilities of the pharmacist. This policy was reversed in 1999 when the House of Delegates moved to support pharmacist's participation in organizations that promote the discretion or professional perogatives exercised by pharmacists in their practice, and supported the rights of pharmacists to negotiate with their respective employers for working conditions that will foster compliance with the standards of pharmaceutical care as established by the profession. However, APhA reaffirmed oppositon to become a collective bargaining unit.

As reported in Chapter 7, *Section for Practicing Pharmacists*, in 1966 APhA inaugurated "a model agreement" for pharmacy owners and employee pharmacists, including hospitalization, disability, and retirement benefits. Eleven years later, APhA added a comprehensive package encouraging pharmacy owners to offer their employee pharmacists various insurance, liability, and retirement options.

In the late 1990s, when the majority of practicing pharmacists were employees rather than employers, APhA initiated a variety of activities to assist employed pharmacists in addressing the stress encountered in the late 20th century practice environment.

CHAPTER 17.

Pharmaceutical Sciences

Commencing with the second annual meeting (1853), scientific papers became an established part of the annual meeting program. William Procter put it this way: "The action of this association should not be limited to the practical, ethical, and educational interests of the profession" and he advocated the offering of prizes for certain investigations. The plan was to have a Committee on Scientific Queries to formulate questions to be answered by members. Virtually every APhA annual meeting from 1853 to 1886 offered a series of responses to questions relating to pharmaceuticals (mainly botanicals). This was continued until 1870 when a revision of the APhA Constitution and Bylaws established a "Committee on Scientific Papers."

Then in 1887, a Section on Scientific Papers was created as one of the first of four APhA sub-divisions "to expedite and render more efficient the work of the Association." During the first five years of the Scientific Section, about forty percent of the papers were devoted to matters of compounding, incompatibilities, and drug standards; thirty percent were

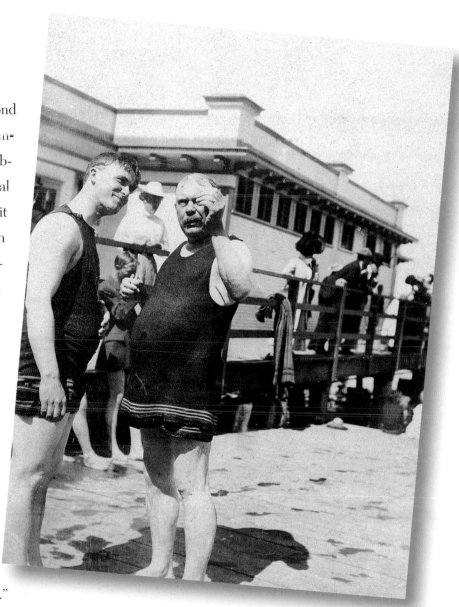

1891-1892 Scientific Section chairman Carl Hallberg is shown enjoying botanizing the Pacific Ocean at Long Beach during the 1909 APhA annual meeting in Los Angeles, California.

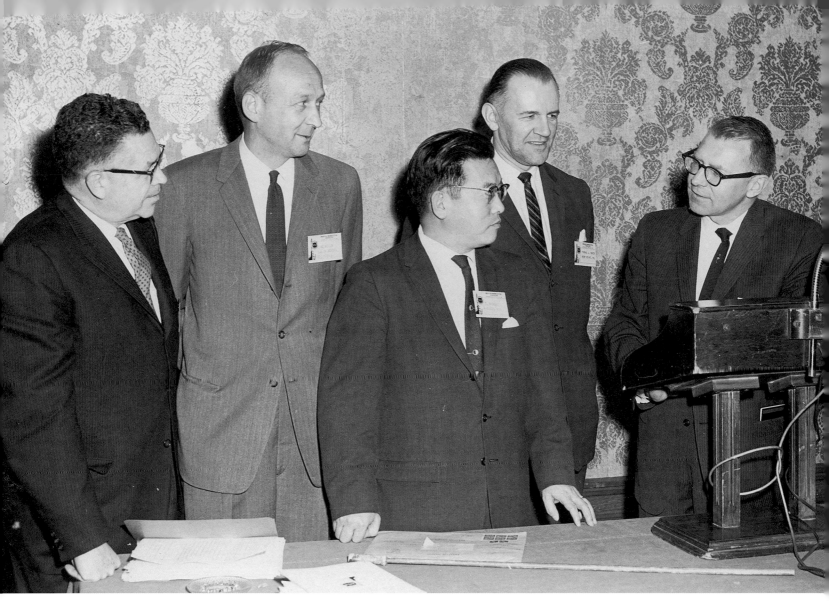

By 1961, the APhA Scientific Section was questioning its organizational structure. Shown here at the 1961 annual meeting are (left to right) 1957-1963 secretary-treasurer Robert Anderson; 1963-1964 chairman Eino Nelson; 1961-1962 chairman Takeru Higuchi; 1962-1963 chairman Thomas Macek; and 1960-1961 chairman Walter Charnicki.

devoted to pharmacognosy, and another twenty-five percent dealt with pharmaceutical chemistry. The number of individual presentations increased from 36 in 1892 to 63 in 1898. From 1887 to 1953, over 2,500 papers were presented before the Scientific Section. A comparative classification of topics discussed in 1891 and 1952 includes:

Classification	1891	1952
Pharmacognosy	30%	12%
Pharmacology	0%	41%
Pharmaceutical Chemistry	25%	40%
Various°	45%	7%

° = Compounding, incompatabilities, drug standards

After World War II, there was an unprecedented flowering of science, including pharmaceutical science. A "new breed" of pharmaceutical scientists and technologists no longer felt that the section structure adequately represented their aims within the framework of APhA.

These concerns were translated into action. Newly installed executive director William S. Apple conferred with his colleagues from the University of Wisconsin, Takeru Higuchi and Joseph V. Swintosky, to plan a new scientific body in APhA. As the plans evolved, it became clear by 1963 that there should be a three-way merger of the original Scientific Section, the Pharmaceutical Technology Section which had been created in 1941, and the Industrial Pharmacy Section which had been formed in 1960. Finally in 1965, the three sections were merged to form the Academy of Pharmaceutical Science, with sections having a much wider scope than the three old sections. They were: Basic Pharmaceutics (the core of the former Scientific Section); Economics and Administrative Science; Industrial Pharmaceutical Technology (a merger of the former Industrial Pharmacy and Pharmaceutical Technology Sections); Medicinal Chemistry; Pharmacognosy and Natural Products (subsequently merged into Medicinal Chemistry); Pharmaceutical Analysis and Control (first named Drug Standards, Analysis and Control); and Pharmacology and Toxicology (first named Pharmacology and Biochemistry).

The founders realized that the participation of pharmaceutical scientists who were not pharma-

cists was essential to make the Academy a viable organization. And yet, the APhA Bylaws seemed to preclude such participation. Thus a new category of APhA membership was created in 1966, that of Scientific Associate. Such members were pharmaceutical scientists who were not pharmacists and did not have full rights to vote or hold office in the parent organization.

In time, these new Scientific Associates were frequently considered by their colleagues as "secondary citizens." And when non-pharmacist Klaus G. Florey was elected 1980-1981 Academy President, he discovered that he was not entitled to a voting seat in the APhA House of Delegates.

Another major concern was whether the Academy could adopt a policy position on an issue in direct conflict with APhA policy. The prime example concerned the APhA white paper on "The Pharmacist's Role in Drug Product Selection." The

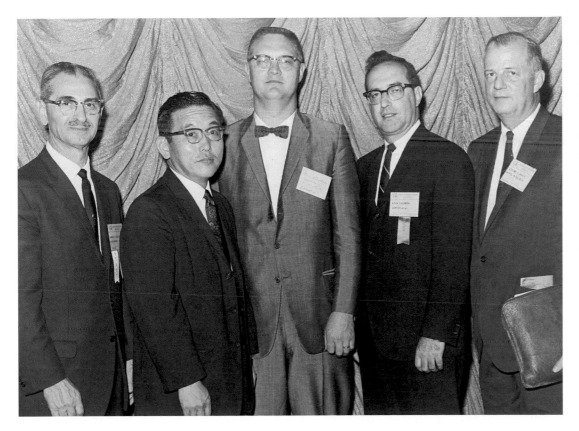

Newly inducted officers of the Academy of Pharmaceutical Sciences in 1967 include (left to right) Samuel Goldstein, secretary; Takeru Higuchi, past president; Joseph Swintosky, president; Leon Lachman, vice president; and George Hager, president-elect.

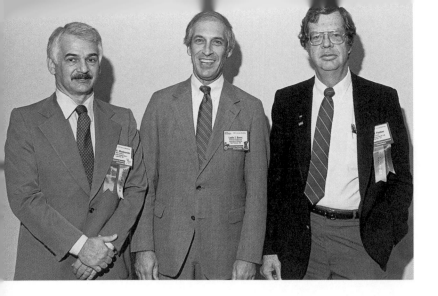

1985-1986 APS president Leslie Benet (center) led the movement to give the Academy of Pharmaceutical Sciences more independence. Benet is flanked by Arthur Mlodozeniec (left) 1984-1985 APS president; and Boyd Poulsen (right), 1986-1987 APS president

Academy's conflict with its parent body intensified, and the 1985 APS Strategic Plan concluded that the Academy "should enjoy a high degree of autonomy within the framework of APhA, essentially managing its own affairs and publications." One of these specific areas was to "maintain operational control of the *Journal of Pharmaceutical Sciences*" which APhA was not willing to grant.

Leslie Z. Benet, the 1985-1986 APS president, led the movement to give APS more independence. In his inaugural address, Benet explored possible alternative structural relationships for the Academy such as a loose federation with APhA or a completely autonomous association. In an effort to avert a threatened withdrawal, APhA appointed a task force to "investigate both the needs of pharmaceutical scientists and the scientific needs of APhA, and to seek such structural organizational arrangements that will accommodate the needs of both groups." Glenn Sonnedecker was appointed as chair of the Task Force which met November 22-24, 1985, and recommended that "the new Academy of Pharmaceutical Sciences be an organization finan-

cially and administratively independent, yet have a strong collaborative relationship with APhA in areas of common interests."

But the window of opportunity had passed, and all the officers of the APhA Academy of Pharmaceutical Sciences resigned at the March 1986 annual meeting and immediately formed their own association called the American Association of Pharmaceutical Scientists. APhA chief executive officer John F. Schlegel contended that "pharmaceutical scientists will always be a vital part of APhA." So in 1986, the APhA Board of Trustees changed the Academy's name to the Academy of Pharmaceutical Research and Science to avoid confusion with the new AAPS. APhA appointed a four-member APhA-APRS executive committee consisting of Jordan L. Cohen and David A. Knapp representing academia, and James H. Hull III and Louis C. Schroeter who were industrial scientists.

The Academy of Pharmaceutical Research and Science held its organizational meeting September 20-21, 1986, in Washington, D.C., with Jordan Cohen as temporary chair. In 1990, the new APRS found its direction under the guidance of executive vice president John A. Gans and APhA staffer Arthur H. Kibbe who organized the end-of-summer science symposia. The science initiative was an integral part of the 1992 APhA strategic plan focusing on the application of science to pharmacy practice.

AAPS continues to flourish as an independent agency with an increasing membership of many non-pharmacists. In 2001, APhA and AAPS entered into an agreement to collaborate on activities of mutual benefit to both organizations.

CHAPTER 18

Advancement of Science

S cience has always been an integral part of the profession of pharmacy. Therefore, discoveries and innovations in science were an important part of the information APhA provided its members from its founding in 1852 to the present. For example, president George Payne described in 1903 how Madame Curie discovered radium from pitch-blende, and he questioned if it was really true that a reported case of cancer in Vienna, Austria, was cured by the rays of radium bromide.

The *APhA Bulletin* for February 1911 featured an article on "Chemotherapy and 606" read before the APhA Philadelphia Branch. The chairman of the Practical Pharmacy and Dispensing Section pointed out that "with the introduction of 606" [Paul Ehrlich's "magic bullet" called Salvarsan], the pharmacist is frequently called on to exercise the profes-

The "Evolution of Materials Used in Medicines" was the theme of the grand prize winner of the 1936 National Pharmacy Week window display contest. The display was entered by Morgan & Millard Pharmacy of Baltimore, Maryland.

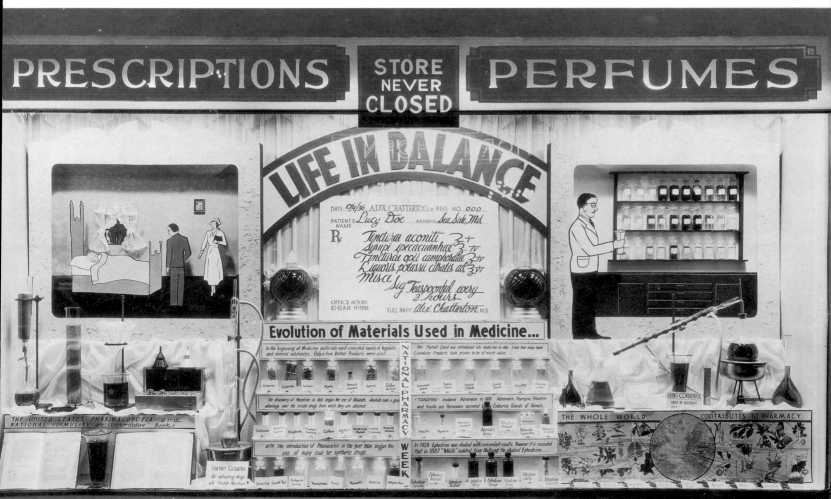

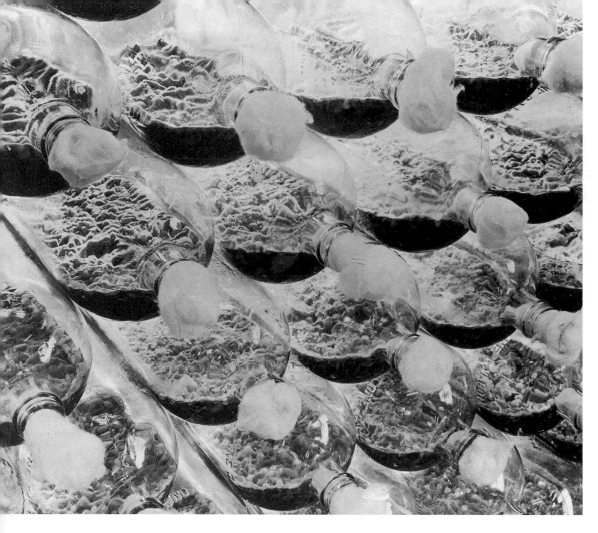

Penicillin was initially produced by surface culture as described in a 1943 issue of the *APhA Journal*. "While stored in these culture bottles, the surface gradually is covered with a penicillin mold."

sional side of his calling." After explaining how the pharmacist prepares "606" in injectable form, Louis Saalbach concluded: "This but emphasizes the fact that the physician needs the pharmacist as much as the pharmacist needs him; and the sooner we can bring about a closer relationship between the sister professions, the better for both of them."

Casimir Funk (whose nutritional studies led to coining the term "vitamine") presented a lecture to the 1923 APhA Scientific Section on progress in vitamin research. Here he described how he had classified vitamine A as antirachitic; B as the antiberiberi vitamin, and C as the antiscorbutic vitamin. Ko Kuei Chen reported in the *APhA Journal* for 1926 how he and his colleagues had isolated ephedrine from the Chinese herb *Ma Huang*.

The *APhA Journal, Practical Pharmacy Edition* described in 1943 the importance of penicillin.

In June 1944, pharmacist John N. McDonnell, chief of the drugs and cosmetic branch of the War Production Board, announced that since production had increased, penicillin would soon be available to pharmacies. The March 1945 issue of the *APhA Journal* announced that "Penicillin Comes to the Corner Pharmacy;" the entire issue was devoted to penicillin, and the issue carried penicillin advertisements by seven different pharmaceutical manufacturers.

Then in November 1945, Selman Waksman authored an article in the *APhA Journal* on streptomycin which he described as a "new antibiotic with low toxicity, and effective against infections not reached by penicillin." Also in 1946, APhA advised its members that new penicillins were partially synthesized, including Benzylpenicillin (Penicillin G).

APhA explained to members in 1947 that the production of radioisotopes in quantity brings med-

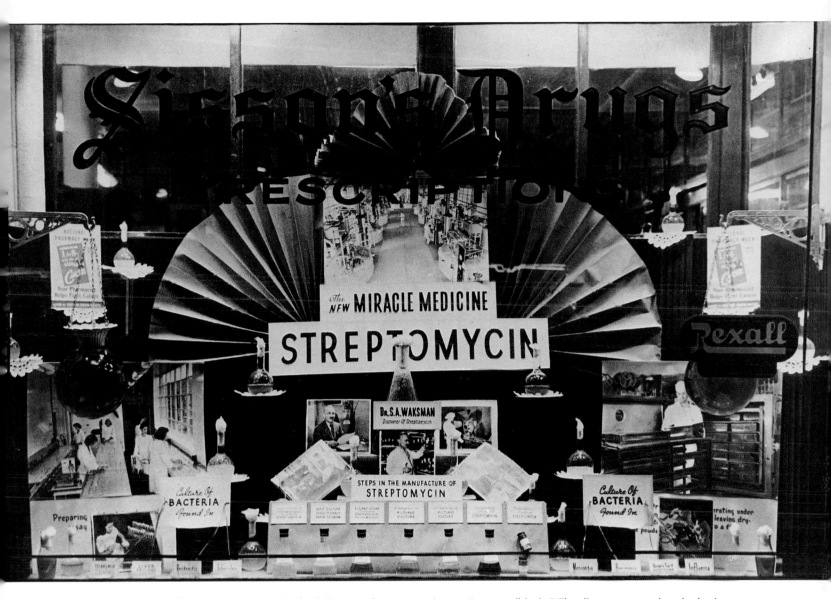

Selman Waksman told APhA in 1945 that he had discovered streptomycin as a "new antibiotic." The discovery served as the basis of a National Pharmacy Week window display installed in 1947 by Sisson's Drugs of Chicago, Illinois.

ical and pharmaceutical science to full-scale development of a new frontier of research. Also diphenhydramine (Benadryl) was described in detail; two years later, antihistamines were described as having promise in the treatment of the common cold.

Aureomycin was described in 1949 as "a new antibiotic for the treatment of bacterial, viral, and rickettsial diseases," while Terramycin was introduced to the market in 1950. APhA members learned in 1951 that cortisone (Edward C. Kendall's Compound E) and corticotropin (ACTH) was available only in hospitals; and hydrocortisone (Kendall's Compound F) was described in 1952. In 1955, APhA outlined the role of pharmacists in the distribution of the Salk Polio Vaccine program.

Pharmacists were introduced by APhA to genetic engineering in 1980, following the submicroscopic manipulations of Watson and Crick's "double

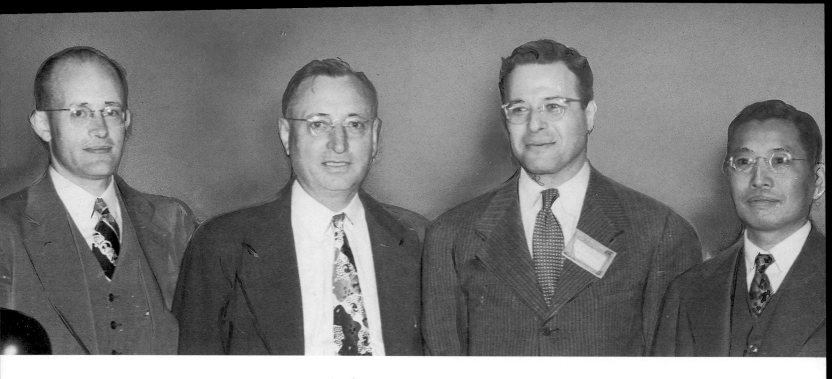

The 1940 program of the APhA Scientific Section featured some noted scientists discussing new drugs. They include (left to right) Mark Nickerson on dibenamine; Walter Hartung on pressor amines; W. H. Hambourger on antispasmodics; and Ko Kuei Chen who had first isolated ephedrine.

helix." This included monoclonal antibody production and recombinant DNA. Then in 1982, members received updates on antiviral agents, antiparasitic agents, new cardiovascular agents, hyperlipidemia agents, antidepressants, and antineoplastic agents.

By 1993, APhA was reminding pharmacists that developments in biotechnology had led to many innovative drug therapies that were now being dispensed by pharmacists. Recombinant DNA technology had yielded 17 protein biopharmaceuticals, beginning with recombinant insulin. The following year, pharmacists were told that three products with interferon activity were already on the market for the treatment of numerous diseases of viral origin.

APhA has kept its members informed of developments vital to the profession in a period which we call, "the Flowering of Science."

CHAPTER 19

State Pharmaceutical Associations

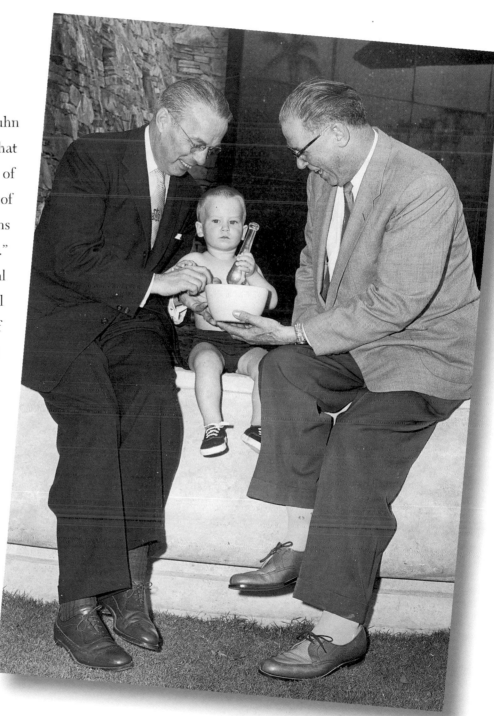

Instructing future pharmacist Jeff Dixon (son of West Virginia Pharmaceutical Association secretary William Dixon) are 1954-1955 president Newell Stewart (left) and 1955-1956 president John Heinz, at the 1955 APhA annual meeting in Miami Beach, Florida.

President Gustavus Luhn observed in 1879 that another achievement of APhA "is the accession of state pharmaceutical associations springing up all over the nation." Five years later, C. Lewis Diehl described the state pharmaceutical associations as "the children of APhA," and indeed, APhA inspired their founding wherever and whenever it could.

When the first state association was established in Maine in 1867, APhA initially considered it to be another local association, but in time, it was recognized as something quite new — the first state pharmaceutical association. Though the Maine association met regularly from 1867 to 1879, no further meetings were held until 1890. The reorganized body seems to have had no connection with the first association, because the report of the

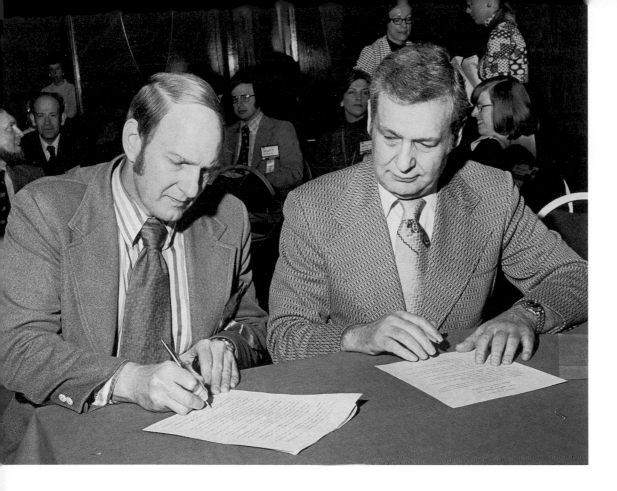

1894 meeting is called the "fifth anniversary meeting."

As evidence of the role of APhA in the founding of state associations, fourteen APhA presidents or vice presidents, and one APhA treasurer served as founding president or secretary of fifteen state associations. They include:

- Vice president Philip C. Candidus (1904-1905), founding president of the Alabama association in 1881-1885.
- Vice president Charles M. Ford (1894-1895), founding president of the Colorado association 1890-1892.
- President George H. Schafer (1881), founding president of the Iowa association 1880-1881.
- Vice president Robert J. Brown (1867-1868), founding president of the Kansas association 1880-1882.
- President Henry T. Cummings (1855), founding president of the Maine association 1867-1873.

- Treasurer Samuel A. D. Sheppard (1886-1908), founding president of the Massachusetts association 1882-1884.
- Vice president Matthew F. Ash (1871-1872), founding president of the Mississippi association 1872.
- President Charles Tufts (1886-1887), founding president of the New Hampshire association 1874-1875.
- President Peter Bedford (1881-1882), founding president of the New York association 1879-1881.
- President Lewis Hopp (1903-1904), founding secretary of the Ohio association 1879-1903.
- Vice president John F. Judge (1881-1882), founding president of the Ohio association 1879-1880.
- President Charles Heinitsh (1882-1883), founding president of the Pennsylvania association 1878-1880.

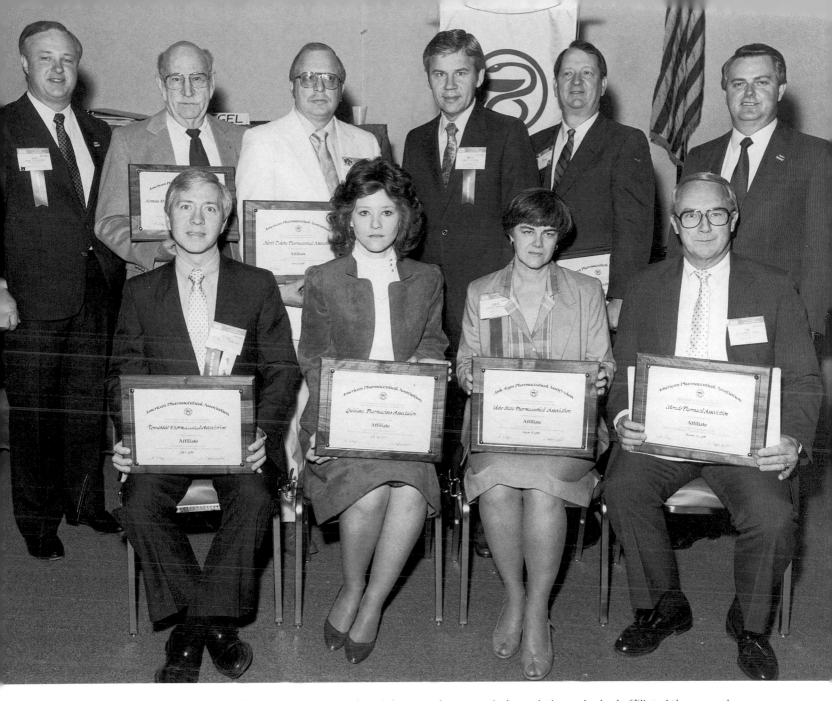

Certificates recognizing APhA affiliation were presented to eight state pharmaceutical associations who had affiliated the year prior to the 1987 annual meeting. They include (seated, left to right) Stephen McDonough (Tennessee); Linda Foreman (Louisiana); Doris Denney (Idaho); and Thomas Gray (Colorado). Standing (left to right) are APhA CEO John Schlegel; Robert Klotzman (Montana); Gordon Mayer (North Dakota); Arvid Liebe (South Dakota); Al Mebane (North Carolina); and APhA president Stephen Crawford.

■ President Gustavus Luhn (1878-1879), founding president of the South Carolina association 1876-1877.

■ Vice president Thomas Roberts Baker (1879-1880), founding president of the Virginia association 1882-1883.

■ Vice president John Alfred Dadd (1884-1885), founding president of the Wisconsin association 1880-1881.

APhA routinely sought opportunities to bring representatives of state pharmaceutical associations into the APhA family. For example, in 1886 president Joseph Roberts proclaimed "a bond of union should exist between state pharmaceutical associations and APhA to identify areas of strength."

It was proposed in 1890 that APhA should hold "a convention of various secretaries of the different states, and that every state association president [should] be made an APhA vice president." Four years later (1894), it was suggested that one member of each state association should be appointed as a "special membership committee."

For decades, representatives of state pharmaceutical associations comprised the membership of the APhA nominations committee for APhA officers. One state association executive continues to serve today on the APhA committee on nominations.

The National Council of State Pharmaceutical Association Executives (NCSPAE) was founded in 1927 as the Conference of Pharmaceutical Association Secretaries which continues to meet at the APhA annual meetings. The Metropolitan Pharmaceutical Association Secretaries was founded in 1928 as the Metropolitan Drug Secretaries Association, but became inactive after 1970.

As early as 1908, president William Martin Searby proposed dual membership for state pharmaceutical associations which would be constituted as a part of APhA. It was not until February 1962 that the effort to get state pharmaceutical associations affiliated with APhA achieved its first success with the affiliation of the Michigan State Pharmaceutical Association. The first joint dues billing was mailed by APhA covering membership for APhA, the Michigan association, and the local pharmaceutical associations.

Delaware affiliated in June 1962, Virginia in July 1962, Wisconsin in October 1962, Iowa in March 1963, Pennsylvania in July 1963. States to follow included Alabama, California, Florida, Illinois, Indiana, Kansas, Kentucky, Maryland, Minnesota, New Jersey, Ohio, South Carolina, Texas, and Utah.

However, by 1975, several states were wavering, and South Carolina was the first to drop affiliation. Then in 1979, APhA offered all states the option of suspending affiliation for 24 months "to permit a rational evaluation of the mandatory reciprocal membership requirement."

The mandatory reciprocal membership provision was eliminated in 1979, even though all state pharmaceutical associations remain as APhA affiliates with voting representation in the APhA House of Delegates.

CHAPTER 20

The APhA Branch Experiment

At the 1903 annual meeting in Mackinac Island, Michigan, APhA approved a motion suggesting that "a branch of this Association be inaugurated and maintained in the City of Philadelphia. Three years later the formation of APhA local branches was approved by the Council with the requirement that each had to have 25 APhA members. The initial proposal, made by Henry Whelpley, was to have the colleges of pharmacy serve as the organizers of the local branches.

The first local branch to be formed was not in Philadelphia, but in Chicago, established in February 1906 with Oscar Oldberg as president and William Baker Day as secretary. Philadelphia was not far behind, organizing Branch #2 in March 1906 with Joseph Price Remington as president. In 1909, the Philadelphia Branch established its own Scientific Section. Joseph Remington served as APhA president 1892-1983; Oscar Oldberg was APhA president 1908-1909; and William Day served as APhA president 1912-1913.

One of the first APhA branches was established in 1906. This postcard photograph of the organizational meeting was used as a Christmas and New Year greeting card. However, the St. Louis Branch was only active for two years and was not reactivated until 1957.

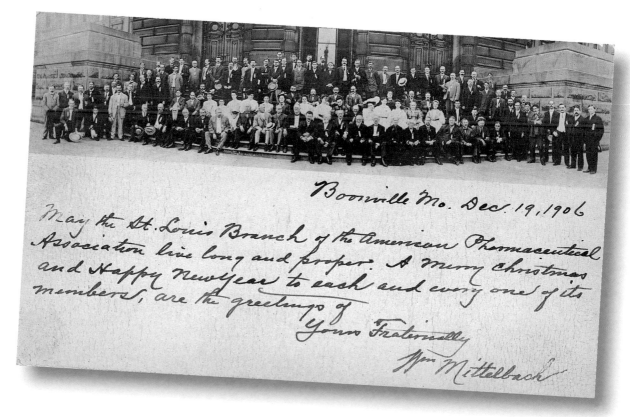

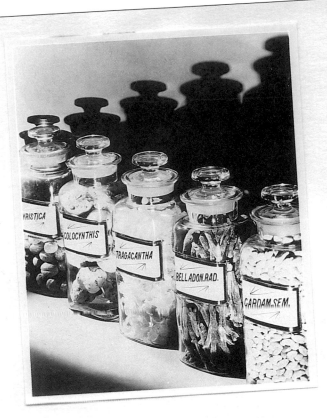

BANQUET
in honor of the institution of the
Northern New Jersey Branch
of the
American Pharmaceutical Association
Elks' Club, Newark   November 20, 1933

The Northern New Jersey APhA Branch was formed in 1933, electing Ernest Little as its first president. Little went on to serve as 1948-1949 APhA president. This is the Banquet Program used in honor of the institution of this Branch.

All other Branches formed during 1906 had APhA presidents as Branch-founding presidents. They included APhA presidents Lewis Hopp (1903-1904) and Henry Vincome Arny (1923-1924) who served respectively as president and secretary of the Northern Ohio Branch (Cleveland); APhA president John Hancock (1873-1874) and general secretary Evander Kelly (1925-1944) serving as founding president and secretary of the Baltimore Branch; APhA president Frederick Wulling (1916-1917) as founding president of the Northwestern Branch in Minneapolis; APhA president Charles Packard (1920-1921) as New England Branch founding president; APhA president

William Alpers (1915-1916) holding the position as the New York Branch president; and APhA president Henry Whelpley (1901-1902) as founding president of the short-lived St. Louis Branch.

APhA Bulletin editor C. S. N. Hallberg editorialized in the April 1907 issue, "When the first APhA Branch was organized some 15 months ago, it was realized that the project was a decided innovation and the program difficult of execution. To those engaged therein, however, it was not a fearful task knowing that their efforts would eventually be crowned with success."

The next Branch to be formed was that of

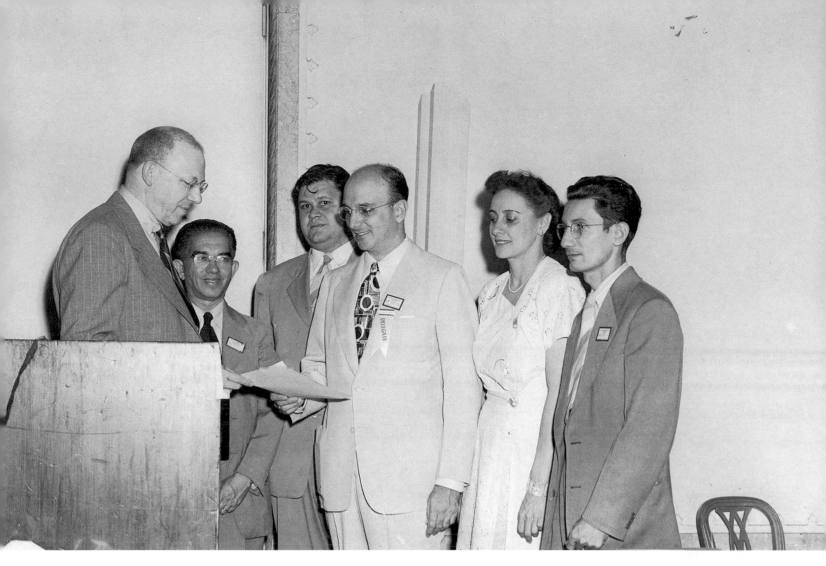

APhA secretary Robert Fischelis charters the Puerto Rico Branch at the 1946 annual meeting. Pictured are (left to right) Robert Fischelis, dean Luis Torres-Diaz, Francisco Hidalgo, Carlos Gonzales, Carlota Badilo, and Rodolfo Escabi. Other APhA branches were also formed in the Canal Zone and in Havana, Cuba.

the City of Washington in 1908, with Harvey W. Wiley as president, and Martin I. Wilbert as secretary. Hallberg described Wiley as, "if not the Moses leading the people of the United States out of the wilderness of poisonous and fraudulent foods and body- and soul-destroying drugs, [he] has at least pointed out the promised land — effective supervision through the Federal Food and Drugs Act."

The next four Branches were organized in 1909 and included the Pittsburgh Branch with 1922-1923 APhA president Julius Koch as founding Branch president; the New Orleans Branch with 1905-1906 APhA third vice president Fabius Godbold as founding Branch president; S. L. Bresler

as founding president of the Denver Branch; and Minor T. Wadell as founding president of the short-lived Indiana Branch. The Nashville Branch was founded 1910 with James Burge as president.

But in 1911, some pharmacists in larger cities were complaining that the formation of APhA branches was competing with their local retail druggists associations. James H. Beal explained in the November 1911 issue of the *APhA Bulletin* that "APhA is not jealous of the success of the other associations. It is the mother of pharmaceutical organizations in the Western Continent, and for more than half a century has urged the formation of organizations to represent the several divisions of the drug trade."

Commencing in the 1920s, APhA reduced the number of APhA members to qualify for organizing a local branch from 25 to 15, which led to the formation of branches in Alabama and Montana. In 1937, the APhA House of Delegates urged that the Association allocate 50 cents to local Branches for each branch member so that they "may more effectively carry out their programs," and each branch should be visited by an Association officer annually.

After the formation of the American Society of Hospital Pharmacists, several APhA branches were jointly recognized as ASHP chapters. Then, stimulated by plans to recognize APhA's centennial, new branches were established variously in California, Florida, Nebraska, New Jersey, New Mexico, Ohio, Oregon, South Carolina, Tennessee, Texas, Utah, Virginia, Washington, and Wisconsin. APhA secretary Robert Fischelis frequently visited founding meetings of these new branches to personally present their charter. During this same period, APhA Branches were also established in the Canal Zone, Puerto Rico, and Havana, Cuba; the latter lasted until Fidel Castro came into power.

In 1962, the name of branches was changed to APhA Chapters, but by this time APhA had launched its campaign encouraging state pharmaceutical associations to affiliate with APhA. So, in 1964, William S. Apple wrote various chapters that "when a state association affiliates with APhA, all APhA Chapters should be dissolved." It was not until 1979 that the APhA Bylaws were amended, terminating the authorization for APhA Chapters. Only two or three of the chapters had on-going programs that had to be transferred to APhA as in the case of the New York Chapter which administered the Remington Honor Medal, and the Philadelphia Chapter which transferred its long-standing Scientific Section to the APhA Academy of Pharmaceutical Sciences.

No comprehensive history of APhA Branches/Chapters has been found, though there is evidence that Robert Fischelis had asked each branch to write its history for the APhA centennial meeting. Only the Philadelphia Branch recorded its history through 1952 for the APhA centennial convention, which now resides in the APhA Foundation Archives.

CHAPTER 21

The House of Delegates Emerges

Perhaps the most important organizational action of APhA in the first half of the 20th century was the creation of the House of Delegates.

On the long train trip to Denver for the 1912 Annual Meeting, general secretary James Hartley Beal and long-time treasurer Henry M. Whelpley discussed the creation of a body within APhA that could represent the thinking of all components of the profession. After a spirited debate in Denver, the APhA House of Delegates was formally organized on August 21, 1912. Two days earlier the APhA Council [now Board of Trustees] adopted an enabling resolution charging the new body "to receive and consider the reports of delegates from the bodies they represent in the House of Delegates."

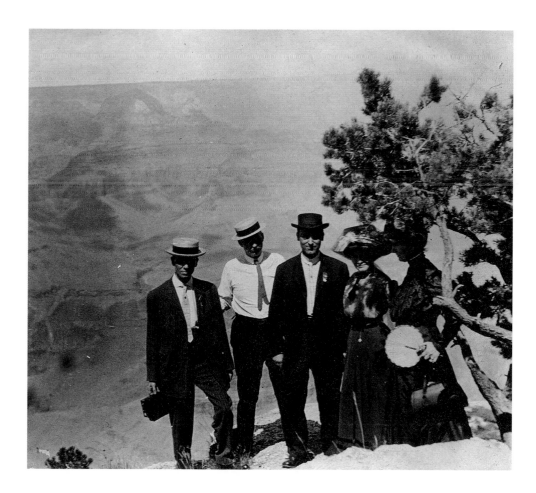

Delegates to the 1912 annual meeting in Denver, Colorado, stop to admire the Grand Canyon. It was on the long trip to Denver that secretary James Beal and treasurer Henry Whelpley drew up plans for the creation of the APhA House of Delegates.

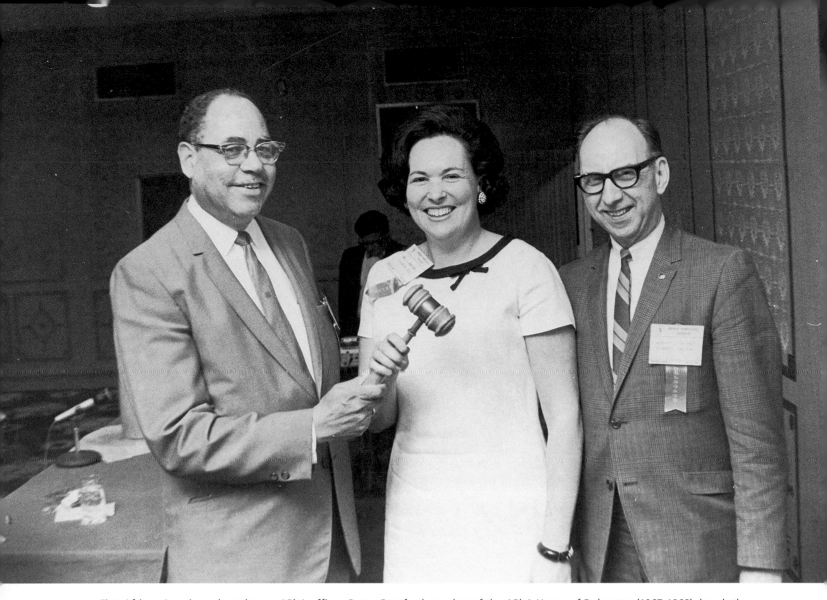

First African American elected as an APhA officer, Byron Rumford, speaker of the APhA House of Delegates (1967-1968), hands the gavel to his successor Mary Louise Anderson, the first woman to serve in the same position (1968-1970). Participating in the installation is past speaker Charles Schreiber (1966-1967). Rumford previously served as vice speaker (1966-1967), while Anderson previously served as APhA second vice president (1967-1968) and was the first woman to be a candidate for APhA president in 1970.

The APhA House of Delegates was not an immediate success; perhaps it was an idea before its time. Evander F. Kelly summarized the state of affairs in his address as 1921 Chairman of the House by concluding that "the House has not fulfilled the expectations of those who established it." Kelly observed that state pharmaceutical associations could not be expected to accept the actions taken in the APhA House of Delegates attended by "the limited few of its members who can attend an annual meeting," and urged the House "to take proper steps to see that the state associations shall have the opportunity to express themselves."

As a result of Kelly's campaign to reorganize the House by expanding "its limited function," the Bylaws were revised in 1924 to give the House additional responsibilities. These included electing, on nomination of the Council, the Association's chief executive officer (known at various times as secretary, general secretary, executive director, president, and executive vice president); treasurer, and honorary president (a responsibility which was retained by the House until 1979 for the Association's chief executive officer and treasurer, and until 1984 for the honorary president). The House was also given the authority to select future sites for Association annual meetings (a responsibility which remained with the House until 1960 when the selection was delegated to the Board of Trustees).

A point of contention existed for decades over the provision that before a House action became official Association policy, it had to be ratified at a general session of the annual meeting. In reviewing this concern, a 1944 Association committee on policy and planning observed that "when the APhA Bylaws were amended to create the House of Delegates, the Council gave the general session veto power over the House fearing the House would usurp many of the functions and decisions of the general sessions." The 1944 committee's conclusion was that "it is time we make actions of the House final." But the Association Bylaws retained the provision that "any action taken by the House of Delegates can be negated at a general session by a majority vote with not less than 50 members present and voting." The House countered in 1956 with a proposed provision that all actions taken by the House were "final until and unless revoked by a three-fourths vote of the Association members present and voting at an official general session of the Association." The provision that "official actions of the House are subject to review and approval of the general sessions" remained a part of the Association Bylaws until 1971.

Conflicts of authority also existed between the House of Delegates and the APhA Council (Board of Trustees). For example, as early as 1913, the Council withdrew the authority of the chairman of the House to appoint its own committee on nominations. In response to delegates who complained that the Council did not act on resolutions adopted by the House, Robert Fischelis explained in 1948

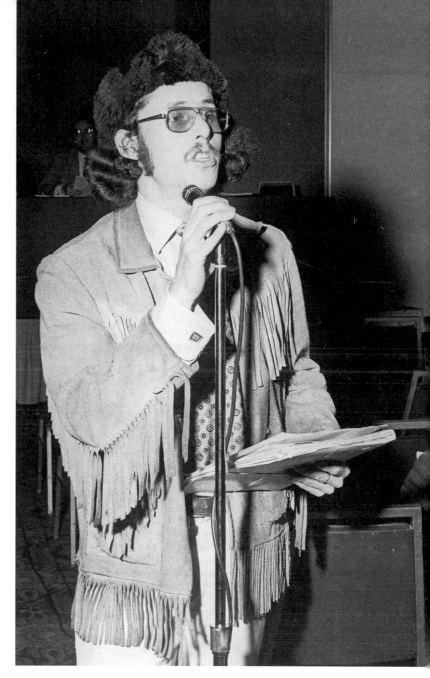

"Rebel Spokesman" Larry Kline sought the legalization of marijuana before the APhA Reference Committee on Public Affairs during the 1971 annual meeting in San Francisco.

that "some resolutions would commit the Association to policies quite outside of its normal range of activities, while others require expenditure of funds which only the Council can authorize."

Twenty-four years later (1972) House speaker Philip Sacks responded to complaints on non-implementation of House actions by noting that it was not always possible to implement policy which required additional staff time and the expenditure of additional funds. Thus the implementation of a policy

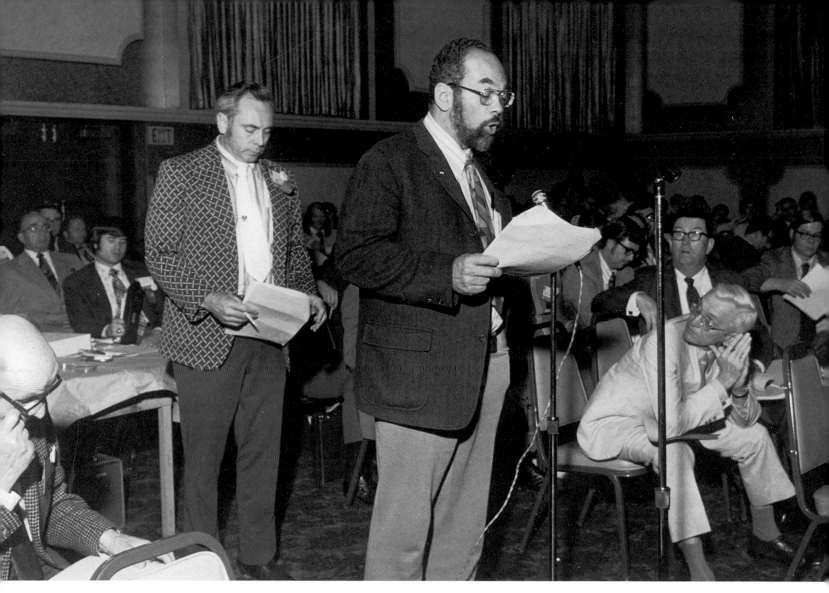

Robert Gibson makes a point during the 1972 APhA Organizational Affairs Reference Committee. Immediately behind Gibson, who was to serve as president 28 years later, is Jim McCoy awaiting his turn at the microphone.

may be possible only with additional income from an expanded membership, and an increase in staffing at APhA headquarters.

"We cannot pretend that there have not been some major disagreements between the APhA Board of Trustees and the APhA House of Delegates," stated 1985 House speaker Lowell Anderson who called for (but did not receive) authorization for the House to override any veto of the Board of Trustees by a two-thirds vote.

1973 House speaker Jacob Miller explained that "the primary function of the House is to provide guidance to the Board of Trustees which has the duty to act for the Association in the interim between meetings [and] to supervise all property, funds, and

finances of the Association. Hence the function of the Board of Trustees is to run the Association." In 1986, House speaker Raymond Roberts re-emphasized that "the function of the House under the Association's Bylaws is as a legislative body in the development of Association policy. While the House is empowered to establish policy, it does not manage the Association."

The House also tackled the question: who does the APhA House of Delegates actually represent? It decided (1973) that: "Policies adopted by APhA are those of APhA alone. Such policies are in no way binding on any other pharmacy organization whether or not affiliated with APhA. Similarly, policies adopted by other pharmacy organizations are in no way binding upon APhA. Other organizations cannot dictate APhA policies, but may influence APhA policy to the extent that they are represented in the APhA House of Delegates."

The initial 1912 Bylaws of the House of Delegates authorized a chairman, two vice chairmen, and a secretary. The Bylaws were revised in 1924 authorizing a chairman and a single vice chairman to be elected in a mail ballot by delegates to the House, and a permanent secretary who shall be the secretary [chief executive officer] of the Association.

The 1946 Association Bylaws gave the House of Delegates chairman a seat on the APhA Council, and 1969 Bylaw amendments changed the title of the House chairman to House speaker, and vice chairman to vice speaker. Commencing in 1971, both the speaker and the vice speaker served as members of the APhA Board of Trustees.

The office of House vice speaker was eliminated in 1979 as a member of the APhA Board of Trustees, after which House speaker Lowell Anderson in 1984 called for abolishing the position of vice speaker "since the vice speaker no longer sits on the Board of Trustees." A special Bylaws committee recommended in 1985 the abolishment of the position of vice speaker "because the office has only limited functions," but the APhA Board of Trustees did not approve the recommendation preferring to "first study the means by which the duties of the vice speaker might be expanded." Then in 1986, the Association's Bylaws were amended deleting the position of vice speaker of the House, and providing for "the election of a speaker *pro tem* in the event the speaker is unable to perform the duties of the office."

Initially, resolutions establishing Association policy originated through recommendations con-

tained in addresses of Association officers, in the reports of Association Sections, and from motions made by individual delegates. Following Evander Kelly's 1921 reorganization, state association delegates were urged by 1925 House chairman Waldemar Bruce Philip "to bring before the House all resolutions adopted by their state that have a bearing on subjects pertaining to Pharmacy." House chairman Robert Swain reported in 1930 that representatives of state associations "confer upon policies of common interest and coordinate their respective policies with each other and with the state societies." This process continued until after World War II.

All resolutions were submitted to a committee on resolutions which was charged with reporting its deliberations to the House. For adoption, "all resolutions shall receive a majority of affirmative votes of those present." The 1948 House Bylaws sought to make the Association's resolutions committee more democratic by requiring nine members, "three of whose terms shall expire in one, two, and three years, respectively."

Over the years, as many as four sessions of the House were held at a single annual meeting to accommodate as many as 29 standing and special committees which submitted their recommendations to the House. In 1957 the House made its first recommendation for the creation of "reference committees to assist in coordinating proposals offered for consideration by the House and translating such proposals into policy decisions;" this was patterned after procedures of the American Medical Association. "The activities of the Association have continued to expand until a full discussion of all of them on the floor of the House has become almost impossible," announced 1965 House chairman Linwood Tice. "In

CHAPTER 22

APhA Foundation

The APhA Foundation, incorporated in the District of Columbia on May 6, 1953, was one of the by-products of the APhA centennial celebration. However, the activity of the Foundation was limited for the first five years. With the election of William S. Apple as secretary in 1959, the Foundation took on a new life. Since the Internal Revenue Service had previously advised APhA that there had not been enough activity by the Foundation to classify it as a charitable, education, and scientific organization, APhA transferred the APhA Library, the APhA Museum, and the APhA Drug Standards Laboratory to the Foundation.

The earliest grants made by the Foundation included a study of the accreditation of hospital pharmacy interns in 1958. A prepaid prescription service study conducted at the University of Pittsburgh, and a study documenting the availability of pharmacy manpower were both supported by the Foundation in 1961. As a result of this new activity, the Foundation was granted tax-exempt status as a 501(c)(3) organization on April 25, 1961.

Over the years, the APhA Foundation funded projects in a wide range of research areas, but in the 1980s most grants involved research in improving pharmacy practice. Then in 1994, the Foundation directed its full attention to a new mission: "To advance the knowledge and practice of pharmacy to optimize therapeutic outcomes through pharmaceutical care." In the summer of 1994, the Foundation launched a new periodical, *Pharmaceutical Care Profiles*. The first "Pharmaceutical Care Networking Directory" was published, and the first seven grants were awarded to help pharmacists design and implement pharmaceutical care programs.

In 1996, the APhA Foundation commenced Project ImPACT (Improve Persistance and Compliance to Therapy), and 20 incentive grants were

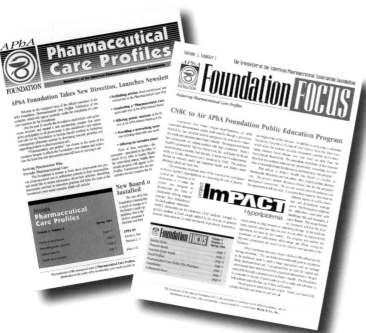

APhA Foundation periodicals launched in the 1990s.

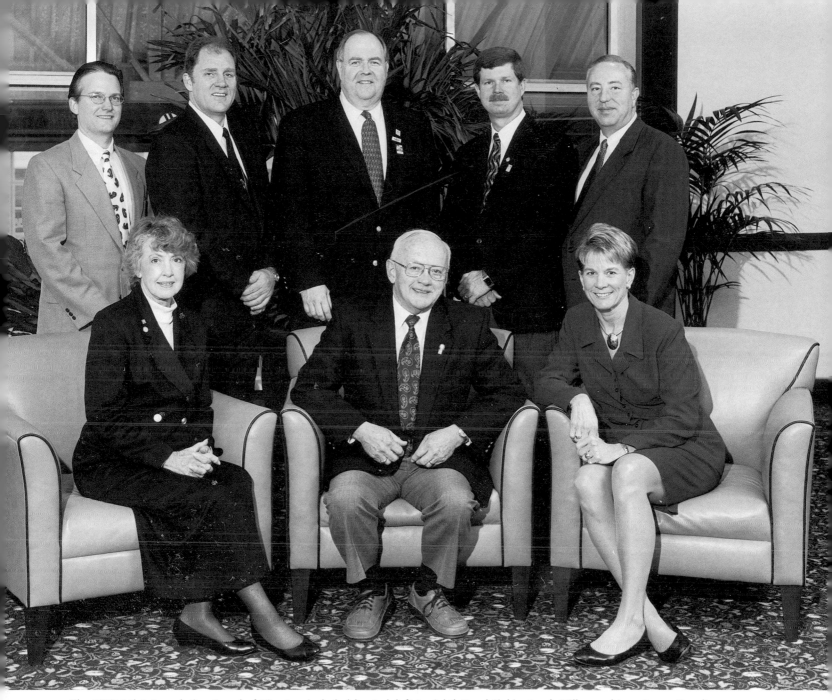

The 1999 APhA Foundation Board of Directors included (seated, left to right) Hazel Pipkin, Jacob Miller, and Jane Jones. Standing (left to right) executive director William Ellis, Brian Isetts, secretary John Gans, Tery Baskin, and Steve Firman.

awarded for innovative projects. William M. Ellis became the first full-time executive director of the APhA Foundation in 1998, and changed the title of the newsletter to *APhA Foundation Focus*. Pinnacle Awards, which had been established by APhA in 1997, were first awarded the following year by the APhA Foundation Quality Center, for exemplary leadership in the improvement of quality in the medication use process by an individual, by a group of individuals, and by a health care organization.

The Advanced Practice Institute was sponsored by the APhA Foundation in 1999 with a three-day program at the University of Florida College of Pharmacy where over 50 practitioners participated in an intensive, advanced learning and skill development experience for pharmacists practicing in ambulatory care settings. The second annual Advanced Practice Institute held in 2000 included new ways to help patients with diabetes, asthma, heart disease, and problems with general medication use.

CHAPTER 23.

American Institute of Pharmacy

In 1858, APhA president John Kidwell operated a pharmacy near the corner of Pennsylvania Avenue and 14th Street in Washington, D.C. He subsequently became known as the "Quinine King" because of the large volume of drugs which he sold to the Union Army during the Civil War. In 1869, Kidwell obtained rights to marshland including part of the property where APhA headquarters was later to be built. The swampy land became known as *Kidwell's Meadows* (later as Potomac Flats) and it remained in the ownership of Kidwell until he died in 1885.

By this time, *Kidwell's Meadows* had been completely filled in, becoming *Potomac Park*, which led Congress to order in 1886 that the Federal government should determine the ownership of the land. In October 1895, the U.S. Supreme Court ruled against more than 50 persons claiming various portions of the land which comprised the whole of *Potomac Flats*. With regard to *Kidwell's Meadows* the Court ruled that it "was undoubtedly acquired for speculative purposes, and for the government to part with its land to promote such purposes was against public policy."

At that time, APhA headquarters moved no less than six times from the office of one secretary to the office of a new secretary. APhA general secretary James Hartley Beal called for "an Association home" in November 1912 to house its archives, library, and a "suitable laboratory for the *National Formulary.*" After APhA moved forward in 1921 with plans for "the securing of a permanent home for the central offices of the Association," Beal was made chairman of the newly appointed Committee on a Permanent Home for APhA. Beal reported that "offers of help were abundant," but by the time of the 1923 annual meeting a scant $21,000 had been pledged for the building. Henry Armit Brown Dunning, chairman of the board of the Baltimore firm of Hynson, Wescott and Dunning Company, described these efforts as "a ridiculous amount considering that there are in the U.S. some 52,000 druggists," and he proceeded to outline a course of action for raising $500,000 "to erect a headquarters building for APhA."

APhA was quick to accept Dr. Dunning's offer, and he was named chairman of the APhA All-Pharmacy Headquarters Building Campaign. Dunning

Opposite Page: The design above was submitted by John Russell Pope in 1907 for Abraham Lincoln's birthplace memorial in Hodgenville, Kentucky, to enshrine Lincoln's original log cabin. Since it was not accepted, Pope resubmitted the design below for the American Institute of Pharmacy. Both the National Park Commission and the District of Columbia Fine Arts Commission accepted the design.

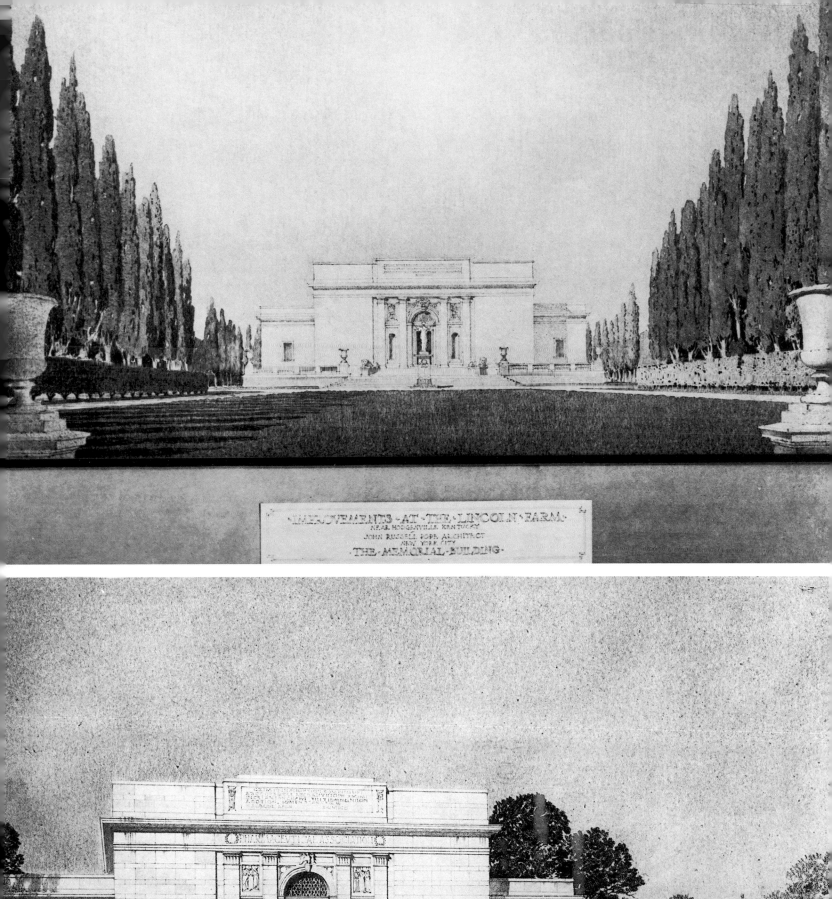

IMPROVEMENTS·AT·THE·LINCOLN·FARM·
NEAR·HODGENVILLE·KENTUCKY
JOHN·RUSSELL·POPE·ARCHITECT
NEW·YORK·CITY
THE·MEMORIAL·BUILDING·

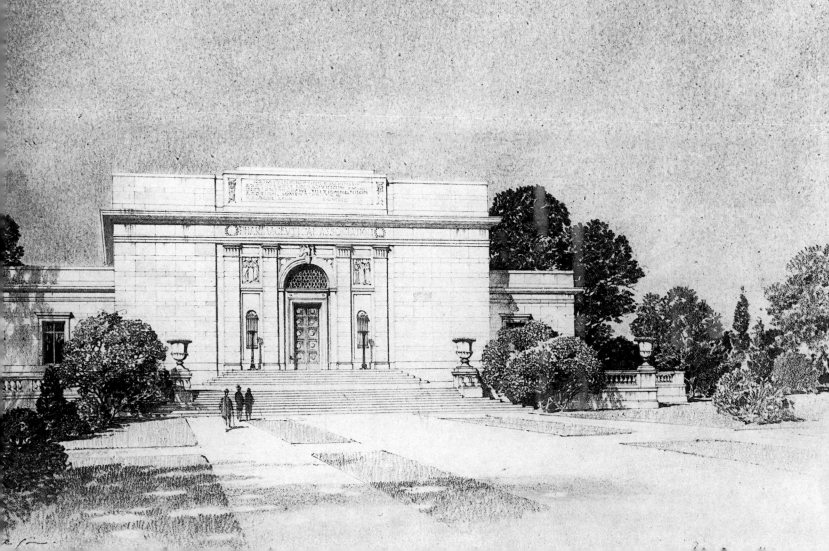

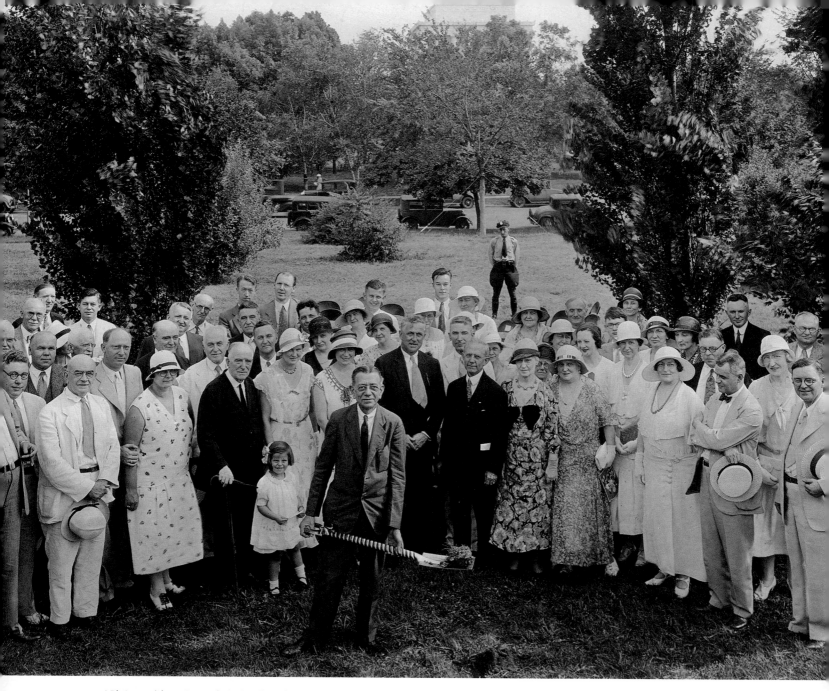

APhA president Samuel Louis Hilton breaks ground for the American Institute of Pharmacy on July 1, 1932. Included in this photograph are Mr. & Mrs. **Walter Adams**; Arthur Boas; G. A. Bunting; H. P. Caemaerer; Dr. & Mrs. Fred Campbell; V. K. Chestnut; Dr. & Mrs. **Frank Delgado**; W. C. Downey; Dr. & Mrs. **Andrew DuMez**; Dr. & Mrs. **Henry A. B. Dunning**; Katherine Dunning; Dr. & Mrs. **Eugene Eberle**; **Robert Fischelis**; Martha Floyd; Carson P. Frailey; Charles Fuhrman; H. C. Fuller; A. F. Gorsuch; Mr. Gardiner; Ida Heilberger; Mr. & Mrs. **Samuel Hilton**; Dr. & Mrs. **Glenn Jenkins**; Esther Jenkins; **Lyman Kebler**; Dr. & Mrs. **Evander Kelly**; Dr. & Mrs. **John Krantz, Jr.**; Minnie Low; Mr. & Mrs. Thomas Moskey; **Edwin Newcomb**; Dr. & Mrs. **W. Bruce Philip**; Mr. Quigley; Ethel Ridway; Miss Rogers; Mr. and Mrs. W. B. Spire; Dr. & Mrs. **Robert Swain**; A. C. Taylor; Sir **Henry Wellcome**; Lee Williamson; and Mr. & Mrs. **Arthur Winne**. [Those with names in bold face served at some time as an APhA officer.]

launched an aggressive program in April 1924, and appointed Edwin Leigh Newcomb, then editor of *Northwestern Druggist*, as director of publicity. By May 1926, $500,000 had been subscribed, and through a succession of three ballots mailed to APhA members over a four-month period in 1927,

Washington, D.C. was selected as the site for a permanent home for APhA.

By the turn of the 20th century, Smithsonian Institution secretary Joseph Henry had prodded a reluctant Federal government to "fill in the canals, drain the marshes, and perfect the roads" in

Washington, D.C. This effort was instrumental in unfolding a plan that in time produced The Mall as we know it today. Construction of the Lincoln Memorial was commenced in 1915, and, it was dedicated in 1922, while the nearby National Academy of Sciences building was started in 1922 and dedicated in 1924.

In February 1928, Dunning personally made a down payment on a plot of land directly opposite the Lincoln Memorial and adjacent to the National Academy of Sciences for the location of the APhA headquarters building. He recommended it to APhA as an "ideal site" for what he was now calling the American Institute of Pharmacy. Meanwhile, the District of Colombia Fine Arts Commission had proposed the creation of The Mall, and announced plans to convert B Street (later named Constitution Avenue) "into a monumental thoroughfare leading from the Capital westward to the Potomac."

There was still an obstacle for APhA to overcome; Upper Water Street cut diagonally across the front of the property that was purchased by APhA. In 1929, APhA officials met with Fine Arts Commission Chairman Charles Moore asking him to urge Congress to close Upper Water Street. Moore appealed to U.S. Senator Henry W. Keyes for such authorization, but before Congress would agree to close Upper Water Street, APhA had to buy the remaining lots to extend the property from 22nd Street to 23rd Street. Within months, APhA purchased the additional lots. In May 1932, Senate Joint Resolution #50 was passed by the House of Representatives and signed into law by President Herbert Hoover authorizing the closing of Upper Water Street and the transfer of a strip of land now owned by APhA to the U.S. government to widen 23rd Street "as an approach to the Lincoln Memorial." The final clause of the Congressional action has since resulted in numerous legal interpretations as to whether or not APhA could ever sell its headquarters building; the 1932 Act of Congress states that the agreement is conditional on the understanding that the use of the building "shall be limited to organizations and institutions serving American pharmacy on a nonprofit basis."

APhA found an architect ideally suited to design the American Institute of Pharmacy. He was John Russell Pope who was responsible for some of the most famous structures in Washington, D.C., including the Jefferson Memorial, the National Archives, the National Gallery of Art, and Constitution Hall. Pope's design was not created expressly for the APhA headquarters building. His first major museum commission in 1907 was to design a memorial for Abraham Lincoln's birthplace in Hodgenville, Kentucky, to enshrine Lincoln's original log cabin. Pope's 1907 design proved too expensive to build, and he was forced to create a less expensive structure that stands today at Lincoln's Farm. Since it was a common practice for architects to re-cycle unused designs, Pope submitted his 1907 design as the plan for the American Institute of Pharmacy.

While government records clearly show the origin of the APhA building design, nary a word is said about it in any APhA publications of the day; some say that pharmacy leaders of the period felt that it was beneath the dignity of pharmacy to reveal that the design was not created expressly for APhA. However, it appears that the original design was the inspiration for of a myth perpetuated for decades by taxicab drivers and tour guides in the nation's capital who told vis-

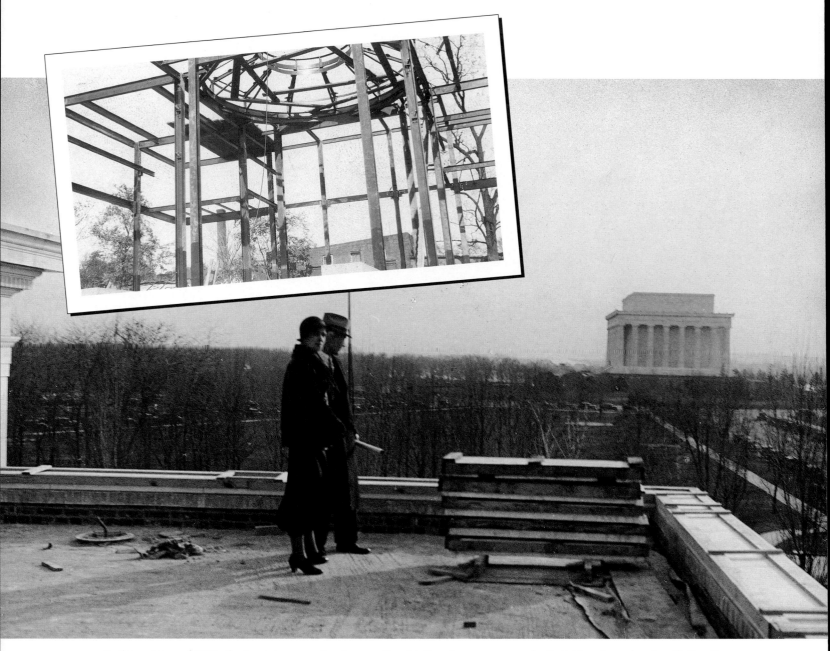

By the summer of 1932, the imposing new structure on Constitution Avenue was gradually taking shape (**see inset**). Shortly before the October 1933 completion of the American Institute of Pharmacy, APhA secretary Evander Kelly and Mrs. Kelly stood on the roof admiring the view of the Lincoln Memorial in the background.

itors that the American Institute of Pharmacy was intended for Lincoln's tomb. Taxicab drivers subsequently called the American Institute of Pharmacy the tomb of "the unknown pharmacist."

Ground breaking for the American Institute of Pharmacy was held July 1, 1932, at which the District of Columbia Fine Arts Commission chairman declared: "We are here today to break ground for a building which shall stand as a symbol of ethics, honesty, and fidelity in ministering to human needs." Construction of

the building took slightly more than one year with a cost override because the government required APhA to use Vermont marble for the building facing.

The American Institute of Pharmacy was not dedicated until May 9, 1934, so that the ceremony could be held during the APhA annual meeting. A highlight of the ceremony was a letter from President Franklin D. Roosevelt reading: "I regret that the press of Executive duties has made it impossible for me to greet you here personally, but through

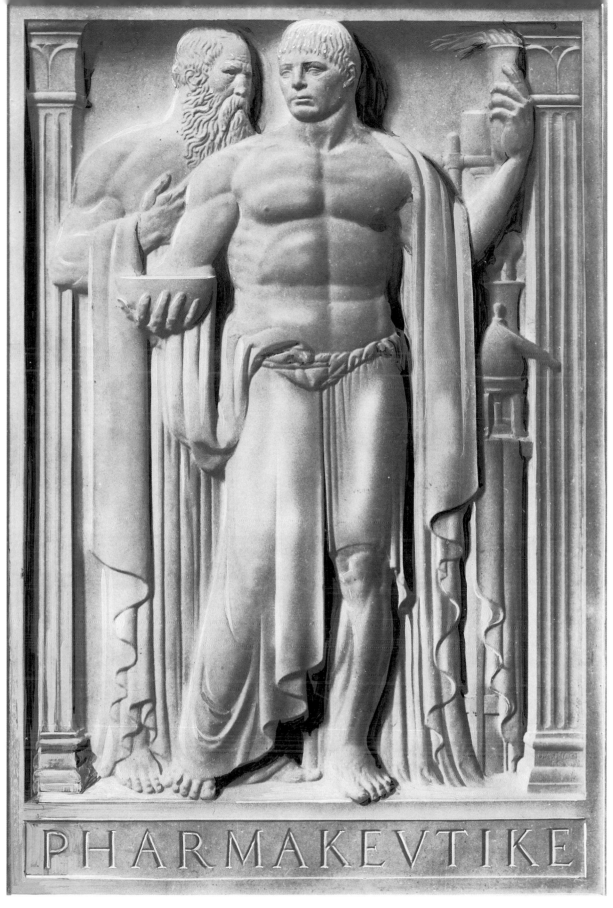

PHARMAKEVTIKE

Above the entrance to the American Institute of Pharmacy is this bas-relief panel entitled PHARMAKEVTIKE representing the profession of pharmacy. The designer, Ulysses Rico, depicts a youth symbolizing progress, and an adult representing "the pioneer who observes the improvements made as fruits of his research."

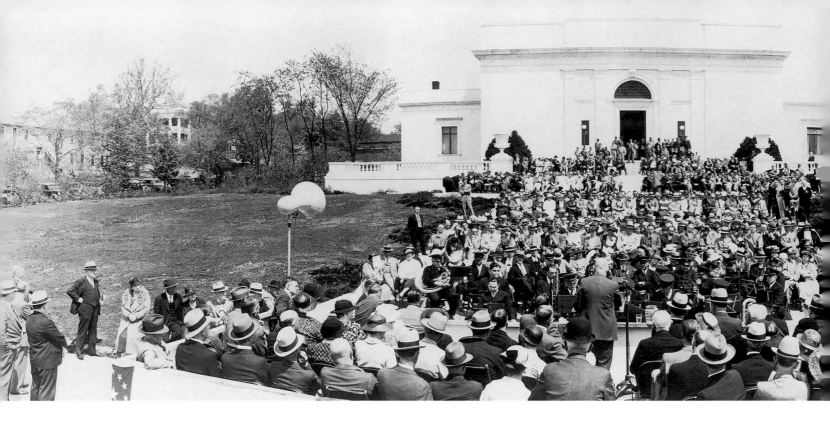

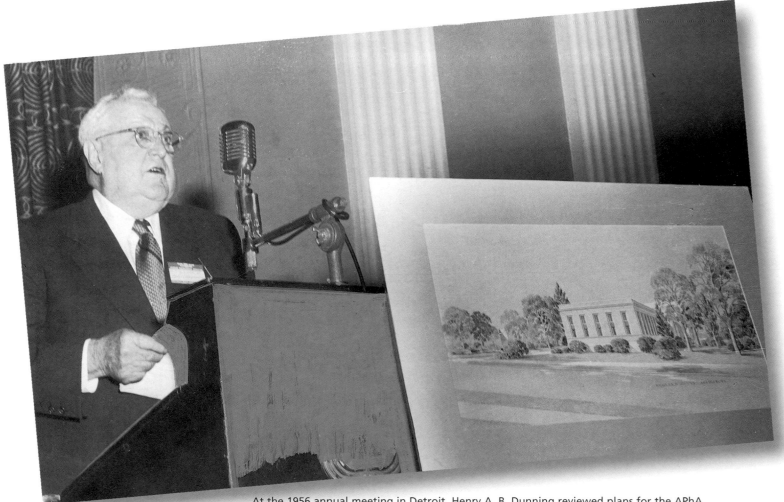

At the 1956 annual meeting in Detroit, Henry A. B. Dunning reviewed plans for the APhA headquarters extension. He reported that his committee had already received $100,000 toward the goal of $300,000 to provide the new wing pictured on the architect's drawing.

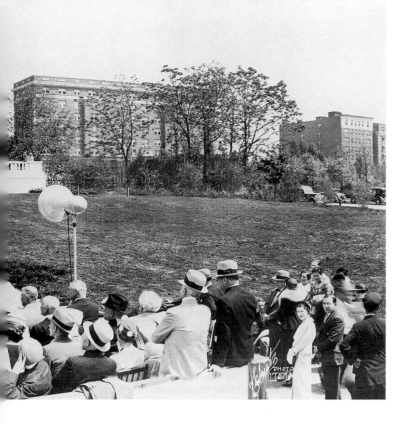

The dedication of the American Institute of Pharmacy was held on May 9, 1934, during the annual meeting in Washington, D.C. A high-light of the ceremony was a message from U.S. president Franklin D. Roosevelt who wrote, "the dedication of this beautiful structure...is an important milestone in the history of the profession of pharmacy."

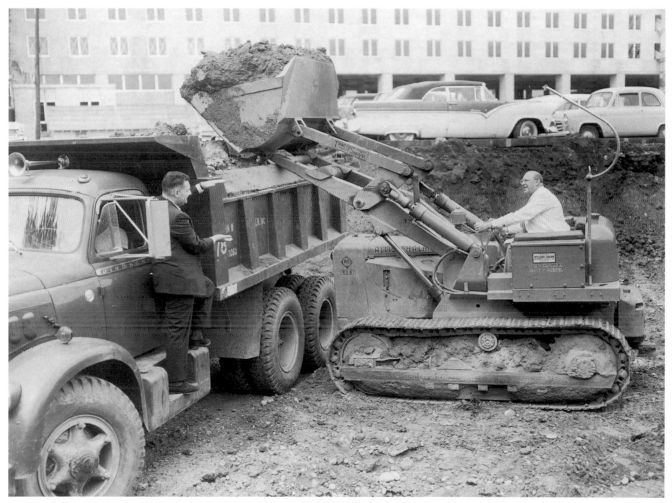

Secretary Robert Fischelis pretends to be the operator of a fork-lift clearing the area in 1959 for the annex to the APhA headquarters building, while secretary-nominate William Apple plays the role of supervisor. Seen in the background is the new Department of State building which had just opened.

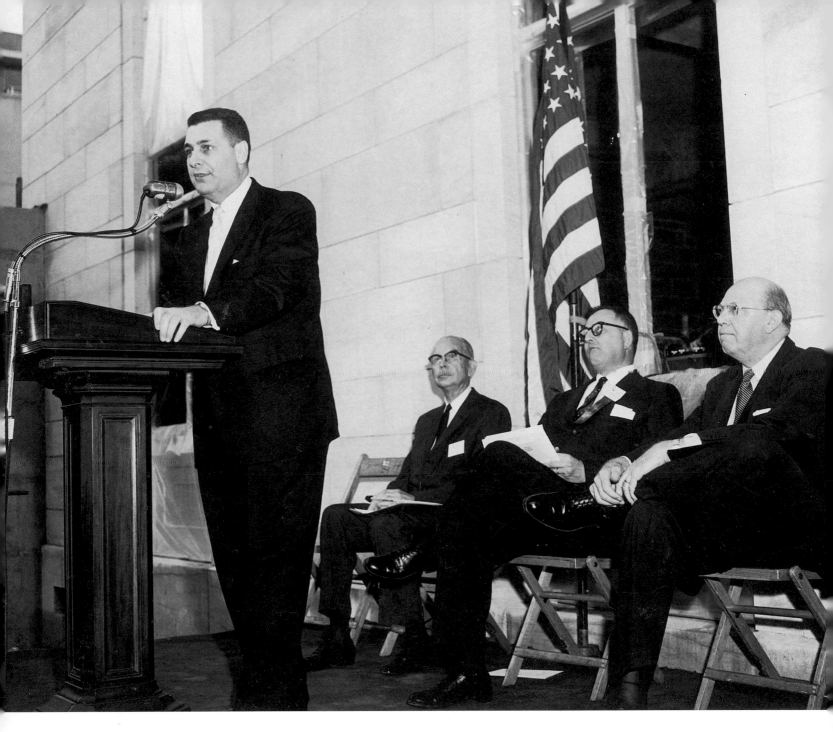

Secretary William Apple speaks at the August 16, 1960, dedication of the APhA headquarters building annex. Seated behind him are president Howard Newton; president-elect George Archambault; and former secretary Robert Fischelis.

this message I express my appreciation of the great work you have accomplished."

National Association of Board of Pharmacy secretary, H. C. Christenson, had earlier recommended that all American pharmacy associations should be housed in the new building. Then in 1936, Patrick Costello urged NABP to "remove its central office" to the American Institute of Pharmacy, and expressed the hope that "the American Association of Colleges of Pharmacy would do

likewise." However, none of the other existing pharmacy associations decided to accept APhA's invitation to move their offices to the American Institute of Pharmacy.

Expansion of the American Institute of Pharmacy commenced in 1956 with plans to build both an east and west wing since the property immediately behind APhA had been purchased by the National Association of Life Underwriters (NALU) to erect their headquarters. When NALU withdrew its plans and sold the lot to the government in 1958, APhA sought and obtained agreement to exchange land with the government to permit the annex to be built immediately behind the original building.

Exchange of land took place in the Fall of 1958, and the government agreed to convert the land immediately behind the original APhA headquarters building into park land as an approach to the new State Department which was dedicated in 1957. Ground breaking for the annex took place on July 14, 1959, but a steel strike delayed construction plans. The annex was dedicated during the 1960 annual meeting on August 16, 1960.

On August 1, 1984, APhA celebrated the 50th anniversary of its headquarters. Four years later, glass front doors were installed so that when the brass front doors are open the Lincoln Memorial can be seen; the reception desk was relocated to the front entry vestibule; and a new lighted sign was placed in front of the American Institute of Pharmacy. Plans were officially unveiled at the 2001 annual meeting to purchase the land behind APhA headquarters and replace the present annex with a new structure.

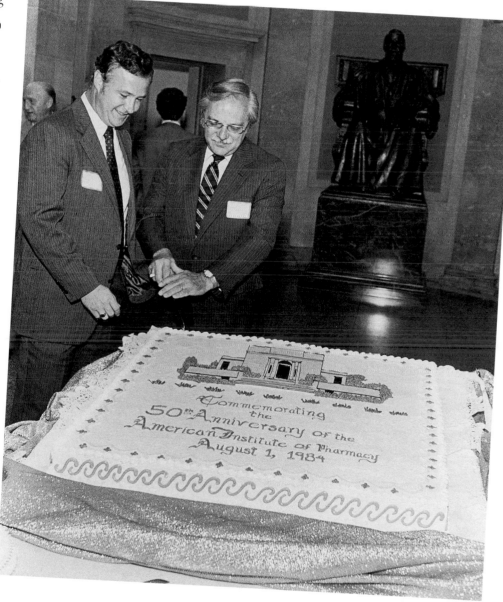

On August 1, 1984, the 50th anniversary of the American Institute of Pharmacy was celebrated. APhA chief executive officer John Schlegel and president Herbert Carlin admire the birthday cake that was served to nearly 500 invited guests.

CHAPTER 24.

Drug Standards Laboratory

While attending the 1934 dedication ceremonies for the American Institute of Pharmacy, Sir Henry Wellcome criticized the proposed location of the laboratory in the basement of the new building, and he offered to have Burroughs-Wellcome construct a "Chemical Biological and Physical Laboratory" if the U.S. government would donate the land from APhA's plots to C Street. The U.S. Congress failed to take appropriate action, and Wellcome withdrew his offer.

In 1935, the *National Formulary* chairman, Edmund N. Gathercoal, opened a drug standards laboratory at the University of Illinois College of Pharmacy. Three years later, the Drug Standards Laboratory was moved to the basement of the American Institute of Pharmacy where it was officially opened on June 15, 1938, with Melvin Green serving as laboratory director. (See Chapter 27. *National Formulary*.)

The APhA Drug Standards Laboratory was revitalized in 1961 with an agreement that the American Medical Association, the United States Pharmacopeial Convention, and APhA would each contribute $25,000 annually to support the activities of the laboratory. A second expansion took place in 1968 when William J. Mader became laboratory director and served until 1971, when he was replaced by Lee T. Grady. In 1972, the Laboratory employed six full-time scientists. One of the most important activities was the issuance of Reference Standards for some 500 drugs. The Drug Standards Laboratory remained in the basement of APhA headquarters until 1974 when APhA sold the *National Formulary* to the *U.S.Pharmacopeia.*

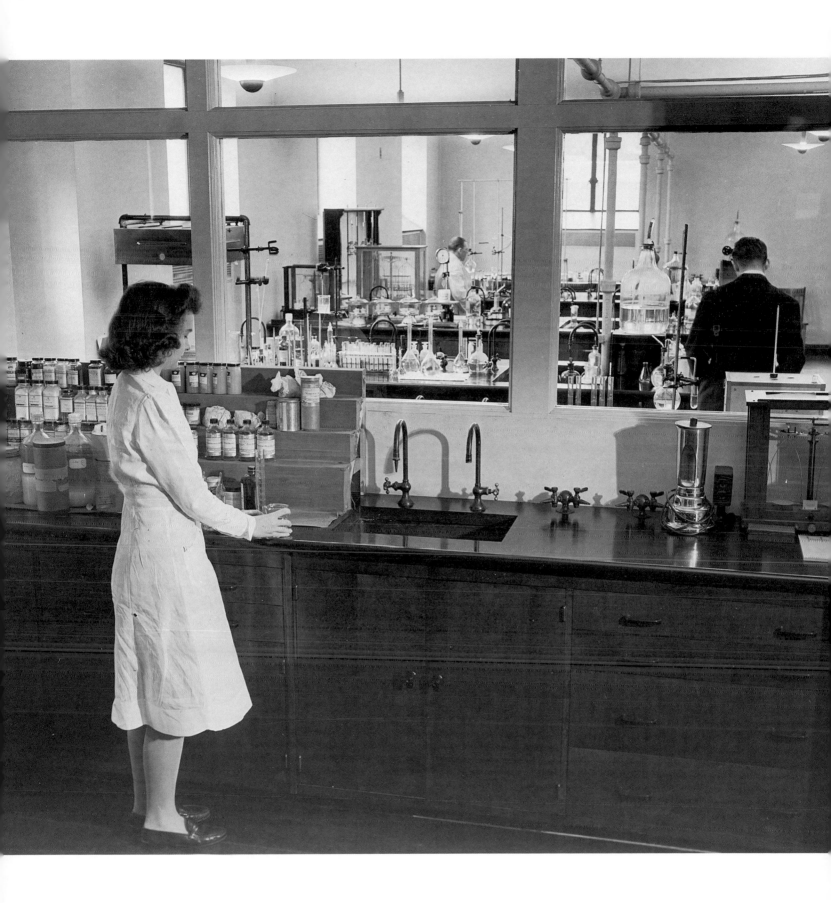

PROCEEDINGS

OF THE

TWENTY-SECOND ANNUAL MEETING

OF THE

American Pharmaceutical Association.

REPORT ON THE PROGRESS OF PHARMACY,

FROM JULY 1, 1873, TO JULY 1, 1874.

BY C. LEWIS DIEHL.

Your reporter aimed to have his report ready to submit to this meeting, but was prevented by his private business engagements from quite finishing it. It is, however, so nearly completed,

Permanent

reports. I

prefers to

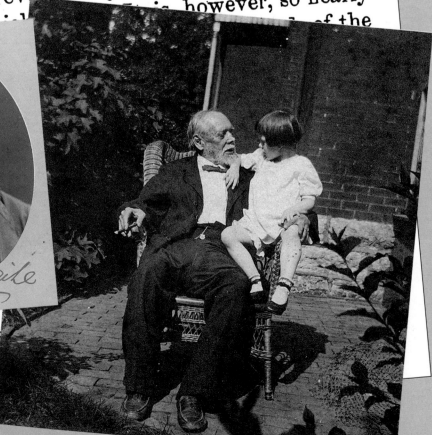

as cannot

which he

The Stat

Europe, has been the

among these are the pa

wortt, on the Status

CHAPTER 25

APhA Publications

Before the founding meeting of APhA in 1852, pharmacists learned about the new association through the pages of the *American Journal of Pharmacy.* After the founding meeting, APhA began to publish the *APhA Proceedings*, its primary publication for 50 years.

In 1856, APhA added a standing Committee on the Progress of Pharmacy to "report annually to the Association on the improvements in Chemistry, Practical Pharmacy and the collateral branches." The first report (1857) was prepared by a committee composed of William Procter, Eugene Dupuy, and James Cooke.

The report on "Progress of Pharmacy" was continued by the committee with varying results, but in 1866, chairman Eino Sander proposed a separate "journal on the progress of pharmacy," and recommended the appointment of "a permanent reporter on the Progress of Pharmacy." Conrad Lewis Diehl was appointed as permanent editor of the *Report on the Progress of Pharmacy* in 1873, succeeding Louis Dohme. The *Report on the Progress of Pharmacy* continued into the 1920s producing what Eugene Eberle described in 1921 as "the most complete pharmaceutical abstracts published in the English language."

One of the actions taken by APhA at its 1902 semi-centennial convention was that APhA should publish "a drug journal." Two years later, APhA president Lewis Hopp called for an APhA news bulletin, not a journal, to be mailed monthly.

The *Bulletin of the American Pharmaceutical Association* began publication in January 1906, stressing association reports, branch and section proceedings, but rarely full length articles. The cover carried the motto *Pharmacia Vera Prevalebit* (True Pharmacy Will Prevail). Some 3,000 copies per month were published with the colorful C. S. N. Hallberg as editor. This burly Swede was described by Harvey W. Wiley as "a rough diamond but a real diamond. His language was strong and incisive, his manner not always those of the polished orator, but his principles were never tainted with wrong. His great characteristic was his fearlessness of purpose." A brain tumor extinguished the life of Hallberg at the age of 54 in 1910.

Opposite Page: Commencing in 1857, the *APhA Proceedings* featured an annual report entitled "Progress of Pharmacy." From 1873 to 1891 and again from 1894 until 1915, this exhaustive review was compiled by Conrad Lewis Diehl. The inset pictures Diehl about the time he commenced service as APhA "Reporter," while the large photo pictures Diehl with his grandson on August 26, 1912. In the background is Diehl's first report which consisted of 300 pages; over the years, Diehl devoted more than 11,000 pages of the *APhA Proceedings* to the "Progress of Pharmacy."

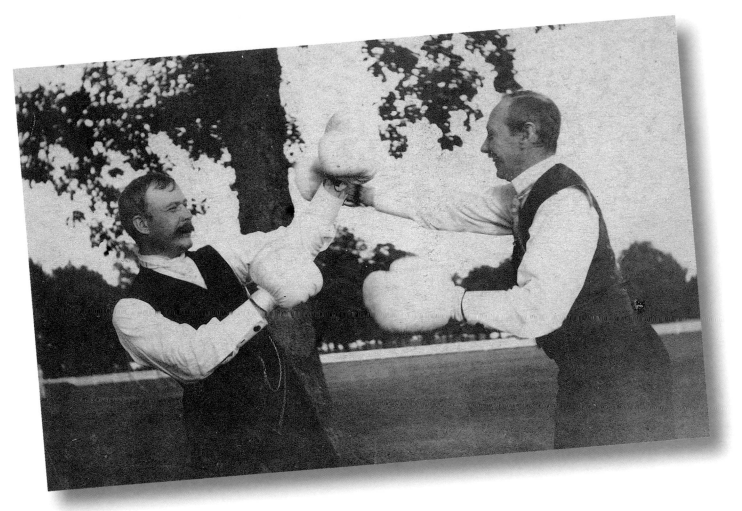

Carl Hallberg served as editor of the *Bulletin of the American Pharmaceutical Association* from its inception in 1906 until his death in 1910. This photo of a feisty Hallberg (on the left) boxing with an unidentified colleague exemplifies the decorum of this burly Swede.

The *Yearbook of APhA*, published from 1912 to 1934, included APhA annual meeting proceedings and reports of the various APhA Branches.

Joseph England reported at the 1910 annual meeting in Richmond, Virginia, that it was decided to "establish a monthly journal of proper size and character to take the place of the *Bulletin*, to be known as the *Journal of the American Pharmaceutical Association*."

The major concern centered on the selection of an editor. In his 1911 presidential address, Eugene Eberle proposed "having the general secretary become editor-in-chief." The timing was fortuitous because Charles Caspary announced his intention to resign from his 17-year service as general secretary. James H. Beal was, therefore, unanimously elected to the twin post as general secretary and editor.

As editor of the new journal, James Hartley Beal proclaimed that no firm could "warp its editorial utterances, or buy space for advertisement of any substance or service considered to be out of harmony with the expressed or plainly implied professions of the association." Under Beal's guidance the *Journal* assumed a personality as well as content different from the old *Bulletin*, which ceased publication with the December 1911 issue. Volume I (1912) provided over 1,400 pages, a bold venture for an association which then had only 2,490 members.

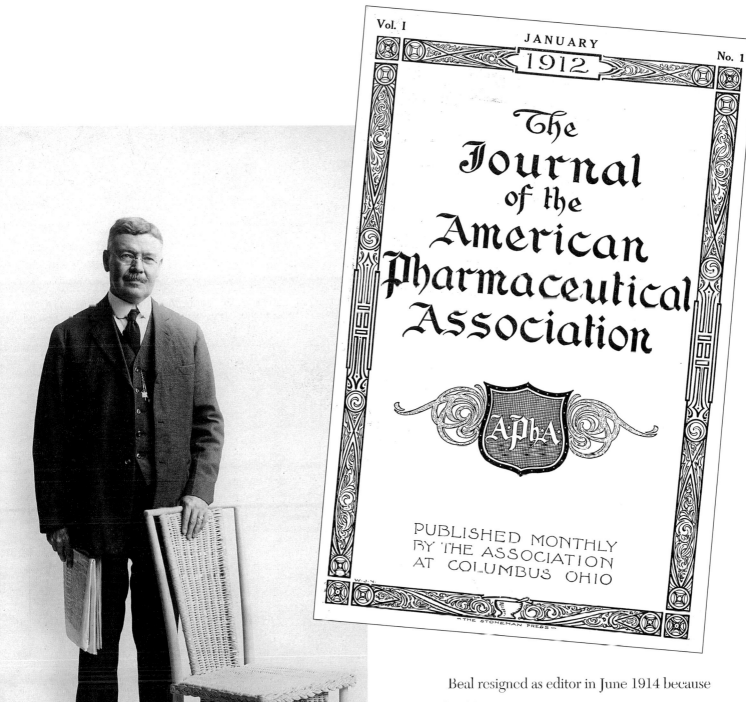

The Journal
of the
American
Pharmaceutical
Association

Vol. I

JANUARY
1912

No. 1

APhA

PUBLISHED MONTHLY
BY THE ASSOCIATION
AT COLUMBUS OHIO

James Beal (seen here in 1902) was selected as the first editor of the *Journal of the American Pharmaceutical Association* (volume 1, number 1, 1912, shown on the right). It was under Beal's guidance that the journal assumed a unique personality.

Beal resigned as editor in June 1914 because of poor health, and after a brief period under the acting editorship of Ernest C. Marshall (June 1914 - May 1915), Eugene G. Eberle assumed the editorial duties for the ensuing 23 years. During Eberle's tenure as editor, the *Journal* clearly assumed a prominent position among professional journals.

After Eberle retired in August 1938, Evander F. Kelly served as acting editor for 16 months. With the rapid increase in the number of scientific papers submitted for publication, over-

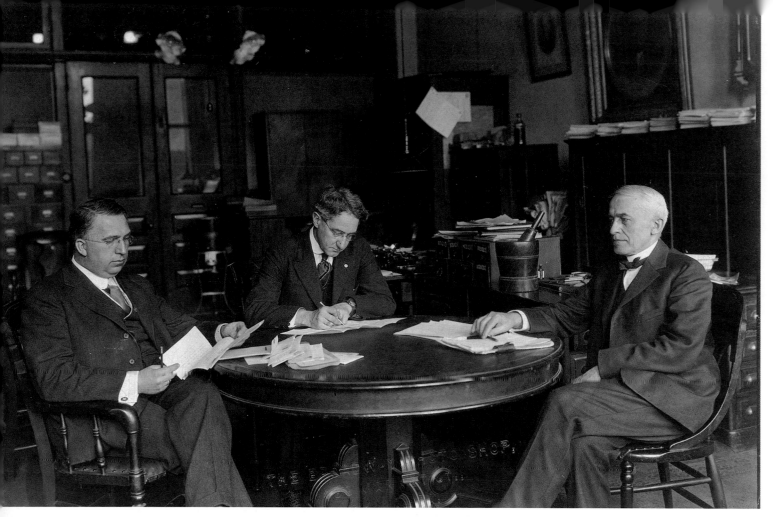

Eugene Eberle assumed editorship of the *Journal of the American Pharmaceutical Association* in 1915. The following year, Eberle (on the right) meets with Charles LaWall (center) and Caswell Mayo (left) in the journal's new office on the second floor of the Philadelphia Drug Exchange.

whelming competition for publishing space soon developed. So in 1940, the *Journal* was divided into two separate editions. The *Practical Pharmacy Edition*, edited by Evander F. Kelly, was designed to appeal to practicing pharmacists while the *Scientific Edition*, edited by Andrew G. DuMez, was designed to appeal to pharmaceutical scientists. Two years later, Robert A. Rodman became editor of the *Practical Edition* in January 1941, while Justin L. Powers took over editorship of the *Scientific Edition* in January 1942.

With the October 1943 issue of the *Practical Edition*, Glenn Sonnedecker took over as editor, serving until October 1948. After several changes in editors (Harold V. Darnell, Robert P. Fischelis, and Bernard Zerbe), Eric W. Martin took over in April 1956, serving to June 1959. Edward G. Feldmann

took over the *Scientific Edition* from Justin Powers in 1960, and merged the *Scientific Edition* with *Drug Standards* (published as the *Bulletin of the National Formulary Committee* from 1938 to 1952 when it changed its name to *Drug Standards*) in January 1961 to form the *Journal of Pharmaceutical Sciences*.

William S. Apple was named editor of the *Practical Pharmacy Edition* in August 1959. When the *Scientific Edition* became the *Journal of Pharmaceutical Sciences*, the *Practical Pharmacy Edition* (January 1961) again became the *Journal of the American Pharmaceutical Association* (*JAPhA* without a sub-title). George Griffenhagen served as editor from 1962 to 1976, developing a significant number of special issues with in-depth reviews of such timely subjects as Clinical Pharmacy, Drug Recalls, Patient Record Systems, the Pharmacist as a

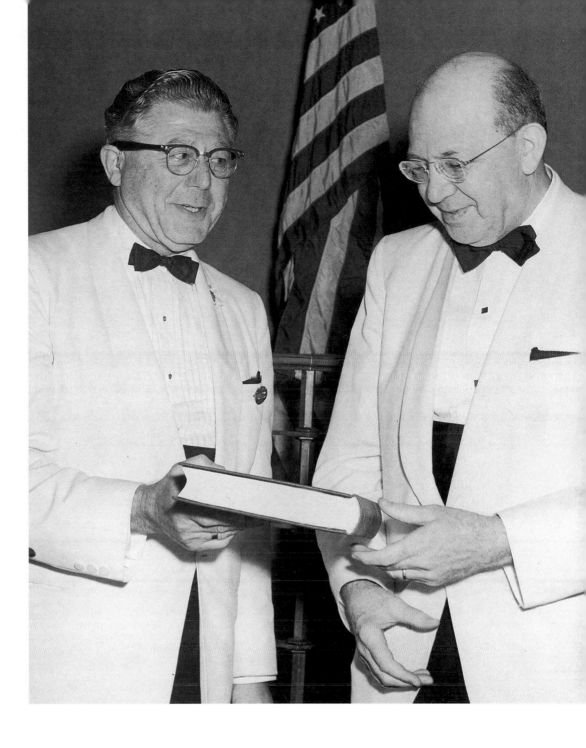

At the 1959 annual meeting in Cincinnati, APhA president Louis James Fischl presented retiring secretary Robert P. Fischelis with a beautifully bound volume containing 15 years of his monthly "Straight from Headquarters" columns appearing in the *APhA Journal*.

Health Educator, and Women in Pharmacy. The most notable was a series of articles from 1964 to 1967 on over-the-counter products that led to the introduction of the Association's most successful publication, *The Handbook of Nonprescription Drugs*. By the third edition, more than 100,000 copies were sold. (See Chapter 37. *Patent Medicines to Nonprescription Drugs*.)

George P. Provost served as editor of the *APhA Journal* from 1976 to 1977 when the APhA Board of Trustees decided to revamp the *Journal* to

compete with trade magazines. In 1978, it was converted to a news periodical called *American Pharmacy* under the editorship of Margaret Eastman, followed by William E. Small (1979-1982).

Realizing that this left a void for those who sought publication of their "practitioner-oriented" contributed papers, the APhA Trustees authorized the publication of a quarterly journal called *Contemporary Pharmacy Practice* which was launched in 1978 with Peter P. Lamy as editor. But it folded in 1982 for lack of subscribers because a sub-

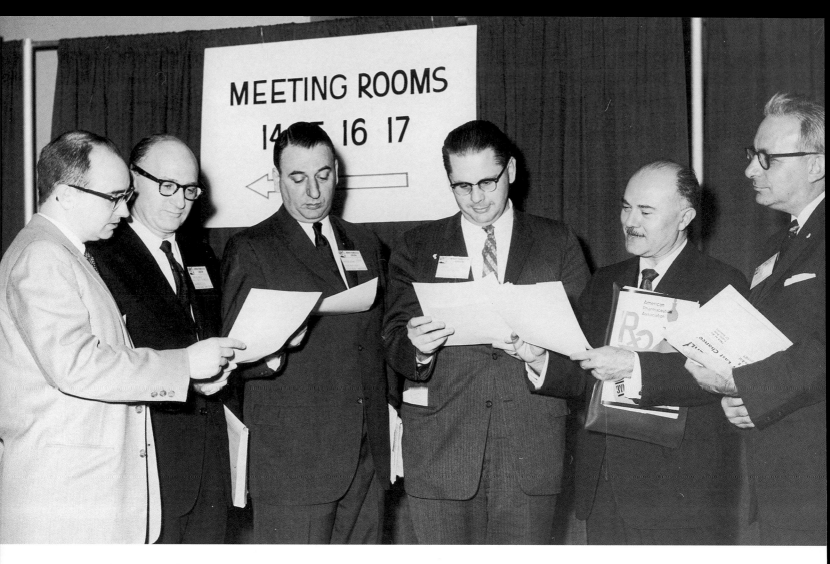

Pharmaceutical editors gathered at the 1962 APhA annual meeting in Las Vegas. They include (left to right) *Journal of Pharmaceutical Sciences* editor Edward Feldmann; *American Professional Pharmacist* editor Irving Rubin; *Drug News Weekly* editor Morton Stark; *JAPhA* editor George Griffenhagen; *American Druggist* editor Dan Rennick; and *Drug Topics* editor Louis Kazin.

scription was not included as an APhA membership benefit. Members had a choice of receiving as part of their membership fee either the *APhA Journal* or the *Journal of Pharmaceutical Sciences*.

With the demise of *Contemporary Pharmacy Practice, American Pharmacy* slowly regained its niche as the vehicle for peer-reviewed, practice-oriented articles. Under the editorship of John Covert (1983-1988), a continuing education series premiered in 1986, and the "Leadership Forum" in 1988 introduced "leaders of the association to communicate their thoughts, their hopes, and their aspirations." Marlene Z. Bloom assumed editorship from 1989 until 1995, when officers of the APhA Academy of Pharmaceutical Research and the Academy of

Pharmaceutical Research and Science reviewed the future of *American Pharmacy*. They recommended, and the APhA Board of Trustees agreed, that a "new path" was needed based on the adoption of pharmaceutical care as the mission of pharmacy practice. Thus the journal returned to its original name, *Journal of the American Pharmaceutical Association*, with the January 1996 issue promising commitment to publishing top quality research articles that directly impact the practice of pharmacy. The new editorial staff included Rick Harding as APhA director of periodicals; L. Michael Posey as pharmacy editor; and Ron Teeter as senior editor. Then in 1997, the *APhA Journal* commenced publishing on a bi-monthly schedule.

The *Journal of Pharmaceutical Sciences* continued under the editorship of Edward G. Feldmann until 1973 followed by Mary H. Ferguson (1974-1982); Sharon G. Boots (1982-1986); Arthur F. deSilva (1987-1991); and Edward G. Feldmann (1992-1994). In 1994, APhA and the American Chemical Society became joint owners and publishers of the *Journal of Pharmaceutical Sciences*, appointing William I. Higuchi as editor. In 2000, Wiley-Liss, Inc., became publisher of the journal, and Ronald Borchardt assumed the position as editor.

In 1962, APhA introduced the *APhA Newsletter* which was edited by Donald E. Prescott until 1973, followed by Judith F. Perruso (1974) and David Bohart (1974-1977). The name of the newsletter was changed in 1977 to *apharmacy weekly* which was edited variously by Alan Steele-Nicholson, Suzanne Stone, Barry A. Muror, David Bohart, Dena Cain, Lindsay Mann, and John Covert. In 1989 the periodical was changed to *Pharmacy Today* with editors Sara Martin (1989-1993); Maureen E. Flanagan (1993-1994); Judy Blanchard (1994); William Blockstein (1995); Daniel A. Hussar (1995-1997); and Susan Easton (2000-). *Pharmacy Update* was also published for two years (1990-1991) with Sara Martin as editor.

The Academy Reporter was published for the Academy of Pharmaceutical Sciences from 1965 to 1996 with the following editors: Samuel W. Goldstein (1965-1969); William C. Roemer (1970-1973); Kathleen Sullivan (1973-1974); William F. McGhan (1974-1976); Lloyd Kennon (1977-1978); Ronald L. Williams (1978-1983); Edward G. Feldmann (1984-1985); Arthur M. Horowitz (1985); Vicki Meade (1986-1988); Sara Martin (1988-1989); and Naomi Kaminsky (1990-1996).

The Academy / GP was published from 1966 to 1975 with the following editors: Richard P. Penna (1966-1972); J. Tina Carriuolo (1970-1972 as co-editor); Ronald L. Williams (1972-1975). The title was changed to *Pharmacy Practice* in September 1975.

Student APhA News / SAPhA News made its appearance in 1971 with Ronald L. Williams as editor, followed by William F. McGhan (1971-1973); Michael I. Smith (1973-1974); Robert E. Henry (1974-1975); John F. Kerege, Jr. (1975-1976); Steven W. Skalisky (1977); Ronald L. Williams (1978-1982); and Constance Johnson Tyler (1978-1982 as co-editor). The name was changed in 1983 to *The Pharmacy Student* with editors James F. Emigh (1983); Stacey Ferguson (1983-1985); Anna Charuk Kowblansky (1985); Vicki Meade (1986-1994); Rick Harding (1995-1999), and Tom English from 2000.

In 1992, APhA introduced a new series of *Special Reports* (also called *New Product Bulletin*), and a *New Therapeutic Bulletin* in 1996 on treatment updates expressly for pharmacists, for which two hours of continuing education credit could be earned. The *Therapeutic Bulletin* was also produced for the American Academy of Physician Assistants commencing in 1997; and the American Academy of Nurse Practitioners commencing in 1998.

In January 2000, APhA introduced a new monthly drug information newsletter for APhA members entitled *APhA DrugInfoLine*. Edited by L. Michael Posey, the newsletter provides "short, timely updates on drug therapy developments." This was followed later in 2000 by a quarterly newsletter entitled *Transitions* for new practitioners.

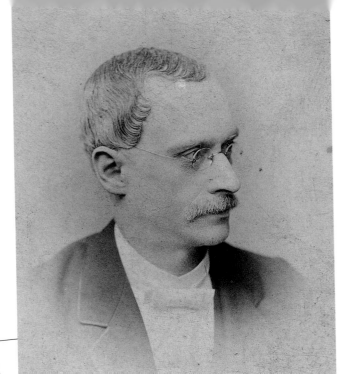

THE

NATIONAL FORMULARY

OF

UNOFFICINAL PREPARATIONS.

FIRST ISSUE.

BY AUTHORITY OF THE
AMERICAN PHARMACEUTICAL ASSOCIATION.

PUBLISHED BY THE AMERICAN PHARMACEUTICAL ASSOCIATION.
1888.

As chairman of the APhA Committee on Unofficinal Formulas, hospital pharmacist Charles Rice laid the groundwork for the development of the *National Formulary*. The first draft was published in the 1886 *APhA Proceedings* designed to encourage physicians to prescribe from this formulary rather than recommend proprietary medicines. The first edition of the *National Formulary* was published in 1888.

1888. C. Lewis Diehl immediately went to work on the second edition (first revision).

The *NF* was revised in 1896 to correct some errors in the first edition, and the second revision coincided with the enactment of the Food and Drug Act of June 30, 1906. This act named the *National Formulary* as one of the official standards for pharmaceuticals. The founders of the *National Formulary* had not anticipated that their book would be adopted as a legal standard. As Glenn Sonnedecker notes, a member of the NF Committee termed the inclusion of the *National Formulary* as an official compendium in the 1906 Food and Drug Act as "an unexpected occurrence...one so great in its consequences that comparatively few realize what it means and how increased importance carries with it increased responsibilities and more exacting requirements."

APhA members seem to have had mixed feelings about the new status for their most ambitious project. In 1909 APhA president Oscar Oldberg felt that Congress made "a ridiculous mistake in adopting [the *NF*] as a legal standard." He, and others, believed that the *NF* would become "less practical, less a manual primarily for the practicing pharmacist." The original concept of the *NF*, as reflected in the first three editions, placed in the hands of pharmacists formulas that could be compounded on a small scale in competition with ready-made preparations.

The *National Formulary* IV (1916) took a giant step in responding to calls for setting "definite standards." *NF* Chairman Edmund N. Gathercoal established a working relationship with the pharmaceutical industry in setting drug standards, and in 1935, he opened a drug standards laboratory at the University of Illinois College of Pharmacy. Three years later, APhA established the Drug Standards

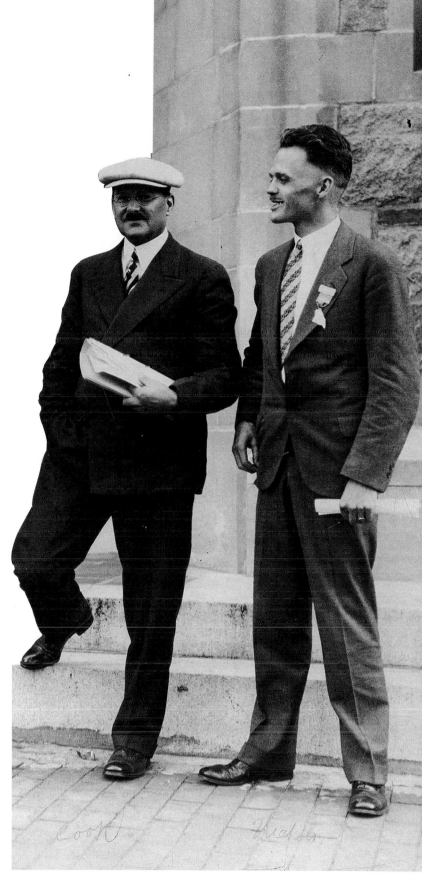

Officers of the *National Formulary* and the *U.S. Pharmacopeia* frequently met to discuss mutual activities. Adley Nichols (right), who had just been elected as *National Formulary* revision committee secretary, stops to chat with E. Fullerton Cook (left), *USP* revision committee chairman, in Cleveland, Ohio, on July 1, 1930.

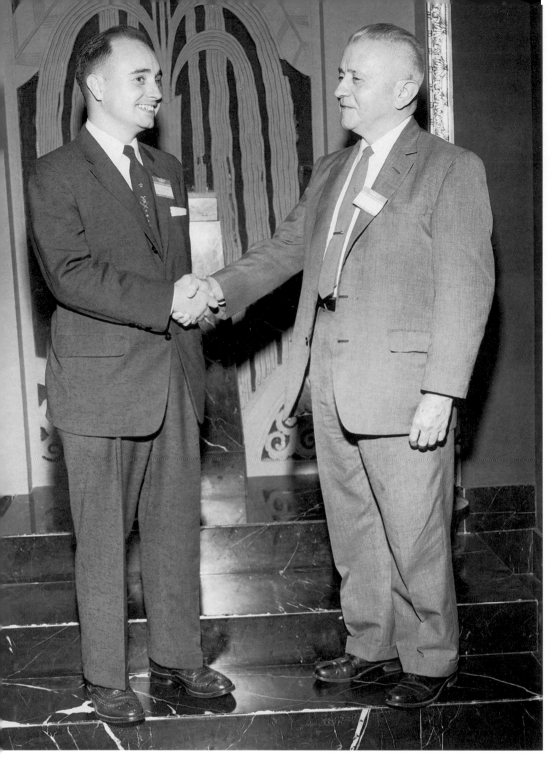

Retiring *National Formulary* director Justin Powers (on the right), who served for *NF* VII to XIV, welcomes the new *National Formulary* director Edward Feldmann in August 1959.

Laboratory at their new headquarters building in Washington, D.C. In the 1960s, the Drug Standards Laboratory at APhA headquarters was revitalized with financial support from the USP which was using these laboratory services, and the American Medical Association which had discontinued its own drug-testing laboratory. (See Chapter 24. *Drug Standards Laboratory*.)

The six chairmen who succeeded Charles Rice and directed revisions of the *National Formulary* from 1889 to 1974 include:

C. Lewis Diehl	1889-1917	*NF* II to IV
Wilbur L. Scoville	1919-1929	*NF* V
Edmund N. Gathercoal	1930-1940	*NF* VI
Justin L. Powers	1940-1960	*NF* VII to XIV
Edward G. Feldmann	1960-1969	*NF* XII, XIII
John V. Bergen	1970-1974	*NF* XIV

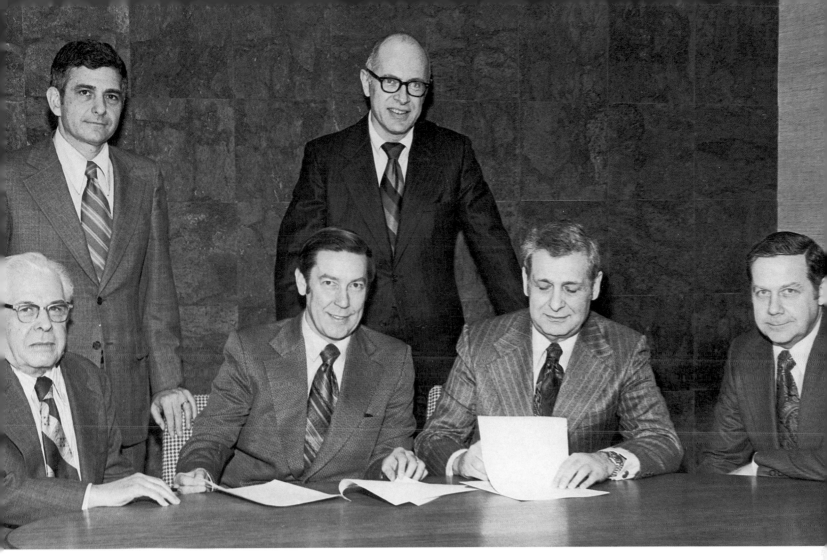

APhA and USPC sign documents in 1974 transferring the *National Formulary* to the U.S. Pharmacopeial Convention as FDA officials observe (standing, left to right) Richard Crout (Bureau of Drugs director) and Alexander Schmidt (FDA commissioner). Seated (left to right) are Paul McLain (USPC Board chairman); William Heller (USPC executive director); William Apple (APhA executive director); and Grover Bowles (APhA treasurer).

As early as 1960, a USP Board of Trustees member, Windsor Cutting, questioned "whether amalgamation of the *USP* with the *NF* would not simplify use and allow economy of format?" But the suggestion lay dormant until 1966 when *USP*'s Lloyd Miller and *NF*'s Edward Feldmann commenced an exploration of a *USP-NF* merger. The 1970 USP Convention adopted a resolution supporting a merger, but it took another four years to reach an agreement whereby the USP would purchase from APhA both the *National Formulary* and the Drug Standards Laboratory. Agreement was announced July 5, 1974, while formal ceremonies to complete the transaction were held on January 2, 1975.

When "unofficial formulas" no longer had a place in the *National Formulary*, a new type of publication emerged, a *Recipe Book* conceived by Henry P. Hynson. In 1909, he presented his proposal to the APhA Council. The following year a committee, chaired by Otto Raubenheimer, was appointed, and brought together and published 114 formulas in installments in the *APhA Journal* for 1912 under "Pharmaceutical Formulas."

A new committee headed by J. Leon Lascoff presented APhA with an unedited collection of 1,500 formulas published by APhA in 1926 under the title, *Pharmaceutical Recipe Book*. A second edition appeared in 1936; a third and final edition was published in 1942.

Code of Ethics for Pharmacists

A *pharmacist* respects the covenantal relationship between the patient and pharmacist.

A *pharmacist* promotes the good of every patient in a caring, compassionate, and confidential manner.

A *pharmacist* respects the autonomy and dignity of each patient.

A *pharmacist* acts with honesty and integrity in professional relationships.

A *pharmacist* maintains professional competence.

A *pharmacist* respects the values and abilities of colleagues and other health professionals.

A *pharmacist* serves individual, community, and societal needs.

A *pharmacist* seeks justice in the distribution of health resources.

adopted by the membership of the
American Pharmaceutical Association
October 27, 1994.

Code of Ethics
American Pharmaceutical Association

he primary obligation of pharmacy is the service it can render to the public in safeguarding the preparation, compounding, and dispensing of drugs and storage and handling of drugs and medical supplies. The practice of pharmacy requires knowledge, skill, integrity; therefore, the state laws restrict the practice of pharmacy to persons with special training qualifications and license to them privileges which are denied to others. Accordingly, the pharmacist recognizes his responsibility to the state and community for their well-being, and fulfills his professional obligations honorably.

relations to the public

The pharmacist upholds the approved legal standards of the United States Pharmacopeia and the National Formulary, and encourages the use of drugs and preparations. He purchases, compounds and dispenses only drugs of good quality. The pharmacist uses every precaution to safeguard the public when dispensing any drugs or preparations. Legally entrusted with the dispensing and sale of these products, he assumes this responsibility by upholding and conforming to the laws and regulations governing the distribution of these substances.

The pharmacist seeks to enlist and to merit the confidence of his patrons. He zealously guards this confidence. He considers the knowledge and confidence which he gains of the ailments of his patrons as entrusted to his honor and does not divulge such knowledge.

The pharmacist holds the health and safety of his patrons to be of first consideration; he makes no effort to prescribe for or to treat disease or to offer for sale any drug or medical device merely for profit; he does not participate in any plan for pharmaceutical service which eliminates the pharmacist-patient-physician relationship.

The pharmacist keeps his pharmacy clean, neat, and orderly and well equipped with accurate measuring and weighing devices and other apparatus suitable for the performance of his professional duties.

The pharmacist is a good citizen and upholds the laws of the states and nation; he keeps the food and drug laws, and other...

the pharmacist's mind regarding the ingredients of a prescription, a possible error, or the safety of the direction, he privately and tactfully consults the practitioner before making any changes. He exercises his best professional judgment and follows, under the laws and existing regulations, the prescriber's directions in the matter of refilling prescriptions, copying the formula upon the label, or giving a copy of the prescription to the patient. He adds any extra directions or caution or poison labels only with proper regard for the wishes of the prescriber, and the safety of the patient.

The pharmacist does not discuss the therapeutic effects or composition of a prescription with a patient. When such questions are asked, he suggests that the qualified practitioner is the proper person with whom such matters should be discussed.

The pharmacist considers it inimical to public welfare to have any clandestine arrangement with any practitioner of the health sciences by which fees are divided or in which secret or coded prescriptions are involved.

relations to fellow pharmacists

The pharmacist strives to perfect and enlarge his professional knowledge. He contributes his share toward the scientific progress of his profession and encourages and participates in research, investigation and study. He keeps himself informed regarding professional matters by reading current pharmaceutical, scientific and medical literature, attending seminars and other means.

The pharmacist seeks to attract to his profession youth of good character and intellectual capacity and aids in their instruction.

The pharmacist associates himself with organizations having for their objective the betterment of the pharmaceutical profession and contributes his share of time, energy and funds to carry on the work of these organizations.

The pharmacist keeps his reputation in public esteem by continuously giving the kind of professional service that earns its own reward. He does not engage in any activity or transaction that will bring discredit or criticism to himself or to his profession.

The pharmacist will expose any corrupt or dishonest conduct of any member of his profession which comes to his certain knowledge, through those accredited by the civil laws or the rules and...

Code of Ethics
OF THE
American Pharmaceutical Association

The Code of Ethics of the American Pharmaceutical Association is a statement of principles adopted by the profession for the self-government of its members.

The primary obligation of pharmacy is the service it can render to the public in safeguarding the preparation, compounding, and dispensing of drugs, and the storage and handling of drugs and medical supplies.

The practice of pharmacy requires knowledge, skill, and integrity; therefore, the state laws restrict the practice of pharmacy to persons with special training and qualifications and license to them privileges which are denied to others. Accordingly, the pharmacist recognizes his responsibility to the state and to the community for their well-being, and fulfills his professional obligations honorably.

The Pharmacist and His Relations to the Public

The pharmacist upholds the legal standards of the United States Pharmacopeia... the distribution of these substances.

NATIONAL PHARMACEUTICAL CONVENTION,

Held at Philadelphia, October 6th, 1852.

CODE OF ETHICS OF THE AMERICAN PHARMACEUTICAL ASSOCIATION.

The American Pharmaceutical Association, composed of Pharmaceutists and Druggists throughout the United States, feeling a strong interest in the success and advancement of their profession in its practical and scientific relations, and also impressed with the belief that no amount of knowledge and skill will protect themselves and the public from the ill effects of an undue competition, and the temptations to gain at the expense of quality, unless they are upheld by high moral obligations in the path of duty, have subscribed to the following *Code of Ethics* for the government of their professional conduct.

ART. I. As the practice of pharmacy can only become uniform by an open and candid intercourse being kept up between apothecaries and druggists among themselves and each other, by the adoption of the National Pharmacopœia as a guide in the preparation of officinal medicines, by the discontinuance of secret formulæ and the practices arising from a quackish spirit, and by an encouragement of that *esprit du corps* which will prevent a resort to those disreputable practices arising out of an injurious and wicked competition ;—*Therefore*, the members of this Association agree to uphold the use of the Pharmacopœia in their practice ; to cultivate brotherly

---

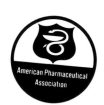

American Pharmaceutical Association

Code of Ethics

CHAPTER 28.

Code of Ethics

The 1852 APhA Code of Ethics, modeled after the one developed in 1848 by the Philadelphia College of Pharmacy, stated:

"The American Pharmaceutical Association, composed of pharmaceutists and druggists throughout the United States, feeling a strong interest in the success and advancement of their profession in its practical and scientific relations, and also impressed with the belief that no amount of knowledge and skill will protect themselves and the public from the ill effects of an undue competition, and the temptations to gain at the expense of quality, unless they are upheld by high moral obligations in the path of duty, have subscribed to the following *Code of Ethics* for the government [i.e. "governance"] of their professional conduct."

One provision of the new Code asked of those who honored it "a discontinuance [of] quackery," including the sale of nostrums. Edward Parrish observed that it is from the sale of patent medicines on which many druggists subsisted, and, in his opinion, these ethical norms had to be the goal and not a condition of membership. So in 1855 APhA dropped the obligation to subscribe to the Code of Ethics as a prerequisite of membership only three years after its founding.

Even though the Code of Ethics was no longer a required code of conduct for membership, APhA members invoked the right to expel members for reasons they considered to be a violation of appropriate professional conduct based on the Code. The first member to be expelled from APhA membership in 1862 was J. L. Hunnewell of Boston. He had used APhA's title and seal "for improper advertising purposes;" and his "improper advertising" appeared on flyers promoting Tolu Anodyne and Eclectic Pills.

The most famous of such actions came in 1869 when Frederick Stearns (an ex-president) was expelled from APhA membership for marketing "Sweet Quinine" which contained no quinine, but cinchonine. Initially in the debate, it was proposed that the Association simply censure Stearns, but that was rejected. After several hours of debate, the roll-call vote was 62 for expulsion and 23 against expelling him. In 1897, APhA reinstated Frederick Stearns membership after he responded to a letter expressing "regret."

It was not until 1915 that the APhA took another look at an APhA Code of Ethics by appointing a special committee of three to revise the 1852

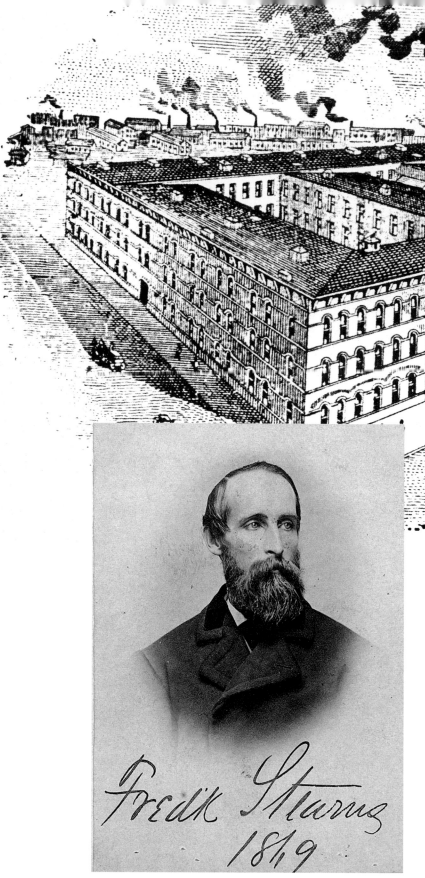

Frederick Stearns, who established a manufacturing firm in 1855, was elected APhA president in 1866. However, he was expelled from membership three years later for marketing *Sweet Quinine* which contained no quinine. In 1897, Stearns' membership was reinstated after he expressed "regret."

Code of Ethics, and to report at the 1916 convention. On August 17, 1922, at the instigation of 1918-1919 president Charles LaWall, APhA adopted a new and rather comprehensive code. The new Code was based on the responsibility of the pharmacist to the public, to the physician, and to fellow pharmacists. LaWall questioned whether the Association should include "a penalizing factor requiring discipline for violations."

This question still confronted pharmacists in 1952. Opinions wavered on procedures to handle violators, especially those pharmacsts who were selling barbiturates and amphetamines without a prescription order. In 1966, APhA established by amendments to the Constitution and Bylaws, a Judicial Board to discipline members, and to render advisory opinions that could lead to reprimanding, suspending, or expelling members for unprofessional conduct.

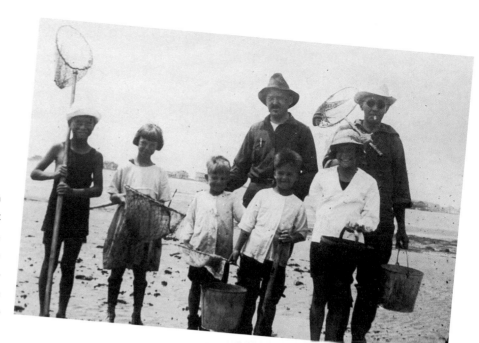

At the instigation of Charles LaWall, a new Code of Ethics was adopted at the 1922 annual meeting in Cleveland, Ohio. During the same meeting, LaWall (right), and vice president E. Fullerton Cook, with their children, enjoy crabbing on the beach.

In November 1967, APhA convened a Conference on Ethics as a result of the consensus that APhA should not settle for a simple revision of the Code of Ethics, but create "an entirely new code, one written in simple, straight-forward and positive language." The responsibility for drafting the new code was turned over to the APhA Judicial Board. The Code was adopted by mail ballot in August 1969, and the Judicial Board commenced to issue disciplinary recommendations.

By January 1970, the Judicial Board had instituted disciplinary proceedings against nine individual pharmacists for alleged violations of the APhA Code of Ethics. Five of these members were expelled and another was reprimanded; however, the actions taken against violators of the APhA Code of Ethics were challenged by the National Association of Chain Drug Stores. On January 11, 1971, the Wayne County Circuit Court in Michigan enjoined the Michigan Pharmaceutical Association and APhA from taking further action against Myron D. Winkelman, director of professional services of the Revco Discount Drug Centers, and Geoffrey Stebbins of Arnold's Pharmacies of Detroit, for advertising prescription services and prescription discount plans. A settlement was reached on April 6,

1973, requiring the Michigan association to withdraw its complaint against Winkelman and Stebbins, and APhA terminated its proceedings pending before the Judicial Board.

On November 24, 1975, the Justice Department filed a complaint against APhA and the Michigan Pharmaceutical Association based on Code of Ethics statements that "a pharmacist should not solicit professional practice by means of advertising..." Even though the Code of Ethics provision was revoked in 1976, both APhA and the Michigan association entered into a Final Judgment on June 18, 1981, agreeing that "it does not oppose price advertising of prescription drugs," and the "Association will not deny membership or take any other action concerning any person because of any type of price advertising of prescription drugs other than false and misleading advertising." APhA also agreed to publish the text of the Final Judgment in its journal for a period of ten years.

The most recent revision of the APhA Code of Ethics was adopted by the membership on October 27, 1994. It consists of eight principles, each based on "moral obligations and virtues established to guide pharmacists in relationships with patients, health professionals, and society."

CHAPTER 29.

Pharmaceutical Education

Two APhA Sections formed in 1887 (Pharmaceutical Education and Pharmaceutical Legislation) merged in 1902. The Section on Pharmaceutical Education was to fill the void created by the lack of an effective organization of schools of pharmacy.

Until the 20th century, the majority of pharmacists gained admission to the profession by apprenticeship, a practice that originated centuries earlier in Europe. Soon after APhA was founded in 1852, there was a call for the national professional society of pharmacists to establish a uniform system of apprenticeship, but this was not fulfilled.

The founding members felt that the "preceptorship of the master should instruct the apprentice in all details of the store and laboratory, and extend to the minutiae of every operation of manufacturing and dispensing." Furthermore, apprentices "should be allowed to leave their employers before the expiration of four years' time for the purpose of completing their education and graduating from some regular school of pharmacy." Other founding members felt that "students could learn practical pharmacy only through the apprenticeship process" because it "kept the control of pharmaceutical education in the hands of pharmacists."

Edward Kremers wrote in 1894 that, "it becomes the duty of schools of pharmacy to raise the standard of their course. Such a procedure would generally do away with the apprentice which would be a matter of rejoice and not of regret." Although some began to follow the 1905 lead of New York in requiring graduation from a college of pharmacy for licensure, many felt that a new college graduate was still not fully competent to practice pharmacy, and that apprenticeship permitted a maturing of skill that could not be aquired in an academic institution.

In 1940, the National Association of Boards of Pharmacy generated the first national guidelines for supervised practical experience required for licensure, but it was not until 1953 that the trade-based term "apprenticeship" was replaced with the profession-based term "internship." In 1935, Harvey A. K. Whitney proposed a plan for pharmacy internship at the University of Michigan Hospitals. Then in 1968, APhA urged that internship (one year subsequent to graduation) be replaced by externship (six months prior to graduation), and in 1974, the American Council on Pharmaceutical Education proposed that "experiences students gain in clinical courses (including clerkships and externships) should be of such caliber so as to serve in lieu of the internship requirement for licensure."

Prior to the Civil War, the number of stu-

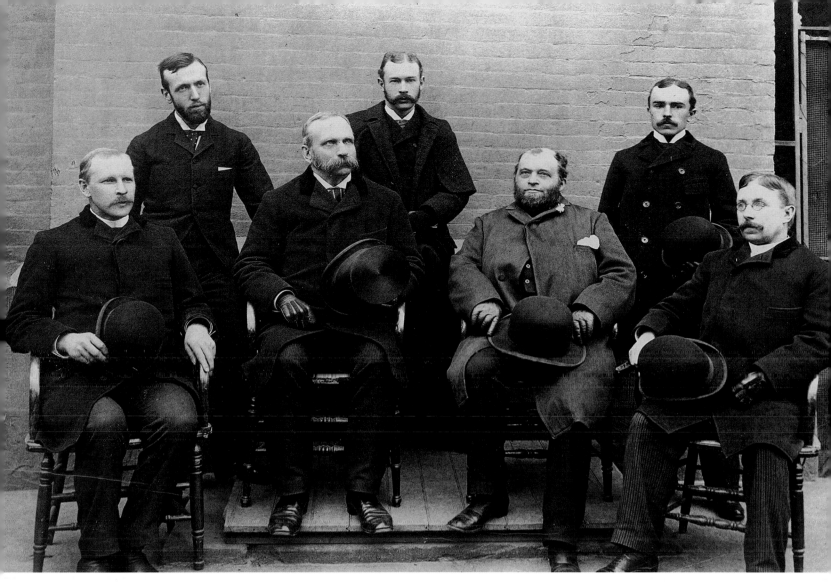

The faculty of the Columbia University College of Pharmacy in 1888 included four who served as APhA officers. They include seated (left to right) **Henry Rusby**, Charles Chandler, **Peter Bedford**, and Arthur Elliott. Standing (left to right) are **Henry Kraemer**, **Frederick Wulling**, and George Ferguson. Those with names in bold type were APhA officers.

dents at the schools of pharmacy (Baltimore, Chicago, New York, Philadelphia, and St. Louis) was small. Of 11,031 "apothecaries and druggists" in the U.S. in 1860, only 514 had graduated from a pharmacy course, most from Philadelphia. By 1873, there were twelve schools of pharmacy with a total attendance of 600 students. APhA president Albert Ebert took note of the fact that, "Much of this is certainly due to the stimulation of our organization."

A convention of delegates from the various colleges of pharmacy met at the annual meeting in 1870 hoping to develop a "uniform standard of qualification for all graduating in pharmacy." The conference directed its first concern to a program estab-

lished by Albert B. Prescott at the University of Michigan that was notable for being the first program at a state-run institution and the first course that did not require apprenticeship experience for graduation.

Prescott, a surgeon during the Civil War and a skilled chemist, challenged the APhA position at the 1871 annual meeting by seeking the right to be seated as delegate from the University of Michigan School of Pharmacy. Objection was promptly raised on his admission as a delegate. A committee composed of a representative of each organization was appointed (including ten past or future presidents), and reported that "the University of Michigan is not,

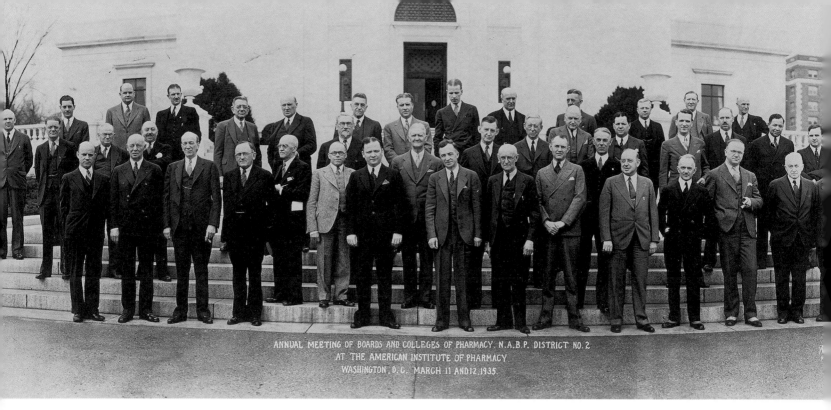

ANNUAL MEETING OF BOARDS AND COLLEGES OF PHARMACY, N.A.B.P. DISTRICT NO. 2
AT THE AMERICAN INSTITUTE OF PHARMACY
WASHINGTON, D. C. MARCH 11 AND 12, 1935.

Members of the American Association of Colleges of Pharmacy and District #2 of the National Association of Boards of Pharmacy assembled on the front steps of the American Institute of Pharmacy in Washington, D.C., on March 11, 1935.

within the proper meaning of our Constitution and Bylaws, a College of Pharmacy; it is neither an organization controlled by pharmacists, nor an institution of learning which insures its graduates the practical training." Thus Prescott was denied a seat as a delegate by a unanimous vote, but admitted as an individual member. Presenting his views at the 1871 meeting, Prescott noted, "All the schools of pharmacy which have been recognized as such by this Association require the completion of apprenticeship before graduating...but it is greatly regretted that no one of these colleges of pharmacy has ever required laboratory training."

By 1874, the Conference of Schools of Pharmacy had agreed that all member schools would issue the "Graduate in Pharmacy" diploma (Ph.G.) for their programs. This further singled out the Michigan program which was offering the "Pharmaceutical Chemist" diploma (Ph.C.). It also led to an 1876 debate by APhA members as to whether to expel the representative of the Tennessee College of Pharmacy

for offering a Doctor of Pharmacy degree, charging that they were not offering any different course than other colleges were offering for a lesser degree, but the motion was defeated.

By 1879, activities of the Conference of Schools of Pharmacy were repeatedly frustrated because their representatives did not have the authority to take positions contrary to those of the practitioner-members of local associations that operated the schools. The Conference held its last meeting at the 1883 APhA annual meeting before dissolving. Thus the APhA Section on Pharmaceutical Education was created in 1887 to fill the void left by the dissolution of the Conference of Schools of Pharmacy.

In 1885, APhA president John Ingalls proposed "systematic instruction beyond the daily routine of manual labor during apprenticeship for instruction," likening it to an 1858 proposal of Procter. In 1892, the APhA Section on Pharmaceutical Education voted to encourage all teaching colleges to adopt a three-year course. Edgar

Patch, 1894 APhA president, recommended the establishment of a scholarship fund, and 1897 president Joseph Morrisson faulted American pharmaceutical education in that "No supervision is exercised over students or apprentices in drugstores."

By the end of the 19th century, James H. Beal and George B. Kauffman were convinced that if representatives of the various schools and colleges of pharmacy "could be brought together where they could speak face to face, their jealousies would subside." So in April 1900, Henry P Hynson sent a circular letter to "all the institutions in the U.S. teaching pharmacy," inviting each to send three delegates to the 1900 APhA convention in Richmond, Virginia. The American Conference on Pharmaceutical Faculties, precursor of the American Association of Colleges of Pharmacy, was thus formed on May 9, 1900, at the APhA annual meeting, with a Constitution mandating that it would meet annually with APhA.

In 1905, the American Conference of Pharmaceutical Faculties and the APhA Section on Education and Legislation met in joint session and adopted recommendations on college degrees as follows: a Ph.G. for graduate in pharmacy; Ph.C. for pharmaceutical chemist; and Phar.B. for bachelor of pharmacy.

APhA also invited both the American Conference of Pharmaceutical Faculties and the National Association of Boards of Pharmacy in 1906 to join in the preparation of the *Pharmaceutical Syllabus* whose objective was to provide uniformity in teaching. In 1910, ACPF approved the general scope of the Syllabus Committee which was composed of seven educators, four of whom had been or were to become APhA presidents. It was decided that the *Syllabus* would be revised every five years,

and the second edition was compiled by the National Committee of the Pharmaceutical Syllabus and published in 1914.

For the first seven years of the existence of the American Conference of Pharmaceutical Faculties, five of the first seven presidents also served in a similar APhA capacity:

	ACPF President	APhA President
Albert Prescott	1900-1901	1899-1900
Joseph Remington	1901-1902	1892-1893
Edward Kremers	1902-1903	————
Henry Rusby	1903-1904	1909-1910
George Kauffman	1904-1905	————
Henry Whelpley	1905-1906	1901-1902
James H. Beal	1906-1907	1904-1905

In addition, an abstract of the proceedings of the ACPF was published in the *APhA Proceedings*, and the *APhA Bulletin* was accepted in 1907 as the official organ of the Conference.

In 1929, APhA recommended that "persons of wealth...be induced to give much needed financial support to a program providing increased education research facilities." Two years later, APhA encouraged the establishment of the American Foundation for Pharmaceutical Education, which was founded in 1942 to guarantee financial support to many colleges during World War II. It contributed largely to the Pharmaceutical Survey of 1946-1949, which pointed the way for the next 50 years.

As early as 1930, APhA sought help "to attract intelligent, industrious young people to study pharmacy." This resulted in the U.S. Office of Education publishing the first of several editions of

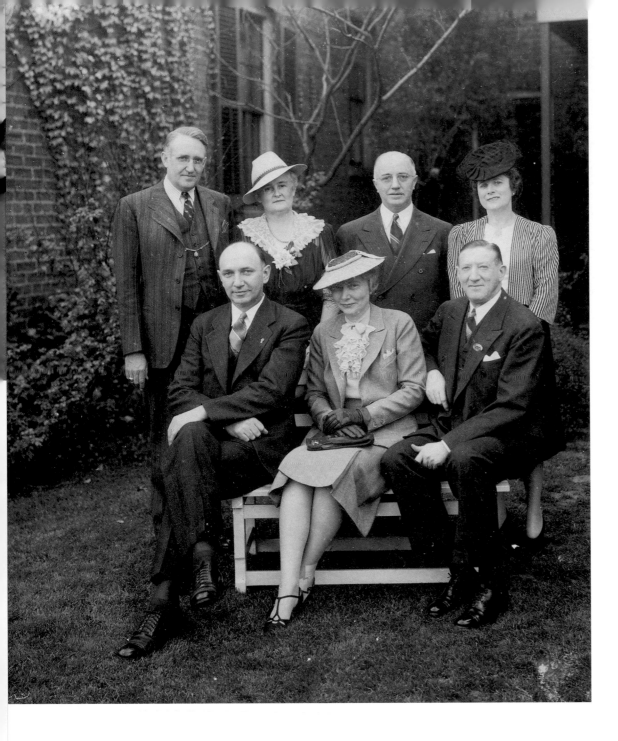

Presidents of three organizations met at the 1940 APhA annual meeting in Richmond, Virginia. They include (seated, left to right) National Association of Boards of Pharmacy president Patrick Costello; Mrs. DuMez and APhA president Andrew DuMez. Standing (left to right) are APhA president-elect Charles Evans; Mrs. Evans; American Association of Colleges of Pharmacy president Charles Rogers and Mrs. Rogers.

legislatures of the different states of the United States."

Maisch then sent the pamphlets to all governors in November 1869, requesting names and addresses of other people who should receive a copy. Most state governors replied with the desired information, and the first state to take action was Rhode Island, passing legislation on March 31, 1870 that was quite close to the model law. Seven other states' proposed laws that initially failed to be adopted. APhA and the young state pharmaceutical associations persisted in their efforts, and by 1878 eight

other states had adopted statutes. At least 21 more states and territories adopted pharmacy laws in the 1880s, and 12 more states enacted pharmacy laws in the 1890s.

In 1879, APhA president Gustavus Luhn proposed that these state boards of pharmacy unite and form themselves into an association similar to that in existence for teaching colleges, then arrange uniformity in the examinations so that licenses in one state would be recognized by all states. So in 1881, various pharmacy boards of the U.S. and Canada met

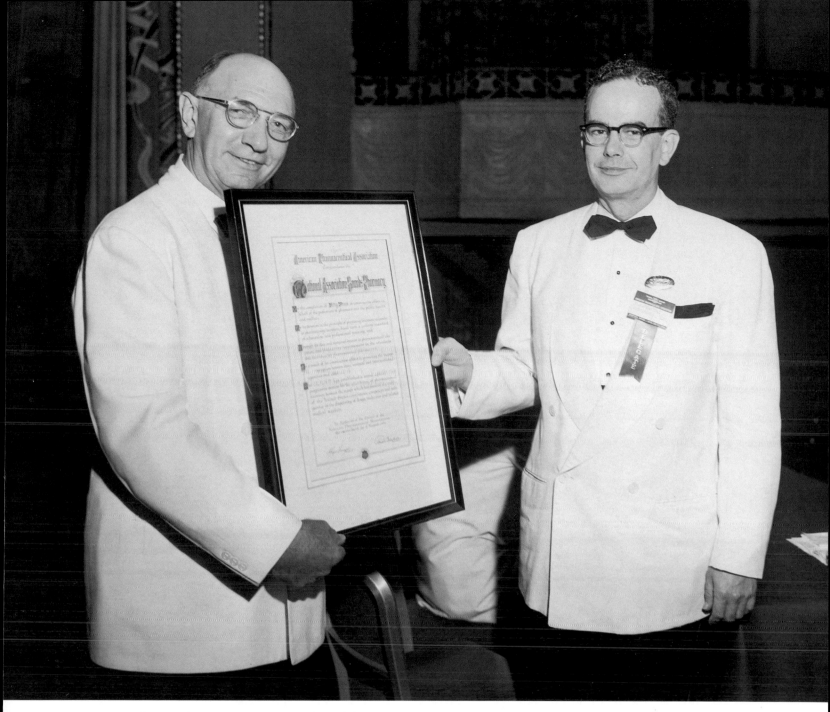

1953-1954 APhA president Royce Franzoni (on the right) presents NABP secretary Patrick Costello with a framed scroll commemorating NABP's golden anniversary at the 1954 APhA annual meeting in Boston.

with APhA "to perfect an organization." The APhA Section on Pharmaceutical Legislation was established in 1887 with attendance by representatives of state boards of pharmacy from Illinois, Iowa, Kentucky, Michigan, Ohio, Pennsylvania, Virginia, and Wisconsin.

As a result of this meeting, the new Section on Pharmaceutical Legislation surveyed state boards in 1888 to determine the possibility of reciprocation of licenses, concluding "the interchange of certificates is coming, perhaps in the near future." Then a resolution was adopted asking the Association to "draw up a general plan for the interchange of certificates of the different Boards."

In 1890 the resulting Association of Boards of Pharmacy and Secretaries of State Associations was formed at the 1890 APhA annual meeting in Old Point Comfort, Virginia, with 16 state boards represented. The following year, 18 boards were represented at the APhA meeting in New Orleans, but nothing more was heard from this group.

Despite this setback, the APhA Section on Legislation persisted.

In 1891, Charles M. Ford told the Section that all state boards should establish reciprocity. In 1900, James H. Beal presented a new model law to the Section on Legislation and Education which was modified and adopted. The goal, according to Henry Whelpley, was to "have states amend their state pharmacy laws to conform to the model law so that the Boards of Pharmacy can soon work out a feasible plan for the interchange of certificates of registration."

Henry Whelpley then urged the Section on Education and Legislation in 1903 to form a sub-section called "Conference of Board of Pharmacy Members" to begin meeting in 1904. A motion was adopted, and a committee of five was appointed to arrange for the conference.

As a result, the National Association of Boards of Pharmacy was established at the 1904 APhA annual convention in Kansas City, and appointed a committee to prepare a constitution and bylaws for approval in 1905 in Atlantic City. The NABP proceedings were published as part of the APhA *Proceedings* for more than two dozen years. According to Melvin Green, since both the Conference of Pharmaceutical Faculties and the NABP were children of the APhA Section on Education and Legislation, and separated by only four years, it is not surprising that the two organizations meet jointly as AACP-NABP districts every year.

CHAPTER 31.

Federal Laws

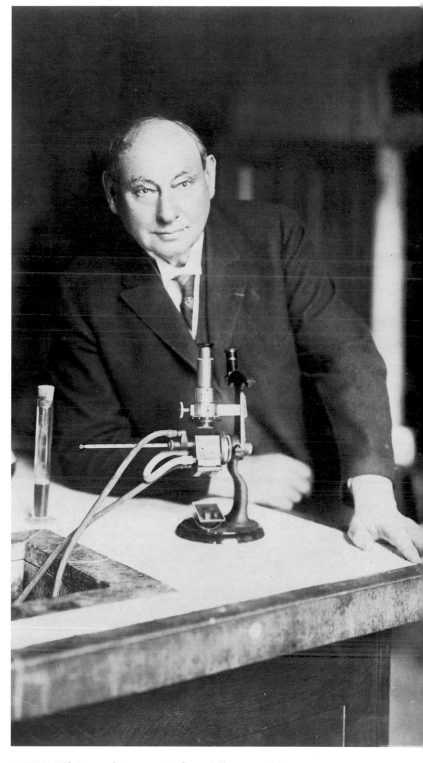

In 1902, APhA urged Congress to financially support the efforts of Harvey Wiley to study the composition and adulteration of drugs; this contributed to the enactment of the 1906 Federal Food and Drugs Act.

As early as 1848, Congress passed "an act to prevent importation of adulterated and spurious drugs and medicines." The Act, as approved June 26, 1848, required examination of products at the port of entry for quality, purity, and fitness for medical purposes. The law was ineffective as it lacked standards for the guidance of the drug examiners and, to some extent, allowed the appointment of unqualified examiners. So in 1851, the New York College of Pharmacy appointed a committee to examine the subject. They concluded that the other Colleges of Pharmacy should take part, and proceeded to invite the colleges of Boston, Philadelphia, Baltimore, and Cincinnati to send delegates to a convention to be held in New York City on April 24, 1851. No delegates arrived, so a subsequent convention was held in New York City on October 15, 1851. This convention recommended the adoption of standards but only for a few drugs. More important was the action to call a convention in Philadelphia a year later to consider the formation of a national association to meet every year. This was the beginning of APhA.

One objective established at the founding meeting of APhA was to "strengthen federal and state laws to curb adulterated drugs." In 1858, APhA presented a petition to Congress describing evasion

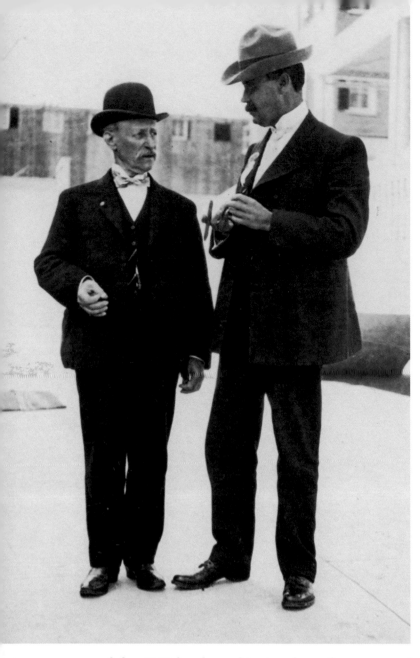

for supplying alcohol used as a medicine. At the same time, APhA took a leading position among U.S. scientific societies, and encouraged Congress to authorize use of the metric system.

Year after year patent-medicine quackery was debated on the floor of APhA annual meetings, and strong resolutions were adopted recommending remedial Federal legislation. The first measure was introduced in 1879, but died in Congress. Between 1880 and 1906, more than a hundred food and drug bills were introduced in Congress without success. At a Pure Food and Drug Congress held in Washington, D.C., January 18, 1898, to formulate legislation, APhA was represented, and Ohio pharmacist Joseph E. Blackburn was elected president.

One man stood out among all others who was seeking national legislation. He was Harvey Washington Wiley, chief chemist of the U.S. Bureau of Chemistry in Washington, D.C. In 1902, APhA urged Congress to financially support the efforts of Dr. Wiley in establishing a laboratory to study the composition and adulteration of drugs; APhA even offered to find a qualified pharmaceutical chemist to become chief of the drug laboratory. The following year, APhA's recommended candidate, Lyman Frederick Kebler, who served as 1923-1924 first vice president, addressed the 1903 annual meeting to describe his new tasks as chief of the drug laboratory at the Department of Agriculture.

A number of forces helped sway public opinion and reverse Congressional opposition to a com-

of the 1848 law by reshipping drugs from ports of rejection to other ports where less vigilance was employed in examination. The petition requested amendments to the law that would change the mode of appointment of examiners, increase their salaries, and furnish chemicals so that examiners might apply chemical tests when necessary. Then, in 1859, APhA appealed to the Secretary of the Treasury to remove a recently enacted prohibition on the publication of a schedule of drugs and chemicals being imported into the U.S. On October 17, 1859. The Treasury Secretary responded favorably.

In 1865, president William Gordon sought relief from the requirement of the Internal Revenue Service for a license and a four dollar per gallon tax

The National Prohibition Act of 1922 required the use of special prescription order forms for medicinal liquor. Since bootleggers regularly forged these forms, a new style was issued by the government every two years. This form used for the first time in 1928 provided both an original and a duplicate copy; one copy for the pharmacist's file and one for the government. The stub was to be retained by the prescriber.

prehensive food and drug law. Chief Chemist Wiley led the way by stumping for the law, pulling together state food and drug officials, the General Federation of Women's Clubs, the American Medical Association, and APhA toward a common purpose. Even though patent medicine interests had long co-opted the press, muckraking journalists published scathing exposés of industry excesses. Most notable among these were Samuel Hopkins Adams' series on the patent medicine industry in *Colliers*, "The Great American Fraud," which began in 1905, and Upton Sinclair's fact-based novel, *The Jungle*, that laid bare the meat packing industry.

Enacted on June 30, 1906, the Food and Drugs Act, among other provisions, outlawed interstate commerce in adulterated or misbranded foods and drugs,

and mandated labeling the quantities of eleven drugs, including heroin, morphine, cocaine, and alcohol. The Act established the *U.S. Pharmacopeia* and the *National Formulary* as official compendia of drug standards.

Immediately after the first Federal Food and Drugs Act was passed, C. N. S. Hallberg reported in the *APhA Bulletin* that "whatever defects may be in portions of the law, the drug trade is to be congratulated upon the full recognition of the *USP* and *National Formulary* as the primary standard of strength, quality, and purity." However, Hallberg warned that "it is fallacious for state legislatures to emulate the example of Congress by attempting to have the various state legislatures at once enact laws on the lines of the Food and Drug Act. There are a number of inconsistencies in the Act which must not

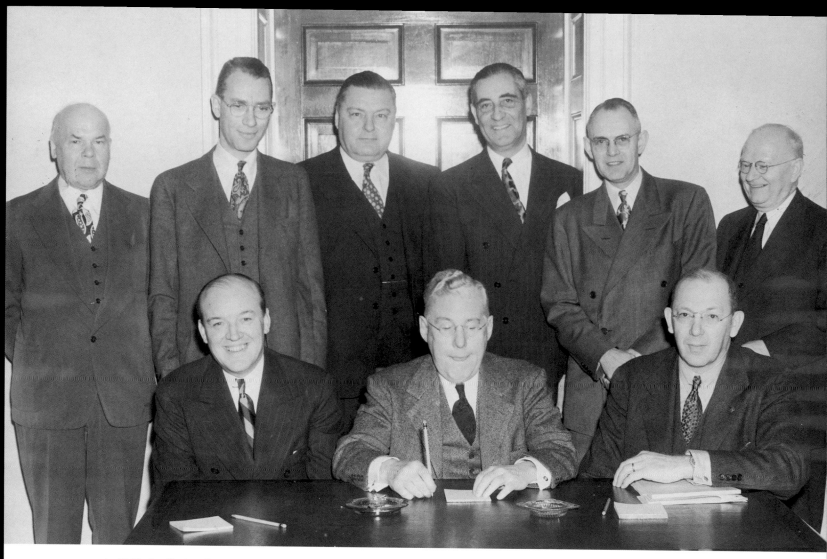

In 1946, the National Drug Trade Conference convened a special legislative committee at APhA headquarters to seek more uniformity in federal and state drug laws. Attending this meeting are (seated, left to right) Ray Schlotterer (Federal Wholesale Druggists' Association); Carson Frailey (American Drug Manufacturers Association); and Robert Fischelis (APhA). Standing (left to right), are Edwin Newcomb (National Wholesale Druggists Association); J. L. Hammer (American Pharmaceutical Manufacturers Association); A. K. Barta (Proprietary Association); George Frates (National Association of Retail Druggists); Lester Hayman (American Association of Colleges of Pharmacy); and Robert Swain (National Association of Boards of Pharmacy).

be allowed to get into any state laws." Hallberg added, "the rigid enforcement of pure food and drug laws reveal possibilities of undue hardship to conscientious druggists, owing to the faulty construction of such laws" and he promised to "cooperate with committees of state pharmaceutical associations...to secure enforcement without subjecting pharmacists to unjust prosecutions."

Following the enactment of the Food and Drugs Act, it appeared that APhA and others believed that it would reform patent medicines by outlawing false therapeutic claims. But in 1911, a divided Supreme Court held that the law did not

prohibit false health claims; only false labeling statements about the ingredients. So in 1912, Congress passed the Sherley Amendment prohibiting false and fraudulent claims of curative and therapeutic effects of drugs. This law proved too difficult to enforce because it required that the manufacturers' intention be demonstrated as fraudulent.

Previously, Congress passed the Biologics Control Act in 1902 to license and regulate serums and vaccines, and APhA adopted a policy in 1903 that the U.S. Public Health Service should establish "a standard antitoxin for determining the strength of anti-diphtheria serum."

Since the control of narcotics was considered a separate issue, APhA and other pharmacy organizations began to think of legislative control even before the final enactment of the 1906 Food and Drug Act. On December 27-29, 1905, APhA, National Association of Retail Druggists, National Wholesale Druggists Association, and Proprietary Association representatives met in Chicago to draft proposed legislation "to lessen the evils due to the improper sale of narcotic drugs." They agreed to APhA's Anti-Narcotic Law Model, developed in 1903 by James Hartley Beal as a guide to state legislatures.

To fulfill the pledges made in an international agreement reached at The Hague in 1912, Congress enacted the Harrison Act of December 17, 1914, to regulate the distribution of narcotics within its own borders. *APhA Journal* editor Eugene Eberle pointed out that "there was a long delay in the issuance of regulations which did not go into effect until May 1, 1920."

In 1932, APhA urged "uniform state narcotic legislation," and in 1938 APhA expressed "its deep concern over the provisions of the federal and state narcotic acts which permit the unregulated and promiscuous retail distribution of exempt narcotics." APhA urged the Commissioner of Narcotics in 1953 "to permit pharmacists to receive codeine prescriptions over the telephone provided they are reduced immediately to writing." The following year APhA commended the Commissioner of Narcotics for assisting in the passage of legislation modifying the Harrison Narcotic Act "so as to permit acceptance of certain codeine-containing prescriptions by telephone." To assist pharmacists in fulfilling the provisions of the Drug Abuse Control Amendments of 1965, APhA published and distributed the *Record*

Book of Stimulant and Depressant Drug Transactions for required inventories by 55,000 pharmacies, and included press-on-labels to be affixed to all controlled drugs.

The Volstead Act (prohibition) in 1922, led APhA to maintain that it has "placed a heavy burden on our calling unnecessarily. If we are to have prohibition, let us see that pharmacists no longer sell liquor which only brings disgrace on our calling." However, illegal sale of liquor by pharmacists does not seem to have been influenced by APhA's action.

In 1934, APhA voiced its support to Congress to include cosmetics in the Food and Drugs Act, and in 1937 APhA believed "any additional delay in the enactment of food, drug, and cosmetic legislation was unjustifiable." In the fall of 1937 a toxic solvent used in a sulfa preparation, called Elixir Sulfanilamide, caused 107 deaths in the U.S.A. That news finally spearheaded Congress to enact the Food, Drug and Cosmetic Act of 1938 requiring that drugs be approved as safe prior to marketing. The stronger drug and food law also included cosmetics and medical devices.

The Food, Drug, and Cosmetic Act was amended in 1941 requiring certification of the safety and efficacy of insulin, and again in 1945 to require certification of the safety and efficacy of penicillin, later extended to all antibiotics. The 1946 Miller Amendment extended the Food, Drug, and Cosmetic Act to safeguard goods in interstate commerce.

In 1948, the U.S. Supreme Court handed down the Sullivan decision confirming that a pharmacist violated the Federal law when he sold a restricted drug without a physician's prescription order. The long-standing confusion, dating back to regulations issued by FDA within weeks of the 1938

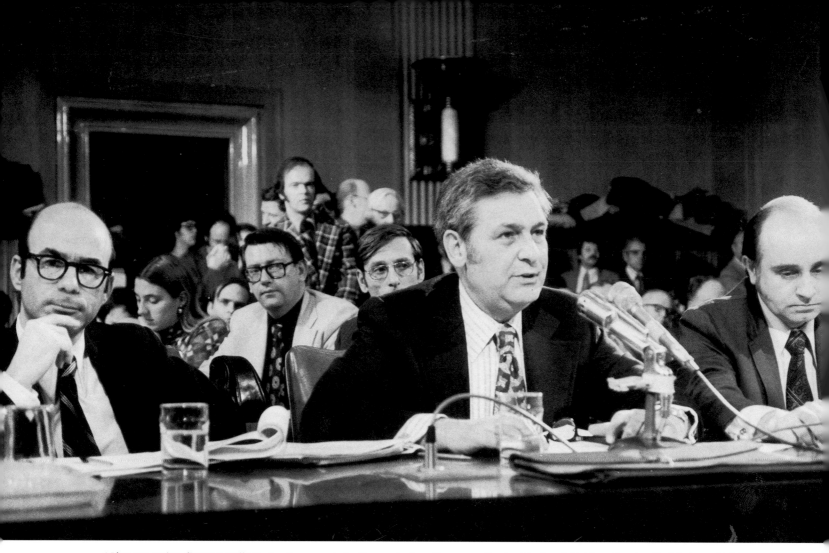

APhA executive director William Apple presents testimony before Congress, flanked by legal division director Carl Roberts (left) and scientific division director Edward Feldmann.

Act, over what constituted a prescription order, who had responsibility for making that determination, and in what manner a prescription could be dispensed, ultimately led to the 1951 Durham-Humphrey amendment, which was signed into law on October 26, 1951. It divided drugs into two classes: prescription (drugs distributed exclusively on an authorized prescription order) and nonprescription (the latter being defined as safe to use without medical supervision if adequately labeled) and established broad parameters for prescription status. It was initially met with concern by APhA. According to APhA secretary Robert P. Fischelis, "if any practicing pharmacist thinks that the passage of this amendment is a great victory, he is apt to have a rude awakening six months from now when the law goes into

effect." To resolve these concerns, the APhA House of Delegates called for a special committee to "evaluate the effects of the Durham-Humphrey Act."

More far reaching, although not so directly involving the practice of pharmacy, were the Kefauver-Harris Amendments. These resulted from nearly three years of Congressional hearings launched in December 1959 by the Senate Judiciary Committee's sub-committee on anti-trust and monopoly, led by Senator Estes Kefauver. The 1962 Drug Amendments, enacted in the wake of the thalidomide disaster, established proof of drug effectiveness, an extended drug clearance provision, enhanced factory inspection authority, increased control over clinical investigations including a requirement for patient consent, the use of nonproprietary drug names, more vigorous standards of good manufacturing practices, and FDA oversight of prescription drug advertising. Since the law required manufacturers to establish safety and effectiveness of all drugs marketed after 1938, the Food and Drug Administration negotiated a contract in 1966 with the National Academy of Sciences and its National Research Council to establish panels of experts to evaluate the effectiveness of all prescription drugs introduced between 1938 and 1962. More than 7,000 prescription drugs were removed from the market, and another 1,500 changed their labels. A similar mass review of nonprescription drugs was also implemented commencing in 1972.

As early as 1938, the APhA House expressed its "profound interest in all plans prepared for extending medical care," but strongly urged "the retention of free choice of physician, dentist, pharmacist and nurse by the patient." Then in 1949, APhA established a comprehensive position on Compulsory National Health Insurance as "unsuited to the American way." The following year, APhA reaffirmed its stand to oppose compulsory national health insurance.

In September 1963, APhA officially recommended the establishment of a "third class of drugs" that would be available only through pharmacies.

The following year, the APhA House of Delegates called for four classes of drugs: (1) prescription-only, renewable only with the prescriber's authorization; (2) prescription-only, renewable only at the pharmacist's discretion; (3) nonprescription, dispensed by pharmacist only at patient's request; and (4) nonprescription, available directly to the public without professional direction or control.

For more than 30 years APhA promoted the concept, but the Food and Drug Administration rejected the idea, claiming they lacked a legislative mandate. Meanwhile the Nonprescription Drug Manufacturers Association objected, claiming that "restriction of products to pharmacy sale would deny consumers the right to buy safe products at convenient locations of their own choice."

In 1984, the House of Delegates revised the concept to focus on a group of drugs "that would facilitate the transfer of drugs from prescription to nonprescription;" and in 1987, the House coined the term "transition class of drugs," calling on pharmacists "to play an active role in consultation, monitoring, and reporting problems associated with the use of drugs included in a transition class of drugs."

In 1991, the Federal Food and Drug Administration announced that it would take action against any community pharmacy that manufactured large amounts of commercially available drugs. So APhA, leading a "compounding working group" of the Joint Commission of Pharmacy Practitioners (JCPP), provided important feedback to FDA that established parameters such as in-house drug supply and the presence of certain equipment that would differentiate drug compounding from drug manufacturing.

At the 1974 APhA annual meeting, 17 pharmacist-lawyers met and decided to create the American Society for Pharmacy Law with Joseph L. Fink III as the founding president.

The Federal Election Campaign Act of 1971, and the establishment of the Federal Election Commission in 1974, led many organizations to form Political Action Committees. A major initiative of John F. Schlegel, newly elected APhA executive director, was to form a Political Action Committee (APhA-PAC) "to influence American health care pol-

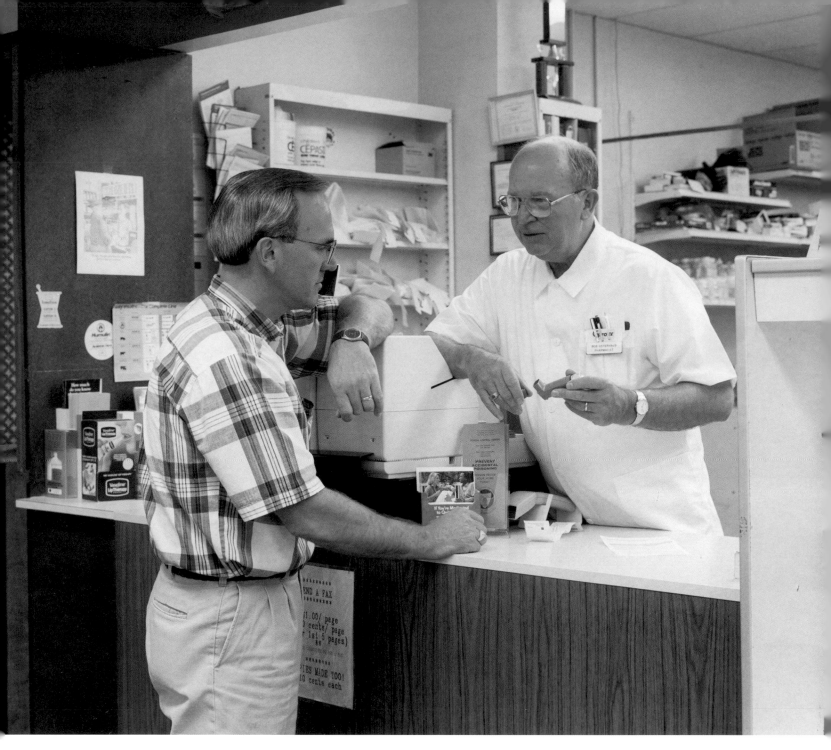

Three APhA past presidents were elected as state legislators. 1886-1887 president Charles Tufts served as a New Hampshire state senator; 1904-1905 president James Beal was an Ohio state legislator; and 1992-1993 president Robert Osterhaus (shown here in his pharmacy) was elected as an Iowa state legislator.

icy as it relates to pharmacy." The Board of Trustees approved its function in May 1985, and appointed Timothy L. Vordenbaumen as the first APhA-PAC president. Meanwhile, Schlegel hired Dorothy Keville, who, on July 2, 1985, registered as APhA's first lobbyist. Some members objected; "the Association should back away from the PAC approach," they wrote, and continue its long-stand-

ing role of furnishing witnesses at legislative hearings and providing Congressional committees with factual information, "not tainted with politics." Bolstered by various members of Congress who addressed annual meetings, APhA-PAC remains active today with Nancy Kalb as chair and treasurer of a Board of Governors.

CHAPTER 32

Women in Pharmacy

ew women engaged in the practice of pharmacy in the U.S. prior to 1860, but the Civil War temporarily opened the practice of pharmacy to women. By 1891, still only two percent of pharmacy students were women. Susan Hayhurst is sometimes reported as the first American woman to graduate from a college of pharmacy (Philadelphia College of Pharmacy, 1883), but this honor appears to go to Mary Corinna Putnam who graduated from the New York College of Pharmacy in 1863. Other women graduates in pharmacy during the 19th century include: Mary Upjohn (University of Michigan, 1871); Louise Baker (Massachusetts College of Pharmacy, 1877); Marion Tirrell (Chicago College of Pharmacy, 1878); Josephine R. Barbat (California College of Pharmacy, 1884); and Zada M. Cooper (University of Iowa, 1897). The latter served as the secretary of the Conference of Pharmaceutical Faculties for 20 years (1921-1941). In 1883, the Louisville College of Pharmacy for Women was established, graduating only 20 students in its 13 years of existence.

Graduation from a college of pharmacy did not always open the door toward equality. For example, Bessie Woods White, a graduate of the University of Michigan, applied to the Kentucky Board of Pharmacy for examination, but was refused.

She appealed to the courts which finally ruled in her favor on December 15, 1886.

The first woman admitted to APhA membership (1882) was Mrs. Ella F. Warren of Bellville, Ohio. Mrs. Eliza Rudolf (1852-1897), described as "the very first woman to own and manage a drugstore in the South," served as secretary of the Louisiana Pharmaceutical Association, and was elected as an APhA member in 1887. Alice Braunworth Halstead of Muscatine, Iowa, joined APhA in 1892, and established a record in 1928 for the longest continuous APhA membership of a woman to that time.

Mrs. Mary Olds Miner was the first woman elected to an APhA office — third vice president in 1895-1896. Her response to the 1895 annual meeting was, "I am mindful of the honor that you have paid me. I receive it not so much for myself but as a tribute you pay to women in pharmacy."

When Miss Josephine Anna Wanous of Minneapolis, Minnesota, was elected 1898-1899 APhA third vice president, Enno Sander described her as a person who "has always shown interest in APhA. I have seen her store in Minneapolis and she is very prosperous. I admire her."

Miss M. C. Dorr was the first woman to present a lecture at APhA in 1898. She discussed women as pharmacists, and observed that, "beautiful

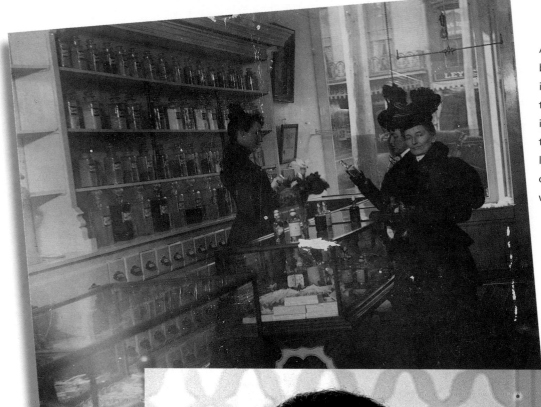

Alice Braunworth Halstead sells a bottle of Solon Palmer's perfume in her Muscatine, Iowa, prescription pharmacy. She joined APhA in 1892 (when this photo was taken) and in 1928 she established a record for the longest continuous membership of any woman to that time.

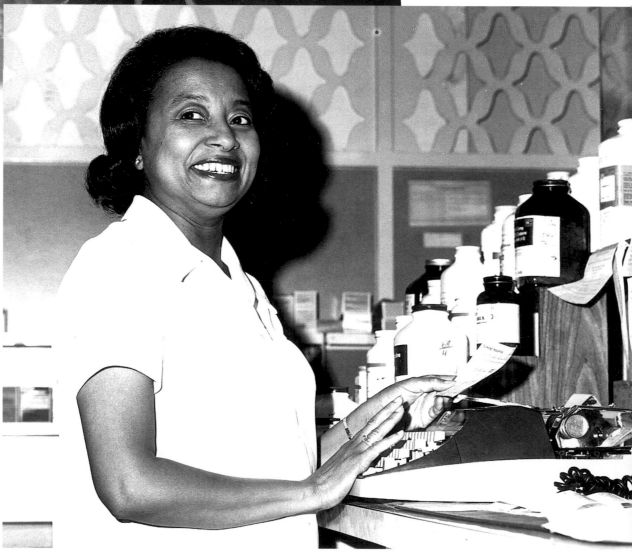

Mary Munson Runge, the first woman to be elected APhA president, checks a prescription order in her pharmacy before her retirement. The number of women pharmacists in the U.S. has increased ten fold since Ms. Runge commenced practicing pharmacy in 1949.

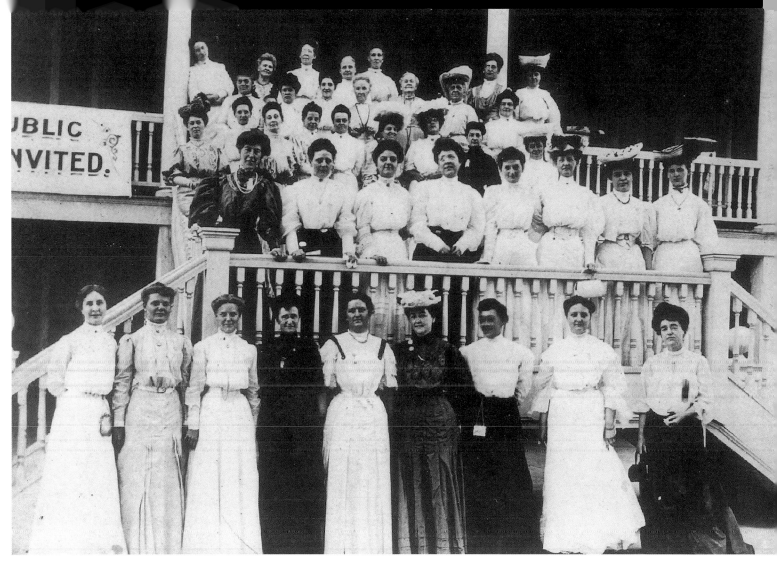

Wives of APhA members and the few women pharmacist members gathered at the 1905 annual meeting in Atlantic City, New Jersey. They chose to call themselves the "Women's Auxiliary." The APhA Women's Section was created seven years later, and the APhA Auxiliary was officially established in 1946.

women can be pharmacists without spoiling their beauty, either of person, disposition, or character." Mrs. Mary Stillwell Hall of Chicago attended the 1901 convention and actively participated in the discussions. Amanda Stahl and Clara Malarkey presented a paper entitled "Women in Practical Pharmacy" before the APhA Section of Practical Pharmacy and Dispensing in 1905. Then in 1906 APhA adopted a resolution encouraging "qualified young women to enter the occupation of pharmacy."

An independent Woman's Pharmaceutical Association was created in 1892 for Illinois pharmacists, and it became national in 1903 with 16 chapters. This was followed in 1905 by the Pacific Coast Woman's Pharmaceutical Association.

An APhA Women's Section was founded in 1912 to "emphasize the right and capability of women to engage in pharmaceutical pursuits [and] to unite the women members of APhA." Pharmacist Zada Cooper served as president 1917-1918, while Anna Bagley served as president 1918-1919 as well as secretary 1912-1916 and again in 1923. However, most of the officers of the Women's Section were non-pharmacist wives of APhA members who worked in their husband's pharmacies as manager or accountant. The Women's Section was dissolved in 1923, much like other women's pharmaceutical associations, to encourage women to join organizations traditionally for men only.

The Women's Auxiliary was organized in

CHAPTER 35.

Interprofessional Relations

When APhA members at the 1853 annual meeting reviewed the results of the Association's survey of pharmacy throughout the country, they found such reports as:

"In the rural districts of Pennsylvania, physicians almost invariably furnish medicine to the patients. In some cases this is unavoidable; in others, it is unjust and injurious to the interests of pharmacy."

More alarming was the 1853 report from Gustavus Simmons of Sacramento, California, who reported: "Two-thirds of all [20] drugstores are kept by physicians...which ruins the legitimate business of apothecaries."

APhA president Samuel M. Colcord presented a lengthy lecture at the 1858 annual meeting entitled "Professional Intercourse Between the Apothecary and Physician." Colcord admitted that this is "a subject upon which pharmaceutists are very much perplexed, each having an opinion peculiar to himself, according to the education and temperament of the individual." But he concluded: "A knowledge of our profession with strict and careful attention to business will assure us success with dignity and standing with the medical profession."

Even though there was an ever increasing number of physicians who sent their prescription orders to pharmacies, it was not until 1890 that official action was taken to enhance professional relations after the American Medical Association created the AMA Section on Materia Medica and Pharmacy (later to become the Council on Pharmacy and Chemistry). Then in 1893, the American Medical Association sent delegates for the first time to the APhA annual meeting, and AMA president Frank Woodbury of Philadelphia told APhA members, "the American medical profession leans on the pharmaceutical profession." The following year, APhA took a position on physician dispensing by recommending the "withdrawal of patronage from all firms engaged in furnishing physicians direct with their manufacturing products."

It was not until 1908 that C. S. N. Hallberg observed in an editorial in the *APhA Bulletin* that "for the first time in the history of pharmacy in this country are physicians not only willing, but anxious, to meet with pharmacists on the common ground of professional conference and to consult about how to escape the thralldom of the proprietary evil."

Liaison between state pharmaceutical associations and state medical societies was advocated by APhA in 1929; ten years later, APhA noted "with great pleasure the many programs being carried out in every state in the country to promote closer relations

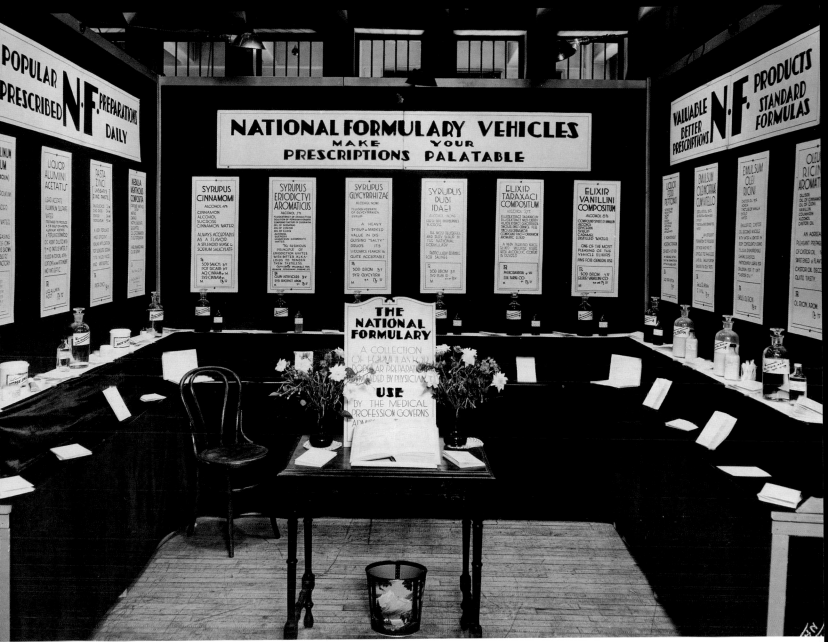

This *N.F.* exhibit was featured at the American Medical Association convention in 1933. The earliest interprofessional relations involved pharmacists working side-by-side with physicians in the revision of both the *U.S. Pharmacopeia* and the *National Formulary*. One of APhA's objectives was to convince physicians to prescribe medication from the *National Formulary* rather than proprietary medicines.

between members of the public health professions."

In 1962, APhA drafted and submitted to the American Medical Association a "Physician-Pharmacist Code of Understanding" declaring physician ownership of pharmacies as unethical. Failing this, APhA took its case to Congress, gaining the support of Senator Philip A. Hart of Michigan. In 1974, APhA and the American Society of Internal Medicine jointly issued a statement on "Prescription Writing and Prescription Labeling," which was revised in 1976.

In 1935, APhA appointed a committee to develop closer relations with dentists, and in 1954

APhA endorsed the position of the American Dental Association in the fluoridation of drinking water. Following the lead of the Connecticut Joint Dental-Pharmaceutical Committee, APhA established in 1968 a liaison committee with the American Dental Association. In 1970, APhA published a booklet entitled *The Dentist & the Pharmacist*.

The APhA Commission on Pharmacy and Veterinary Medicine was created in 1965, and the following year the Association developed with the American Veterinary Medical Association a Code of Interprofessional Relations.

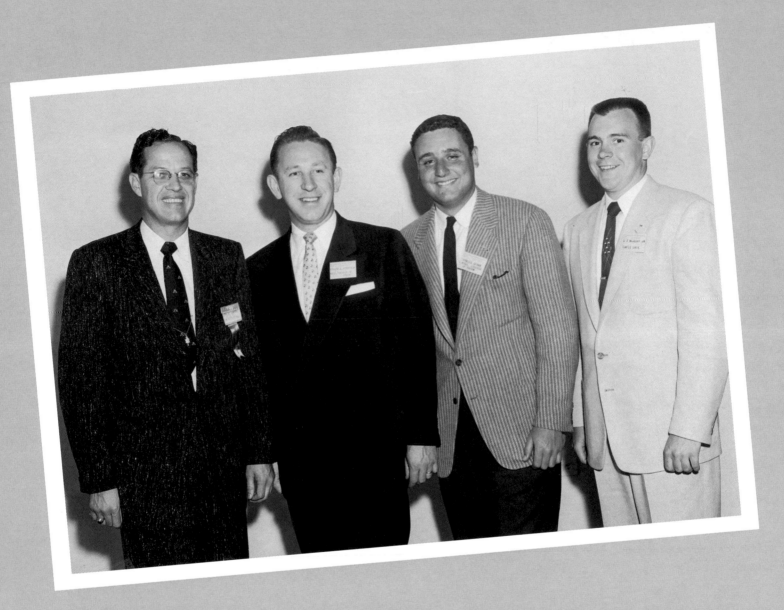

The first APhA Student Section officers (1954-1955) include (left to right) John Sanders (delegate to the House of Delegates); Edward Perednia (chairman); Harold Sparr (secretary-treasurer); and Stuart Westbury, Jr., (alternate delegate to the House of Delegates).

CHAPTER 36.

Pharmacy Students

Clarence B. Jordan presented a paper in 1921 proposing the creation of Student Branches of APhA. Following the suggestion of Jordan, on November 22, 1922, the University of North Carolina organized a combination local and student branch and then petitioned the APhA Council for recognition. Students at two other universities followed North Carolina's example. In 1923, a local branch was formed at the University of Washington, and in 1929, 337 students at the University of Pittsburgh petitioned the APhA Council to form a branch.

The achievements of these early unofficial student branches aroused the interest of many pharmacy leaders, and in 1928, the APhA president appointed a committee of three to determine the possibility of establishing student branches in all schools of pharmacy. At the 1931 annual meeting, the Bylaws were amended to authorize the formation of student branches. Three student branches were formed that year at the University of Pittsburgh, the State College of South Dakota, and Washington State College. Student Branches were formed in 1932 at the University of Florida and the University of Wisconsin. St. John's University followed suit in 1934.

The number of student branches grew steadily; as the number increased, it became traditional for students to meet informally at APhA annual meetings to discuss mutual problems and issues facing the profession. By 1956, there were 74 Student Branches in the 75 accredited colleges of pharmacy, with a total APhA Student membership of 13,100.

Recognizing the need for a more official forum, student representatives, their faculty advisors, and members of the APhA Committee on Student Branches encouraged the 1951 session of the APhA House of Delegates to grant students one voting delegate in the House of Delegates. The following year, the House recommended the establishment of a Section for Pharmacy Students, and authorized such a section in 1953.

The APhA Student Section was founded in 1954, and for the first time pharmacy students were authorized to send a single delegate to the House of Delegates. A total of 167 pharmacy students attended the founding meeting at the 1954 annual meeting, presided over by Linwood F. Tice, chairman of the APhA Committee on Student Branches. Bylaws were approved, officers were elected, and the new Student Section was declared officially organized.

In 1969, the association converted its Student Section to the Student American Pharmaceutical Association which was known as

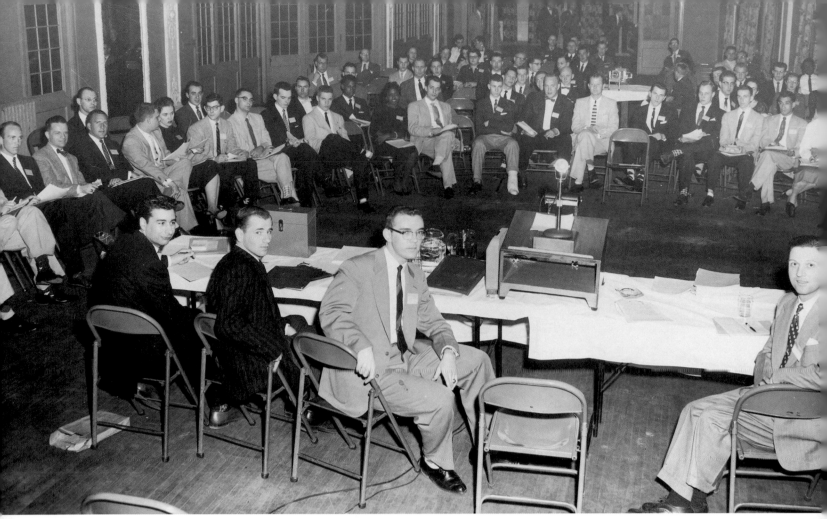

Only three women pharmacy students attended the 1956 Student Section meeting at the Tellar Hotel in Detroit.

Student APhA from 1969 to 1972, and SAPhA from 1972 to 1983, during which time students established their own House of Delegates. To increase participation of recently graduated pharmacists in APhA, an unofficial group called the Young Pharmacists' Caucus was created in the late 1970s which published a newsletter entitled *The Grapevine*. It was edited variously by Luan Dodini, Donna Walker, Michael Smith, Lucinda Maine, and Brian Bullock.

In 1986, SAPhA became the Academy of Students of Pharmacy, gaining 28 delegates to the APhA House of Delegates, and became known as APhA-ASP.

In 1992, the "New Practitioner Initiative" was launched to provide timely information to recent pharmacy school graduates. Then in 1997, students achieved a goal they had sought in the 1970s — a seat on the APhA Board of Trustees — by an amendment of the APhA Bylaws making all three Academy pres-

idents voting members of the APhA Board of Trustees. As early as the 1968 annual meeting, students were encouraged to help combat the drug abuse problem; three years later, Student APhA launced an interdisciplinary "Project SPEED" (Student Professionals Engaged in Education on Drugs) supported by a three-year grant from the National Institute of Mental Health. The "National Patient Counseling Competition" was established in 1983, based on a concept developed by the Philadelphia College of Pharmacy and Science. Until 1998, the competition was co-sponsored by Student APhA and the U.S. Pharmacopeial Convention, and continues to be held annually by the Academy of Students of Pharmacy. "Operation Immunization" was launched in 1997 by the Academy of Students of Pharmacy and the Student National Pharmaceutical Association (see Chapter 33 for details on SNPhA).

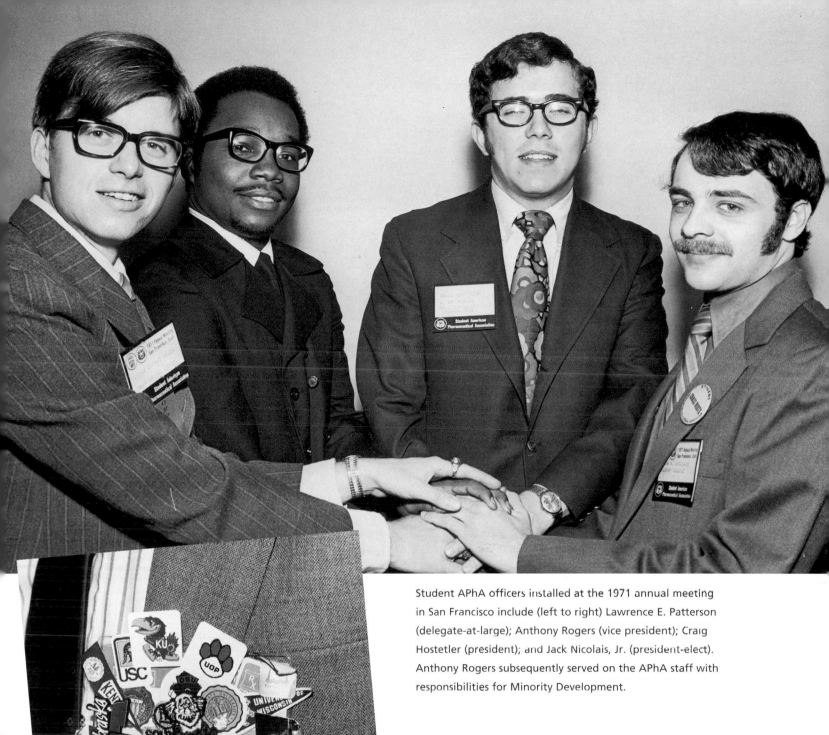

Student APhA officers installed at the 1971 annual meeting in San Francisco include (left to right) Lawrence E. Patterson (delegate-at-large); Anthony Rogers (vice president); Craig Hostetler (president); and Jack Nicolais, Jr. (president-elect). Anthony Rogers subsequently served on the APhA staff with responsibilities for Minority Development.

By the 1988 APhA annual meeting, the trend for collectng and displaying lapel pins from various colleges of pharmacy was well underway.

CHAPTER 37

Patent Medicines to Nonprescription Drugs

Long before APhA was founded, the American "patent medicine" promoters were already busy at work, profiting from the "patented" nostrums from England. But these "patent medicines" were actually secret remedies. After American independence, the trek to the U.S. Patent Office commenced. A study made in 1849 by a U.S. Congressional committee revealed that there were no less than 600 different patent medicines on the U.S. market, and one entrepreneur alone was spending a hundred thousand dollars a year in advertising his purgative. The expanding market for patent medicines and the expansion of the American newspaper went hand-in-hand since the popular press provided a good medium for promoting the sale of these nostrums; this fostered the birth of the advertising industry in America.

By this time, APhA had come onto the national scene, and one of the first objectives set forth at the organizational meeting was to investigate these nostrums. A committee was appointed to "act efficiently in abating this great evil," and the following year, Charles Guthrie told the pharmacists gathered at the 1853 annual meeting, "from a small beginning, quackery has grown to a great monster of which we are afraid." Quite a debate ensued in which many arguments (to be heard again and again) were put forth. "Some physicians were endorsing certain patent medicines, so why shouldn't apothecaries sell them," some contended. "Further, if apothecaries didn't sell them, the grocers and other shop keepers would," they added. Even Edward Parrish expressed the view that the "public sentiment was not yet ready for the abolition of patent medicines."

By a split vote of 13 to 8, APhA officially resolved in 1853 "that pharmaceutical brethren discourage by every honorable means the use of these nostrums; to refrain from recommending them to their customers; not to manufacture any medicine the composition of which is not made public; and to use every opportunity of exposing the evils attending to their use."

Two years later (1855), APhA dropped the obligation to subscribe to the Code of Ethics as a prerequisite of membership because it intimated that members were required to discontinue the sale

Opposite Page: This illustration from Ayer's *Book of Emergencies* (Lowell, Massachusetts, 1888) presents an image of the way patent medicine king James Cook Ayer hoped every pharmacy would look — filled with advertisements for *Ayer's Sarsaparilla* and *Ayer's Almanac*. Ayer also introduced many manufacturing innovations such as a pill mass mixer and the mechanical pill machine.

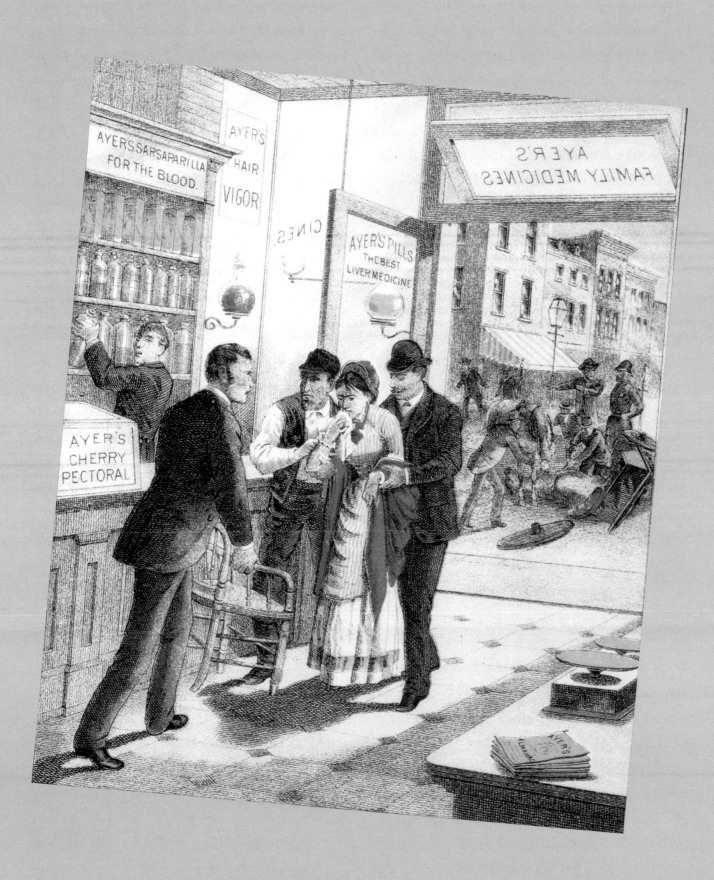

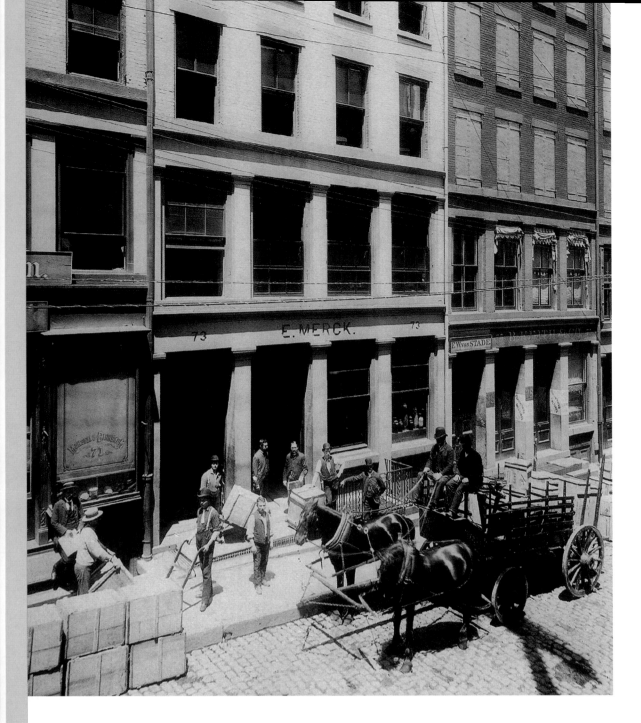

Merck & Company was founded in the Engel Apotheke (Angel Pharmacy) in Darmstadt, Germany. The firm opened its first office in the U.S. in February 1887, located at No. 73 William Street in New York City (shown here). By 1896 the firm had moved to the new *Merck Building* at University Place.

Concern over the rapidly expanding drug manufacturers led William Procter, Jr. to tell APhA members at the 1858 annual meeting that, "pharmacy may be defined to be the art of preparing and dispensing medicines, and embodies the knowledge and skill requisite to carry them out in practice. But if the preparation of medicines is taken away from the apothecary, and he becomes merely the dispenser of them, his business is shorn of half its dignity and importance, and he relapses into a simple shopkeeper."

The following year, Robert Battey, 1859 APhA president *pro tem*, admitted that "there is doubtless much to be gained by the introduction of zealous and rising investigating men who are manufacturing chemists." But he expressed concern that these "manufacturing chemists [are] neither pharmaceutists nor druggists as required by our Constitution, [and yet] we are opening the door of our citadel to a dangerous extent if we admit them."

It was during the Civil War that the American pharmaceutical industry took decisive steps into maturity as they provided the medicinal

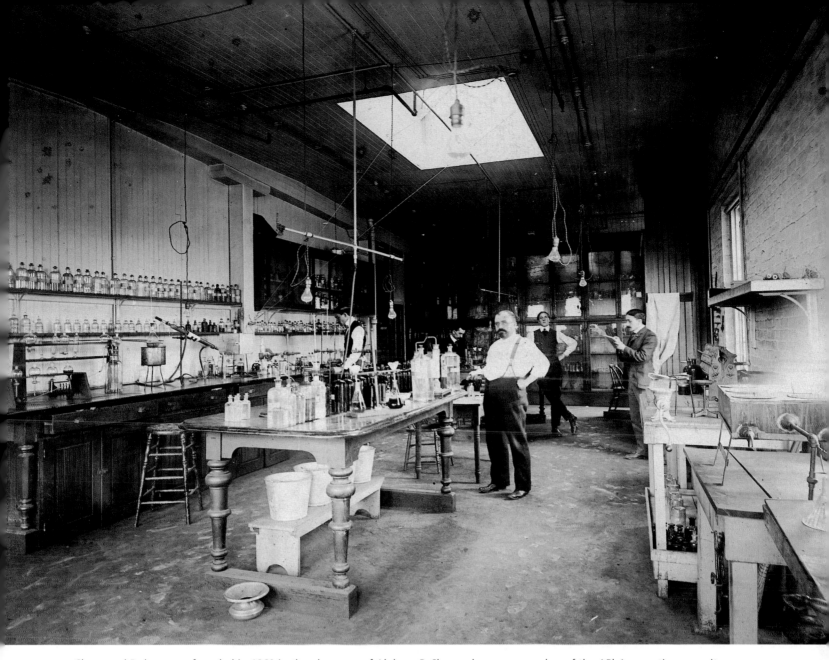

Sharp and Dohme was founded in 1860 in the pharmacy of Alpheus P. Sharp who was a member of the APhA executive commit-tee in 1863 and 1870. Subsequently, Louis Dohme, Alfred Robert Louis Dohme, and Charles Emile Dohme were all APhA officers. This photograph portrays the Sharp and Dohme Research and Control Laboratories in 1900.

needs of the military. After the Civil War, APhA sought closer ties with industry leaders, and Frederick Stearns was elected APhA president in 1866. The following year Edward R. Squibb was nominated as APhA president, but Squibb declined stating that the stress of business prevented him from accepting. He also pointed out that "I am not a prac-tical pharmaceutist" but added, "I am willing to work for the Society, and can, as chairman of the Business Committee." He did serve as chairman of the APhA business committee from 1863 to 1868.

Other prominent 19th-century industry pio-neers who held positions as members of APhA included:

Burroughs Wellcome & Company: Henry S. Wellcome was a member of the APhA busi-ness committee 1876-1877.

Eli Lilly & Co.: Eli Lilly was APhA local secretary 1878-1879.

Lloyd Brothers (subsequently purchased by Hoechst Pharmaceuticals): John Uri Lloyd served as APhA president 1887-1888.

McKesson & Robbins: John McKesson was an

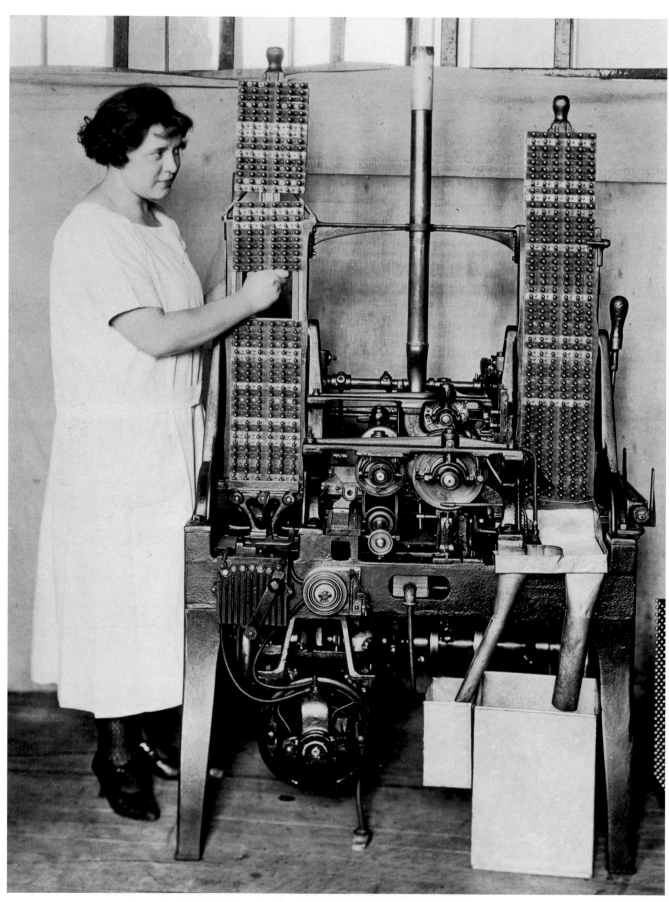

By the 1920s, new equipment was introduced by the prescription drug industry for the mass production of pharmaceuticals. This 1926 photograph shows the *Wilkie Machine* used for producing capsules.

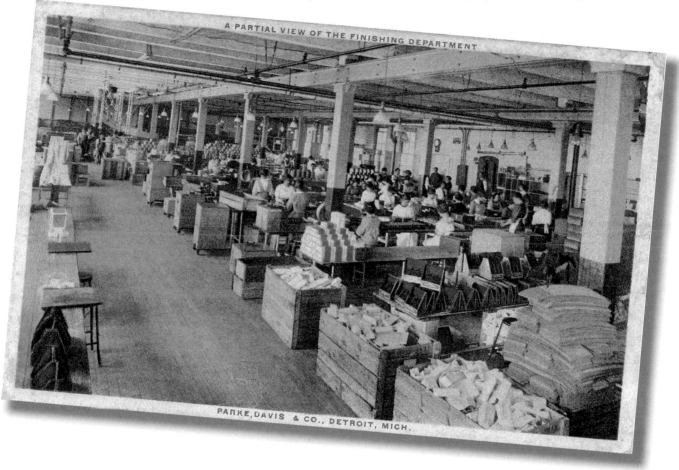

This picture postcard is described as "a partial view of the finishing department of Parke-Davis & Company of Detroit, Michigan," circa 1930.

1871 member of the APhA committee on the drug market.

Parke, Davis & Co.: Samuel P. Duffield was a member of the APhA committee on scientific queries in 1866.

W. H. Schieffelin & Co.: William A. Brewer served as president 1853-1854.

Seabury & Johnson: George J. Seabury was first vice president 1891-1892.

Sharp & Dohme (subsequently became a division of Merck & Company): Alpheus P. Sharp was a member of the executive committee in 1863 and 1870; Louis Dohme was second vice president 1882-1883; Alfred R. L. Dohme was chairman of the Scientific Section 1894-1895; and Charles Emile Dohme was president 1898-1899.

Smith Kline French Co.: Mahlon N. Kline

was a member of the APhA committee on the drug market from 1883 to 1886.

John Wyeth and Brother: Conrad Lewis Diehl served as president 1874-1875.

In 1884, APhA adopted a resolution seeking legislation "to secure a sufficient statement of the composition of all medicines to be put on each package." Two years later, president Joseph Roberts noted, "Since the rapid multiplication of proprietary medicines works serious evils to legitimate pharmacy, pharmacists should use their best efforts to induce physicians when prescribing to give preference to official *USP* remedies."

By the turn of the century, newer pharmaceutical compounds were "flooding the market," according to Joseph Remington, and as early as 1897, Canadian

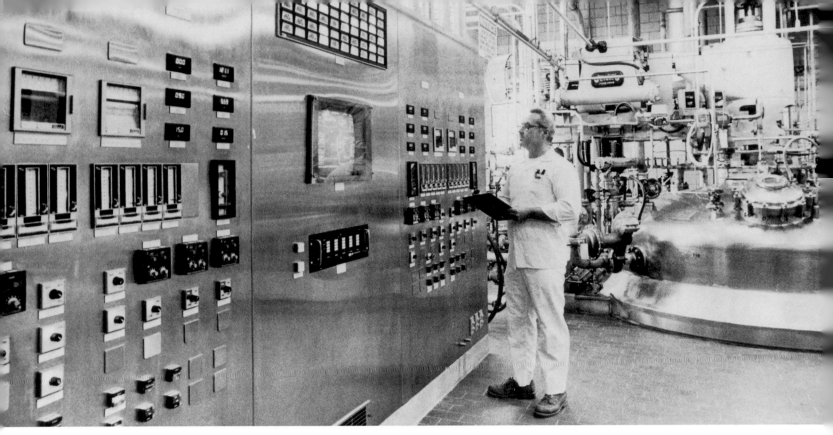

By the second half of the 20th century, pharmaceutical manufacturers were using the latest technical advances and producing pharmaceuticals in enormous quantities.

resident and APhA president Joseph Morrison identified very high prices for new drugs in the U.S. compared to the prices in Canada (an enduring theme). According to Morrison, Phenacetin cost $1.00 in the U.S. but only 35 cents in Canada; and Sulfonal cost $1.35 in the U.S. but only 30 cents in Canada.

Unlike the manufacturers of patent medicines who had organized in the 19th century, there was no concerted effort for the prescription drug industry to organize into an association. However, the first half of the 20th century saw a proliferation of associations of pharmaceutical manufacturers. The American Association of Pharmaceutical Chemists was founded in 1907, and changed its name in 1920 to the American Pharmaceutical Manufacturers Association. The National Association of Manufacturers of Medicinal Products was founded in 1912, and changed its name in 1917 to the American Drug Manufacturers Association. It wasn't until 1958 that these organizations merged to form the Pharmaceutical Manufacturers Association, later

known as the Pharmaceutical Research and Manufacturers of America.

The Parenteral Drug Association was founded in 1946; the National Association of Pharmaceutical Manufacturers in 1955 (formerly the Drug and Allied Products Guild); and the Generic Pharmaceutical Industry Association in 1981. The latter two associations merged in 2001 as the Generic Pharmaceutical Association. The National Pharmaceutical Council was established in 1953 as a trade association conducting public relations for the major research-oriented pharmaceutical manufacturers.

To find better procedures for drug recalls, APhA and the Pharmaceutical Manufacturers Association undertook a survey of recall methods used in various countries around the world. Proposals made by APhA included the development of a system providing that pharmacists and wholesalers would promptly receive the notification of any drug recall.

CHAPTER 39.

Pharmaceutical Wholesalers

When APhA was founded, many "druggists" were serving as a retailer as well as a wholesaler. After the Civil War, some of these druggists closed their retail business so that they could devote their full attention to wholesaling. One early example was George A. Kelly of Pittsburgh.

As more exclusive drug wholesalers were established, a group in the middle west met in Cincinnati in 1876 to found the Western Wholesale Druggists' Association to "correct excessive and unmercantile competition" and remove "evils and customs that are against good policy and sound business principles." The organization changed its name

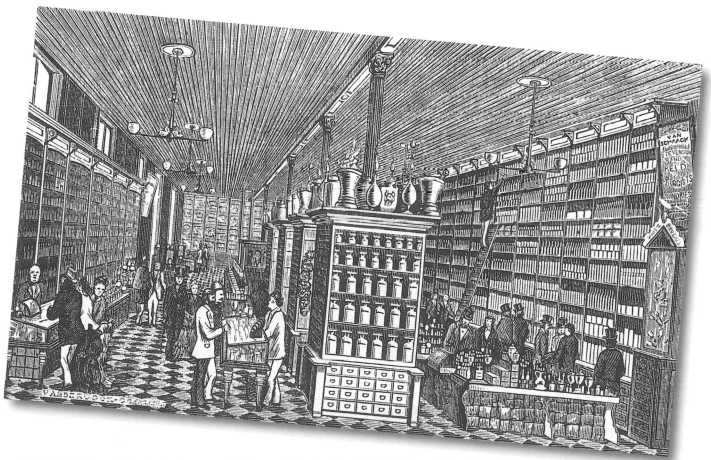

This depicts the well-stocked salesroom of Chicago wholesale druggists Van Schaack, Stevenson & Reid in 1875. The firm supplied medicines, dyes, paints, oils, glassware, proprietary medicines, perfumery, toilet articles, and chemical products.

in 1882 to National Wholesale Druggists' Association to reflect its national scope. Relations with APhA got off to a good start.

APhA came to the support of the Western Wholesale Druggists Association in 1880 by seeking repeal of the stamp tax on proprietary medicines that Congress had imposed during the Civil War; two years later, a delegation from the Western Wholesale Druggists Association received permission to participate in the deliberations of the APhA annual meeting, but without the right to vote. In turn, James Richardson of the wholesaler group (also an APhA member) invited APhA to send a similar delegation to the wholesalers meeting in Cleveland. In response, Charles Bullock observed that "many of our founders were men who were engaged in [wholesaling] although some combined it with retailing or dispensing of drugs." Delegations between APhA and the National Wholesale Druggists Association continued to be exchanged for the remainder of the 19th century, and many of the wholesale delegations were chaired by APhA members. In 1895, George Seabury told APhA members that there were 662 wholesale druggists with 200 exclusive wholesalers servicing 28,000 pharmacies.

Many pharmacists felt that they could save money by group purchases from wholesalers and manufacturers, and they established what were called "buying clubs." The first U.S. pharmacy-owned co-op organized in 1888 when Philadelphia pharmacists formed a buying group. From 1896 to 1907 one buying club after another was formed. By 1905 there were so many "buying clubs" that they organized as the American Druggists Syndicate, and as the Associated Drug Companies of America the following year. Both associations were succeeded by the Federal Wholesale Druggists' Association in 1915, which for years limited its membership to these "buying clubs" (later termed "pharmacy-owned cooperatives"). However, the Federal Wholesale Druggists' Association opened its membership in 1940 to other exclusive wholesalers.

The Pharmaceutical Distributors International (DPI) was founded in 1956, and the International Pharmaceutical Distributors Association (IPDA) was established in 1974 by merger of FWDA and DPI. Then in 1984, they were absorbed by the National Wholesale Druggists Association which changed its name in January 2001 to the Healthcare Distribution Management Association.

CHAPTER 40

Exhibitions

A s early as 1853, APhA president William Brewer exhibited a "cabinet of specimens of indigenous medicinal plants" at the annual meeting. The first exhibit featuring products of commercial firms was shown at the 1855 annual meeting. It included exhibits by Powers & Weightman; Tilden & Co.; and three other firms. By 1859, there were 23 firms exhibiting their wares, including Powers & Weightman, Edward R. Squibb, and the New England Glass Company.

The 1874 APhA annual meeting exhibition hall was decorated with "bunting and evergreen wreaths suspended from the wall," and the 57 exhibitors included Mallinckrodt, McKesson & Robbins, Powers & Weightman, Schieffelin, William R. Warner, and John Wyeth.

There were no exhibits at the 1876 APhA annual meeting. Instead members visited the Philadelphia Centennial Exposition celebrating the centenary of the signing of the Declaration of Independence. Pharmaceutical preparations were exhibited by Bullock & Crenshaw; Hance Brothers & White; Seabury & Johnson; Frederick Stearns; and

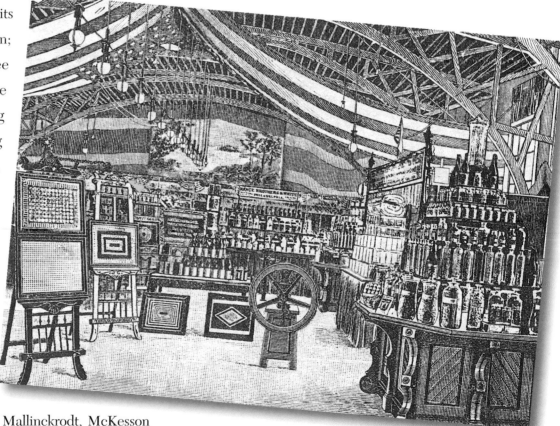

The first APhA exhibition was held in 1855. This exhibit of Hance Brothers & White was awarded a gold medal as the best display at the 1888 APhA exhibition.

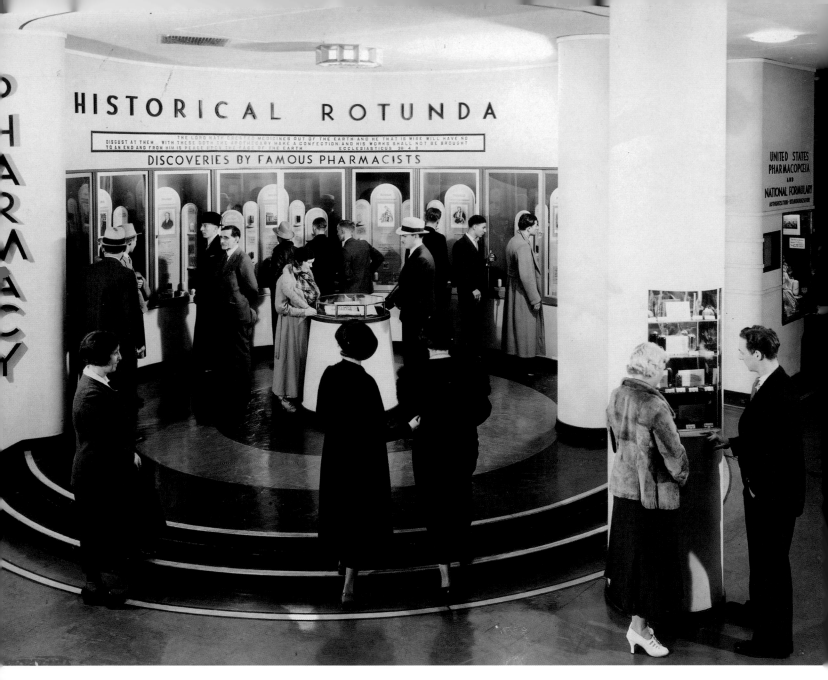

APhA sponsored an exhibit at the 1933-1934 *Century of Progress* in Chicago. The exhibit included a case (in the center of this photograph) containing a reproduction of the *Papyrus Ebers*, the earliest pharmaceutical document that survives from ancient Egypt.

John Wyeth & Brother; plus equipment by Henry Troemner (scales); and Whitall Tatum (glassware).

The 1888 APhA annual meeting exhibition included 75 exhibitors with Hance Brothers & White receiving an award "for the best general exhibit" (see illustration). In addition to pharmaceuticals, firms exhibited cash registers, safes, tobacco products, and even vehicles produced by the Columbus Buggy Company.

In 1893, two full days were set aside for APhA members to visit the Columbian Exposition in Chicago commemorating the 400th anniversary of the discovery of America. APhA members were amazed by the spectacular "White City" that used electricity for the first time on a lavish scale. Major pharmaceutical firms presented elaborate exhibits, including Merck in its own exposition building.

APhA voted to discontinue exhibits at the annual meeting in 1890 "because some abuses crept in," but they subsequently voted to "revive the aban-

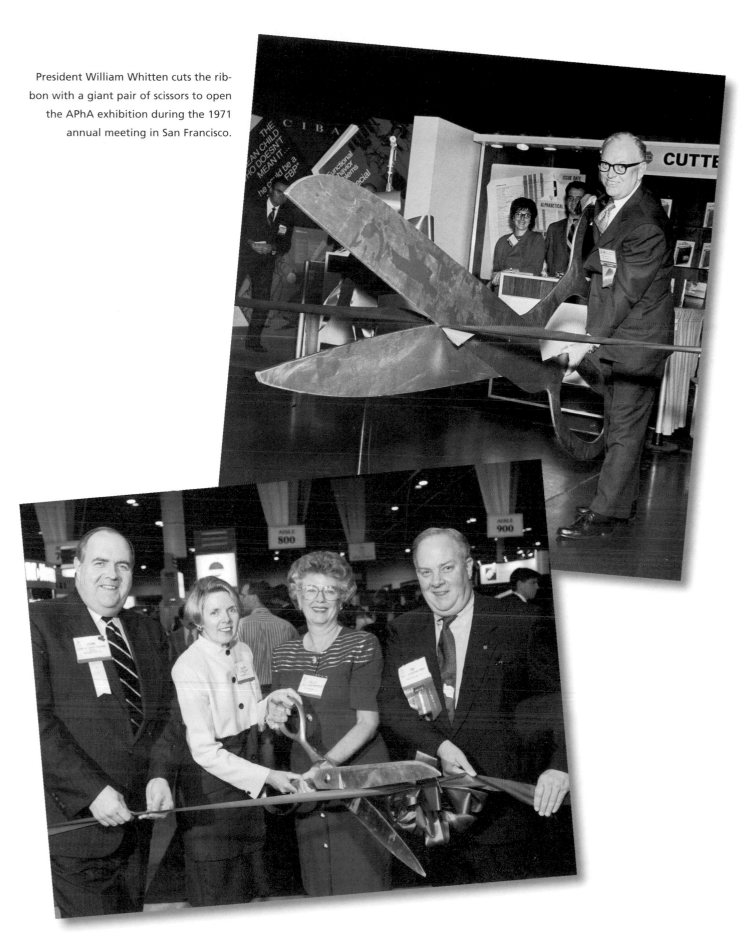

President William Whitten cuts the ribbon with a giant pair of scissors to open the APhA exhibition during the 1971 annual meeting in San Francisco.

President Tim Vordenbaumen (right) and executive vice president John Gans (left) hold the ribbon while their spouses (Eilene Gans and Sally Vordenbaumen) use a giant pair of scissors to open the exhibition during the 1995 APhA annual meeting in Orlando, Florida.

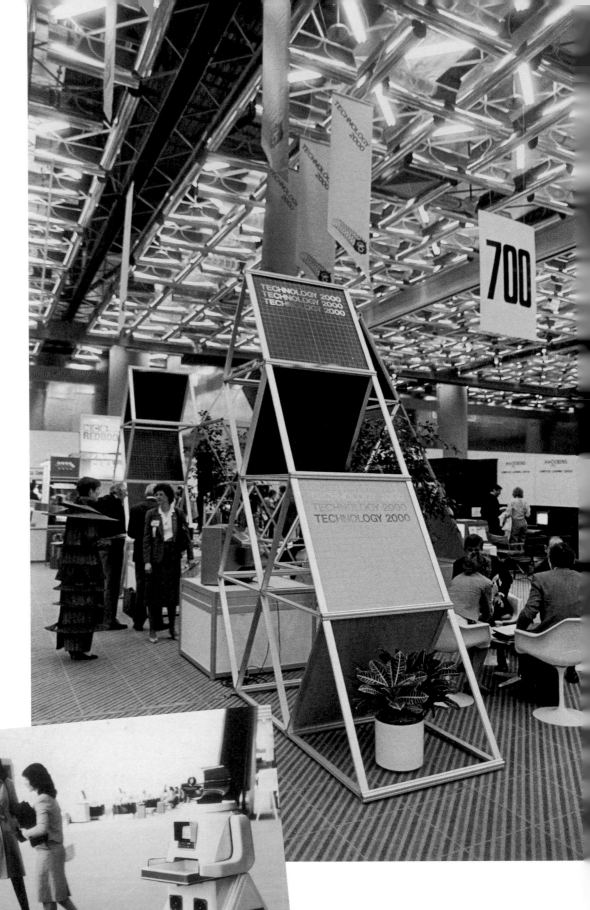

The 1984 annual meeting in Montreal went high-tech. With a theme of *Technology 2000*, a young lady dressed as a visitor from outer-space roamed the exhibition hall while a robot (see inset photo) greeted attendees arriving at the convention center.

doned custom" at the 1898 meeting that also included formal lectures by exhibitors. Among the firms participating were American Soda Fountain Co.; Johnson & Johnson; Mallinckrodt Chemical Works; Merck & Co.; William S. Merrell; H. K. Mulford (who exhibited diphtheria antitoxin); Parke Davis & Co.(who exhibited adrenalin); Rosengarten & Sons; Sharp & Dohme; Smith Kline & French; and E. R. Squibb & Sons.

Pharmacists attending the 1904 annual meeting in St. Louis visited the Louisiana Purchase Exposition to see exhibits of many pharmaceutical firms displaying innovations in dosage forms. APhA members who traveled to San Francisco for the 1915 annual meeting were treated to several visits to the Pan Pacific International Exposition including the president's reception. The fair celebrated the completion of the Panama Canal. The 1905 annual meeting exhibition featured 27 firms including Eli Lilly;

McKesson & Robbins; Merck & Co.; and Smith Kline & French.

APhA sponsored an impressive pharmacy exhibit at the 1933-1934 Chicago Century of Progress; here the public learned of discoveries by famous pharmacists. The exhibit also featured a restoration of the Philo Carpenter Apothecary Shop, and a scale model of the APhA headquarters building in Washington.

Again annual meeting exhibits were discontinued because many of the firms participating were offering products or services inconsistent with APhA's goal of promoting professional pharmacy. However, in 1960 APhA launched an exhibition program featuring 50 scientific and technical exhibits. By the 1990s, the APhA annual exposition included more than 200 different exhibitors, and continues as an integral part of each annual meeting.

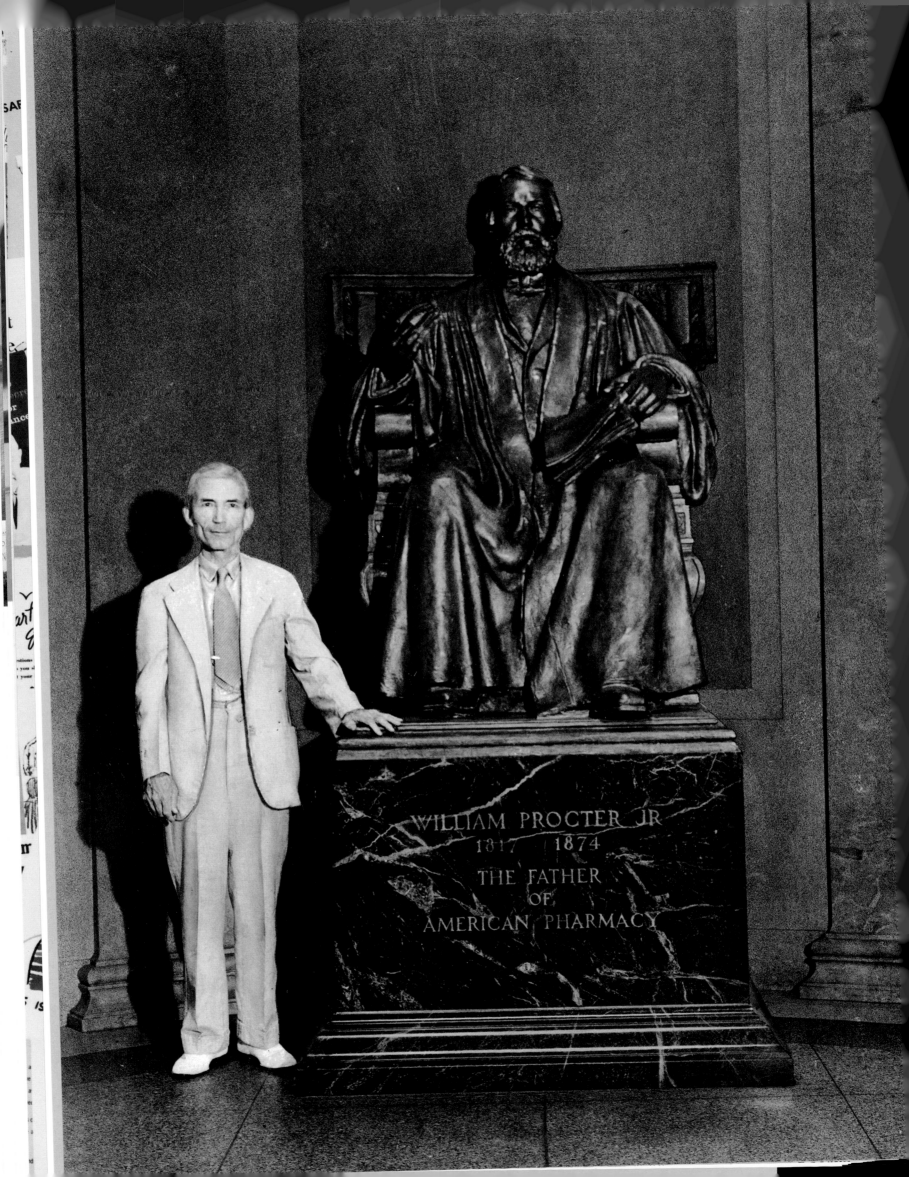

WILLIAM PROCTER JR
1817   1874

THE FATHER
OF
AMERICAN PHARMACY

bronze base depicts in bas relief the pharmacists who served in the Revolutionary War, the Civil War, the Spanish American War, World War I, and World War II, surrounded by pharmaceutical equipment and drugs of choice used during each war. General J. Lawton Collins, deputy chief of staff of the U.S. Army, was the principal speaker at the 1948 dedication ceremony.

The memorial flag pole was updated on May 25, 1993, with a sculptured bronze plaque honoring pharmacists who served in the Korean, Vietnam, and the Persian Gulf conflicts. The 1993 ceremony featured the U.S. Navy Ceremonial Band, remarks by the surgeons general of the Army, Navy, and Air Force, and a keynote address by U.S. Senator John McCain who was a prisoner of war during the Vietnam conflict.

Other APhA awards named for individuals include pharmacy's most prestigious award, the [Joseph P.] Remington Honor Medal introduced in 1918 for lifetime achievement; the Hugo H. Schaefer Award for outstanding voluntary contributions introduced in 1964; the Daniel B. Smith Practice Excellence Award in 1964; the Hubert H. Humphrey Award for government and/or legislative service in 1978; the Takeru Higuchi Research Prize in pharmaceutical sciences in 1981; the H. A. B. Dunning Award for industry support in 1984; the Linwood F. Tice Friend of ASP Award for pharmacy student support in 1988; the Gloria N. Francke Leadership Mentor Award for pharmacy leadership in 1994; and the William H. Briner Distinguished Achievement Award in Nuclear Pharmacy Practice in 1997.

Opposite Page: On May 3, 1941, a bronze statue of William Procter, Jr. was unveiled in the American Institute of Pharmacy rotunda. Secretary Evander Kelly stands beside the statue which was designed by William Simpson of Baltimore, Maryland.

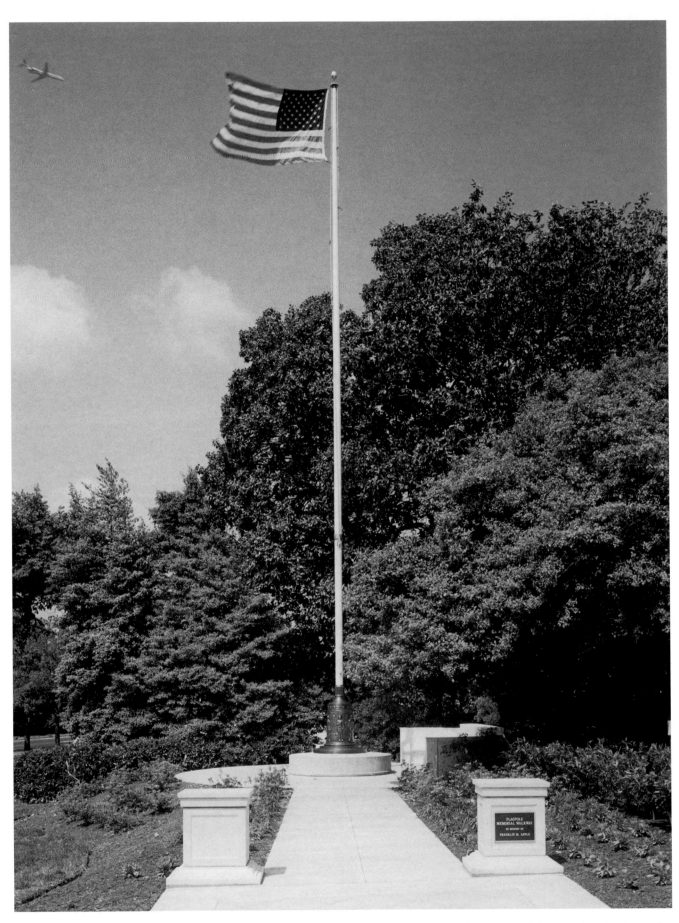

On May 7, 1948, a memorial flagpole, gift of Henry A. B. Dunning, was dedicated on the front lawn of the American Institute of Pharmacy to honor those who served in conflcts through World War II.

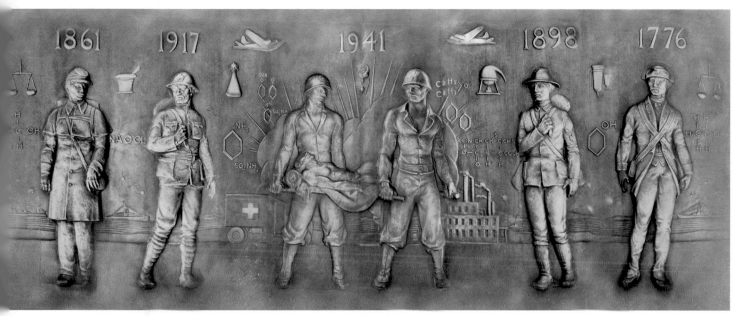

The base of the war memorial flag pole is a sculptured bronze drum (shown here as a flat panel) depicting uniformed American soldiers of the Civil War, World War I, World War II, the Spanish American War, and the American Revolutionary War. Between the uniformed figures are laboratory equipment and chemical formulas to symbolize the production and use of significant drugs of the various periods in military medicine.

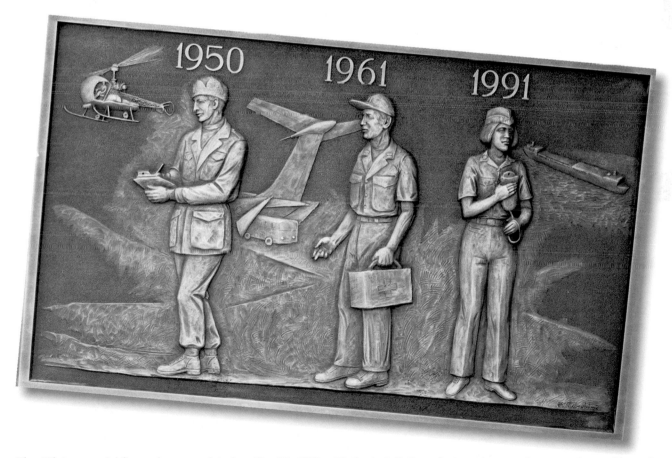

The APhA memorial flag pole was updated on May 25, 1993, with the installation of a large bronze plaque on the marble wall facing the flag pole. The sculpture depicts a U.S. Army male pharmacist checking out medical supplies during a helicopter medical evacuation during the Korean conflict; a U.S. Air Force male pharmacist observing the loading of casualties on a *Starlifter* during the Vietnam conflict; and a U.S. Navy female pharmacist holding a parenteral solution during the Persian Gulf conflict. The hospital ship in the background symbolizes the *USS Mercy* and the *USNS Comfort*.

Petition

For Reason that pharmacy is a health profession of major importance, serving the public in every town and city throughout the nation as the compounder and dispenser of physicians' prescriptions, the custodian and dispenser of narcotics and other potent drugs necessary for the treatment of disease; and

For Reason that this service is rendered as a matter of professional duty for an average of fifteen hours a day throughout every day of the year; and

For Reason that pharmacists, in cooperation with physicians and other medical scientists, in order to assure dependable therapeutic agents, have, at regular intervals issued the United States Pharmacopoeia in which are set up high and exacting standards for drugs and medicines, and which have been adopted as public standards through Acts of Congress and the legislatures of each of the forty-eight states; and for reason that a new revision of this authoritative work was begun in 1940.

We, The Undersigned, respectfully request the United States Post Office Department to design and issue

A NATIONAL PHARMACY STAMP in Recognition of the Public Health Significance of the Profession of Pharmacy

Pharmacists throughout the land sell across their counters each year a minimum of one hundred million postage stamps as a community service and Government cooperation.

This 1940 petition, distributed by Parke-Davis field representatives, sought half-a-million signatures urging the U.S. Post Office to issue a postage stamp "in recognition of the public health significance of the profession of pharmacy."

CHAPTER 46

Pharmaceutical Philately

Sylvester Dretzka introduced a resolution adopted by the 1934 APhA House of Delegates calling for "a U.S. commemorative stamp for the dedication of the American Institute of Pharmacy." Then in 1939, both APhA and NARD adopted resolutions seeking a stamp commemorating the 120th anniversary of the *U.S. Pharmacopeia*. A national committee was formed by APhA which proclaimed April 21-27, 1940, as National Pharmacy Stamp Week, and Parke-Davis launched a nationwide drive to obtain half-a-million signatures on a petition to endorse the move.

But the campaign failed in its objective, as did efforts in 1952 to commemorate the APhA centenary, and in 1965 to recognize William Procter, Jr., on the 150th anniversary of his birth. Proposing that prior

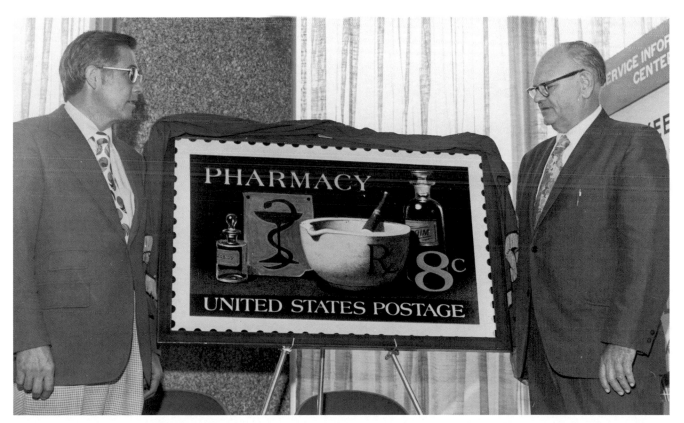

Philatelic recognition was achieved with the unveiling of the pharmacy stamp design by APhA president Clifton Latiolais (left) and NARD president Crawford Meyer (right) at a Detroit, Michigan, ceremony held August 14, 1972.

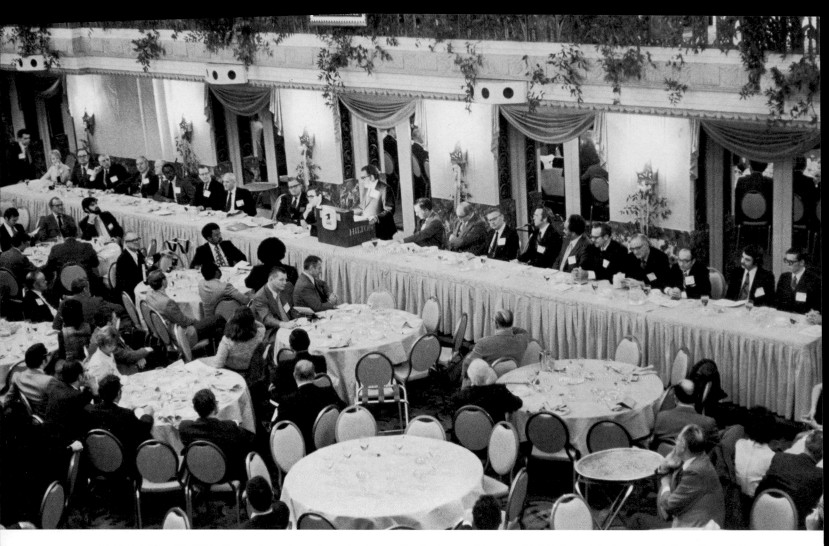

On November 10, 1972, the postage stamp honoring the nation's pharmacists was officially issued during a special meeting of the APhA House of Delegates in Cincinnati. Shown here are representatives of every U.S. national pharmacy organization seated at the head table during the first day of issue ceremonies.

failures "contained the seeds of later success," Irving Rubin launched a campaign which resulted in the U.S. Postal Service announcing (1971) that "a postage stamp in tribute to the service role played by the nation's 100,000 pharmacists will be issued next year."

On November 10, 1972, the eight-cent postage stamp honoring the nation's pharmacists was officially issued during an interim meeting of the APhA House of Delegates in Cincinnati. The first day of issue ceremonies included a luncheon at the Netherlands Hilton Hotel in Cincinnati attended by over 500; at the head table were seated representatives of every U.S. national pharmacy organization. First day postmarks were affixed to over 800,000 pharmacy pieces of mail franked with the pharmacy stamp, and featuring more than 85 different "cachets" (illustrations on the left side of the envelope) sponsored by dozens of different organizations and firms

CHAPTER 47

International Relations

The First International Pharmaceutical Congress was held in Brunswick, Germany, in 1865; even though an invitation was sent to APhA, no U.S. pharmacist was present. William Procter, Jr., attended the Second International Pharmaceutical Congress held in Paris in 1867. Procter's report of the Congress observed that "some of the speakers had alluded to pharmacy in America in a way calculated to give a wrong impression [so I] prepared a statement and obtained permission to read it in English so that it might go on the record." Procter was speaking of the divergence of opinion between Europe and the United States on the compulsory limitation of pharmacies.

APhA extended a series of invitations to hold an International Pharmaceutical Congress in Philadelphia during the 1876 Centennial Exposition, and then in Chicago during the 1893 Columbian

APhA hosted the Seventh International Pharmaceutical Congress at the *Columbian Exposition* August 21-23, 1893, immediately following the 1893 annual meeting in Chicago. Joseph Remington was elected president and Oscar Oldberg served as secretary of the international congress, attended by delegates from 11 countries.

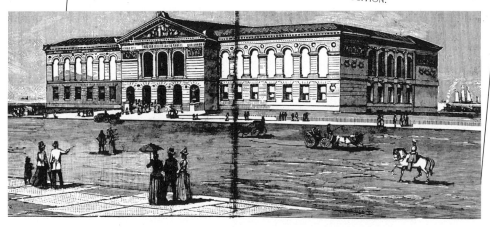

REFERENCE GUIDE

TO

THE WORLD'S FAIR

(ILLUSTRATED)

THE GRANDEST INTERNATIONAL EXPOSITION IN THE HISTORY OF THE WORLD

for the use of those attending the 41st Annual Convention

OF THE

AMERICAN PHARMACEUTICAL ASSOCIATION

AND WHO PROPOSE TO VISIT THE EXPOSITION.

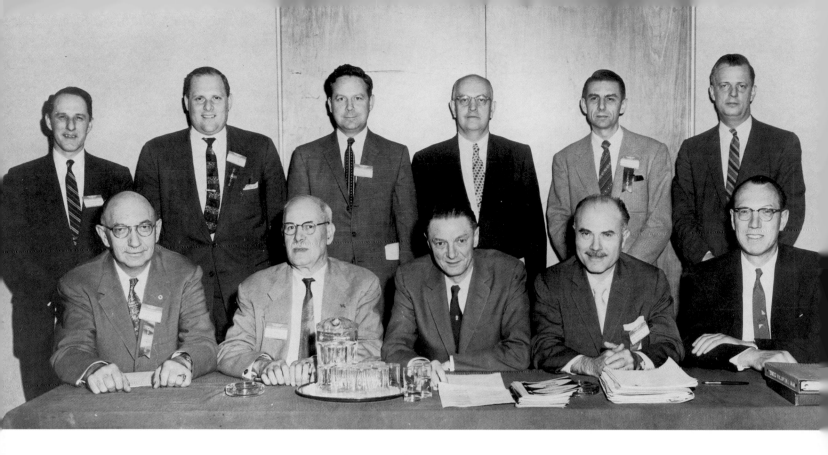

Section secretaries for the Fourth Pan American Congress of Pharmacy held in Washington, D.C., in 1957 include (seated, left to right) Patrick Costello; James Munch; Adolph Tiesler; Dan Rennick; and Lloyd Miller. Standing (left to right) are Heber Youngken, Jr.; Robert Abrams; Grover Bowles; Melvin Green; Glenn Sonnedecker; and George Hager.

Exposition. The first invitation was not accepted, but success was achieved when the Seventh International Pharmaceutical Congress was held on the fairgrounds of the Chicago Columbian Exposition, August 21-23, 1893. Joseph P. Remington was elected Congress president and Oscar Oldberg was seated as secretary. Delegates came from 11 countries including 120 U.S. pharmacists.

It was not until the Tenth International Pharmaceutical Congress held in Brussels in 1910 that it was agreed to support a proposal from the Dutch Pharmaceutical Association to create the International Pharmaceutical Federation (FIP) which held its first General Assembly in The Hague in 1912. In 1923, president Julius Koch recommended that APhA "should assume full membership in FIP," and in 1925, APhA became an FIP member. Official contact between FIP and APhA was lost during World War II, but FIP re-organized afterward.

Meanwhile, the Pan American Federation of Pharmacy (FEPAFAR) was created at a meeting in Havana, Cuba, in 1948 attended by a U.S. delegation that included Don E. Francke, who subsequently urged greater participation by U.S. pharmacists in both Congresses of FIP and FEPAFAR. As a result, the Fourth Pan American Congress of Pharmacy was held in Washington, DC, in November 1957, with Robert A. Hardt serving as president and George Griffenhagen as secretary general. Nearly 1,200 pharmacists from 22 American countries as well as 18 European and Asian countries attended.

The 31st International Congress of Pharmaceutical Sciences was held in Washington, DC, September 7-12, 1971, hosted by APhA and sponsored by the International Pharmaceutical Federation (FIP). A total of 1,209 registrants was recorded, 745 of whom were from 45 foreign countries. Thomas J. Macek served as chairman of the organizing committee.

At the request of General Douglas MacArthur, Supreme Commander for the Allied Powers, five APhA members left for Japan in 1949 to help the Japanese restore their pharmaceutical industry after World War II. The APhA team was headed by Glenn L. Jenkins as APhA president; others included Troy C. Daniels, Don E. Francke, F. Royce Franzoni, and Hugh C. Muldoon. During the four week stay in Japan, they visited pharmacy schools, community pharmacies, hospital pharmacies, and pharmaceutical manufacturing facilities.

The next major cooperative venture with Japan convened in Honolulu, Hawaii, as the joint Japan and United States Congress of Pharmaceutical Sciences (JUCPharmSci), December 1-7, 1987. Co-hosted by APhA and the Pharmaceutical Society of Japan, this congress was attended by 2,845 pharmaceutical scientists. It featured 1,145 poster presentations, 715 by Japanese, 361 by Americans, and 69 by pharmaceutical scientists from 21 other countries. This is the largest number of posters ever presented at any international pharmacy conference.

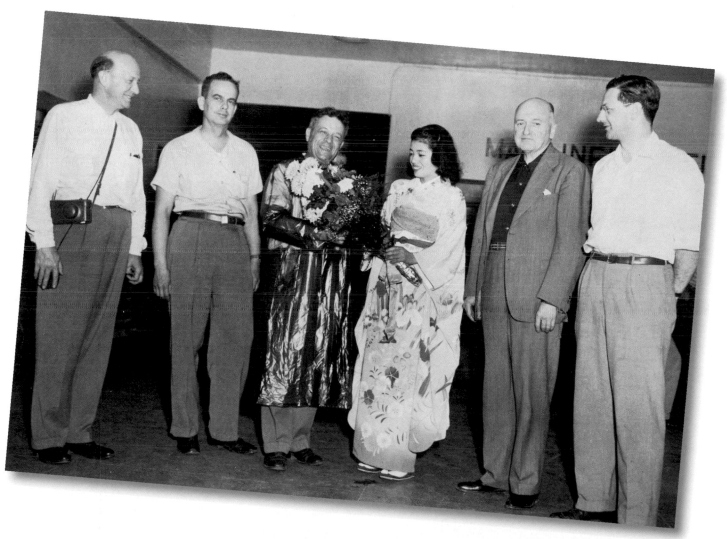

At the request of General Douglas MacArthur, five APhA members traveled to Japan in 1949 to study post World War II pharmacy conditions. They include (left to right) Troy Daniels, Royce Franzoni, Glenn Jenkins, host Miss Tokulu Hattori of the Japanese Pharmacists Association who is presenting flowers, Hugh Muldoon, and Don Francke.

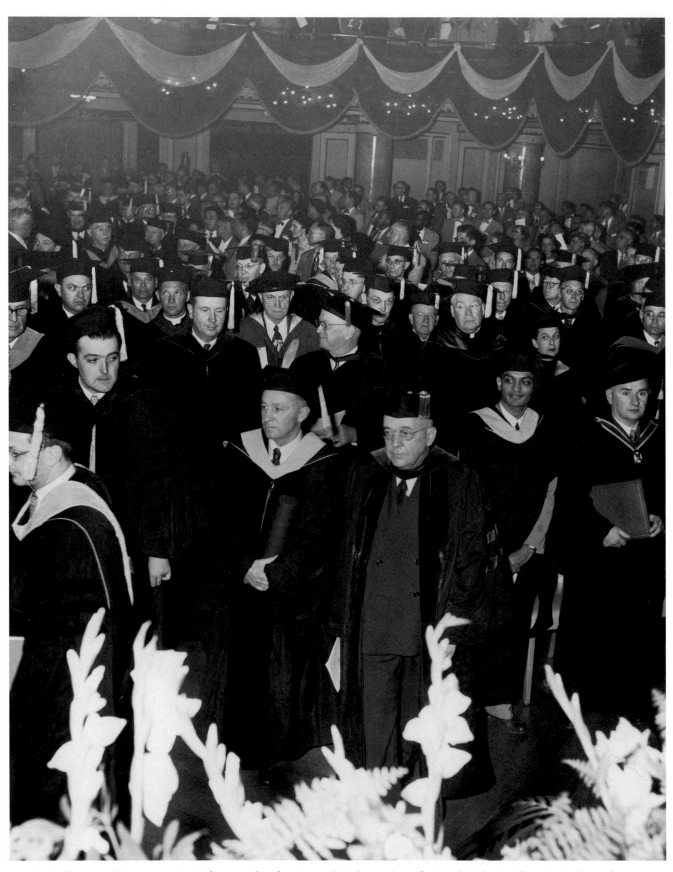

Academically gowned representatives of twenty-five foreign and 86 domestic professional and scientific societies brought greetings to APhA at the 1952 centennial session. While primarily a tribute to APhA, the greetings were a reflection of the high regard in which U.S. pharmacists have been held.

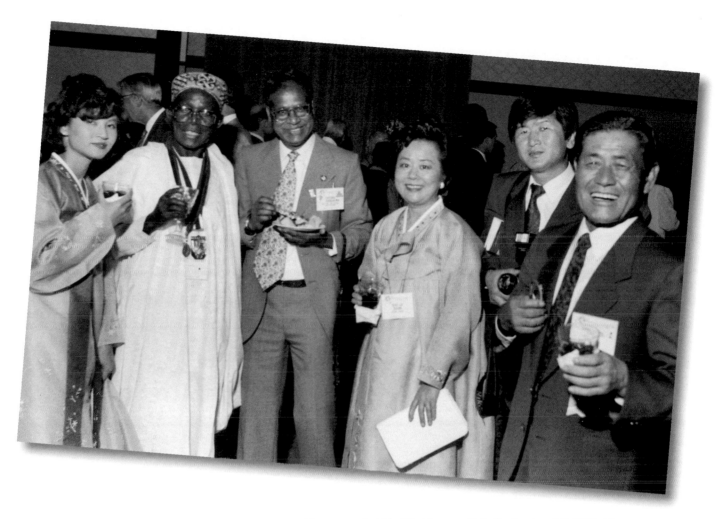

Pharmacists from 93 countries attended a Pharmacy World Congress held in Washington, D.C., September 1-6, 1991. Many came in native costumes to a reception serving only food and beverage that originated in America.

As a member of both the International Pharmaceutical Federation (FIP) and the Pan American Federation of Pharmacy (FEPAFAR), APhA was asked once again to host congresses of both groups. The result was the convening of Pharmacy World Congress in Washington, D.C., September 1-6, 1991; it consisted of the 51st Congress of Pharmaceutical Sciences (FIP), the 14th Pan American Congress of Pharmacy (FEPAFAR), and the 19th Central American and Caribbean Congress of Pharmaceutical Sciences (FFCC). A total of 1,535 pharmacists attended from 93 countries, the largest number of countries represented at any international meeting held in the U.S.A.

When APhA executive vice president John A. Gans was elected as a vice president of both the International Pharmaceutical Federation and of the Pan American Federation of Pharmacy, it was the first time that anyone had held this dual role.

CHAPTER 48.

Other Organizations

By the mid-1970s, pharmacists were seeking specialized membership services. One of the first was a convenient source of life insurance. The Druggists' Mutual Benefit Society had been founded in 1876, and the Western Druggists Mutual Benefit Association in 1879. Both were created exclusively to provide life insurance to their members, but were short-lived because pharmacy groups could not compete with the evolving private insurance companies.

As the APhA semi-centennial convention approached, the only other new national pharmacy associations involved recreational pursuits such as the American Drug Trade Bowling Association,

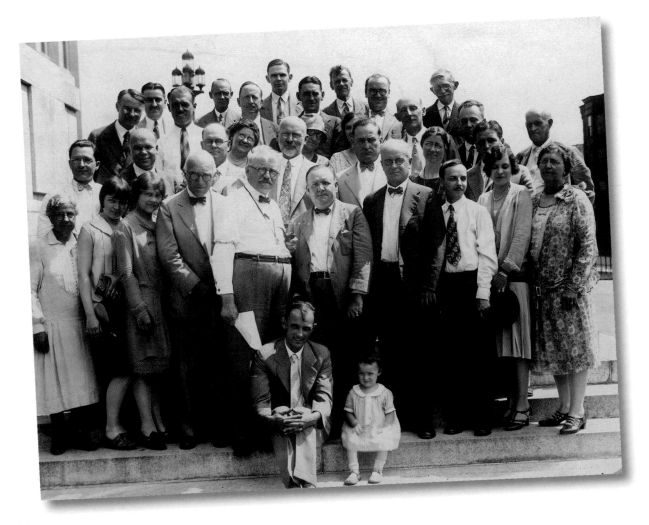

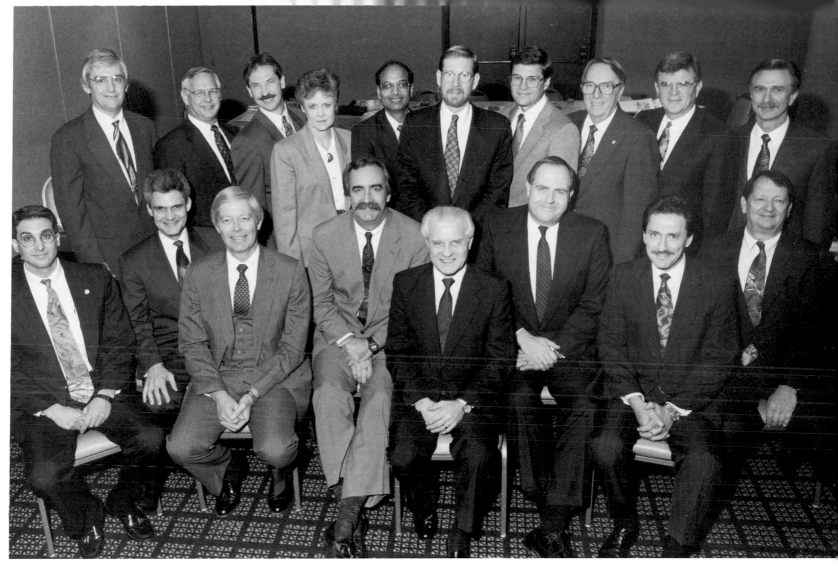

Attending the 1991 meeting of the Joint Commission on Pharmacy Practitioners on behalf of APhA were president Marily Rhudy (standing fourth from left); Academy of Pharmacy Practice and Management president Calvin Knowlton (seated, second from right); and executive vice president John Gans (seated, third from right).

founded in 1897; and the Apothecaries' Bicycle Club, founded in 1898.

APhA convened a conference in 1913 so that the chief executive officers of the national pharmaceutical associations could exchange views on legislative and other activities that might affect both the profession of pharmacy and the drug industry. The first

Opposite Page: The Plant Science Seminar, established in 1923 for teachers of pharmacognosy, met in Boston for their sixth annual meeting. Among those included in this 1928 photograph are Bernard Christensen, William Day, Ivor Griffith, Edwin Newcomb, Robert Wilson, and Heber Youngken. The group became the American Society of Pharmacognosy in 1959.

meeting, which chose as its name the National Drug Trade Conference (NDTC), included representatives of APhA, the National Association of Retail Druggists, the National Wholesale Druggists Association, the National Association of Manufacturers of Medicinal Products, and the American Association of Pharmaceutical Chemists. APhA resigned from NDTC in 1975, but rejoined in 1985. In 1996, the group changed its name to the National Conference of Pharmaceutical Organizations.

Another group bringing together only representatives of national professional pharmacy organizations is the Joint Commission of Pharmacy

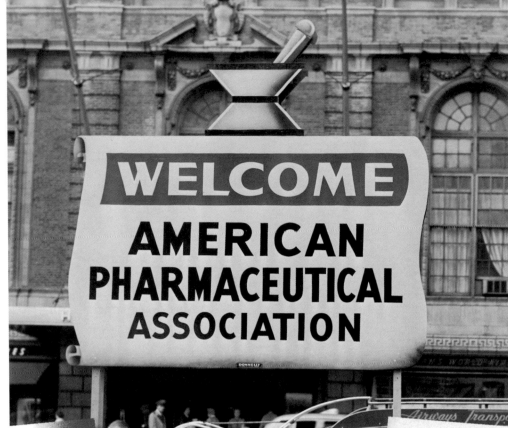

Members are welcomed at the 1954 American Pharmaceutical Association Annual Meeting.

Program

OF THE
91ST ANNUAL MEETING
AND

War Conference

OF THE

AMERICAN
PHARMACEUTICAL
ASSOCIATION
AND
AFFILIATED ORGANIZATIONS

DESHLER-WALLICK HOTEL
COLUMBUS, OHIO
SEPTEMBER 9-11, 1943

Program

One Hundred and Fourth Meeting*

American
Pharmaceutical
Association

and

Affiliated Organizations

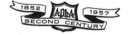

1852 APhA 1957
SECOND CENTURY

HOTEL STATLER
NEW YORK, N. Y.
April 28-May 3, 1957

Consult Daily Bulletin for additional
events and possible changes
in program

*The Association was organized in 1852. This
is the 104th meeting of the Association. Meetings have been held annually except 1861
and 1945.

1902	September 8-15	Philadelphia, PA		1912	August 19-24	Denver, CO
1903	August 3-8	Mackinac Island, MI		1913	August 18-23	Nashville, TN
1904	September 5-9	Kansas City, MO		1914	August 24-29	Detroit, MI
1905	September 4-9	Atlantic City, NJ		1915	August 9-13	San Francisco, CA
1906	September 3-8	Indianapolis, IN		1916	September 5-9	Atlantic City, NJ
1907	September 2-7	New York, NY		1917	August 27-Sept. 1	Indianapolis, IN
1908	September 7-12	Hot Springs. AR		1918	August 12-17	Chicago, IL
1909	August 16-20	Los Angeles, CA		1919	August 25-30	New York, NY
1910	May 2-7	Richmond, VA		1920	May 5-10	Washington, DC
1911	August 14-19	Boston, MA		1921	September 5-9	New Orleans, LA

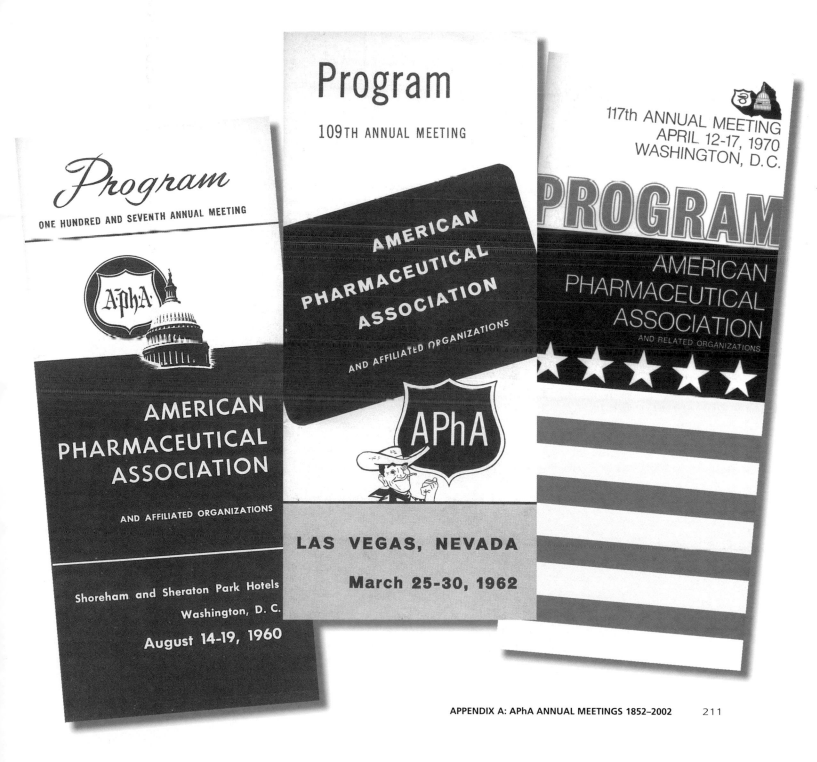

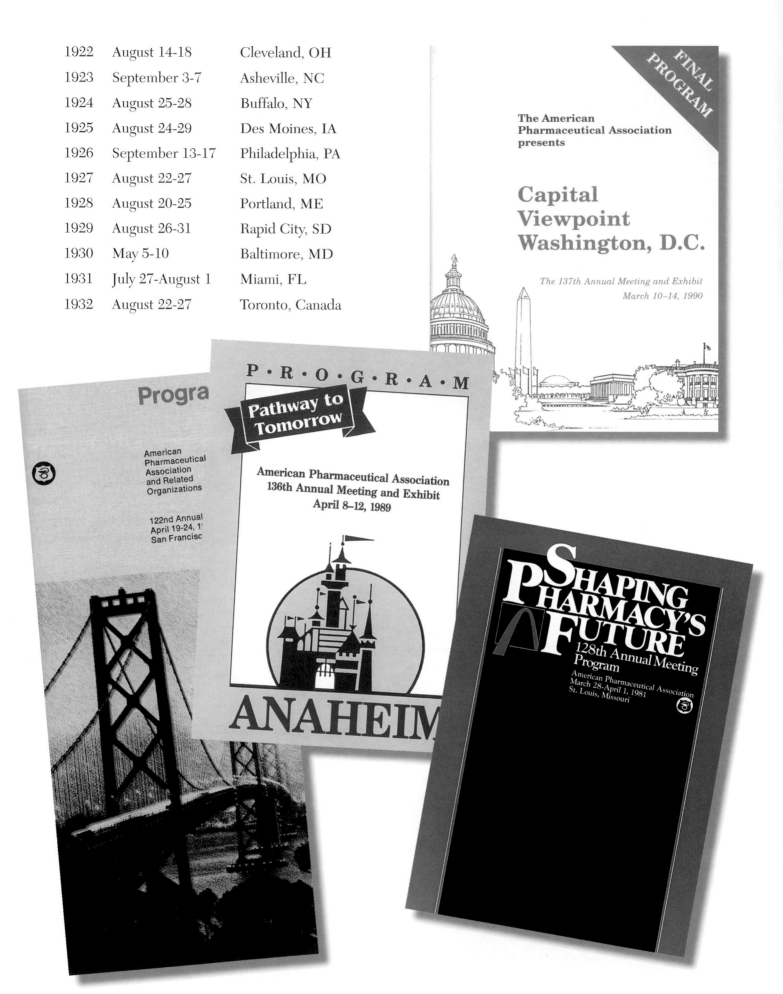

1922	August 14-18	Cleveland, OH
1923	September 3-7	Asheville, NC
1924	August 25-28	Buffalo, NY
1925	August 24-29	Des Moines, IA
1926	September 13-17	Philadelphia, PA
1927	August 22-27	St. Louis, MO
1928	August 20-25	Portland, ME
1929	August 26-31	Rapid City, SD
1930	May 5-10	Baltimore, MD
1931	July 27-August 1	Miami, FL
1932	August 22-27	Toronto, Canada

FINAL PROGRAM

The American
Pharmaceutical Association
presents

Capital
Viewpoint
Washington, D.C.

The 137th Annual Meeting and Exhibit
March 10–14, 1990

Progra

American
Pharmaceutical
Association
and Related
Organizations

122nd Annual
April 19-24, 1
San Francisc

P·R·O·G·R·A·M

Pathway to
Tomorrow

American Pharmaceutical Association
136th Annual Meeting and Exhibit
April 8–12, 1989

ANAHEIM

SHAPING
PHARMACY'S
FUTURE
128th Annual Meeting
Program
American Pharmaceutical Association
March 28-April 1, 1981
St. Louis, Missouri

1933	August 26-Sept. 1	Madison, WI	1945	No Meeting	
1934	May 5-12	Washington, DC	1946	August 27-30	Pittsburgh, PA
1935	August 5-10	Portland, OR	1947	August 26-30	Milwaukee, WI
1936	August 24-29	Dallas, TX	1948	August 8-14	San Francisco, CA
1937	August 16-21	New York, NY	1949	April 24-30	Jacksonville, FL
1938	August 22-27	Minneapolis, MN	1950	April 30-May 5	Atlantic City, NJ
1939	August 20-26	Atlanta, GA	1951	August 26-31	Buffalo, NY
1940	May 4-11	Richmond, VA	1952	August 17-23	Philadelphia, PA
1941	August 17-23	Detroit, MI	1953	August 16-21	Salt Lake City, UT
1942	August 16-22	Denver, CO	1954	August 22-27	Boston, MA
1943	September 9-11	Columbus, OH	1955	May 1-6	Miami Beach, FL
1944	September 7-9	Cleveland. OH	1956	April 8-13	Detroit, MI

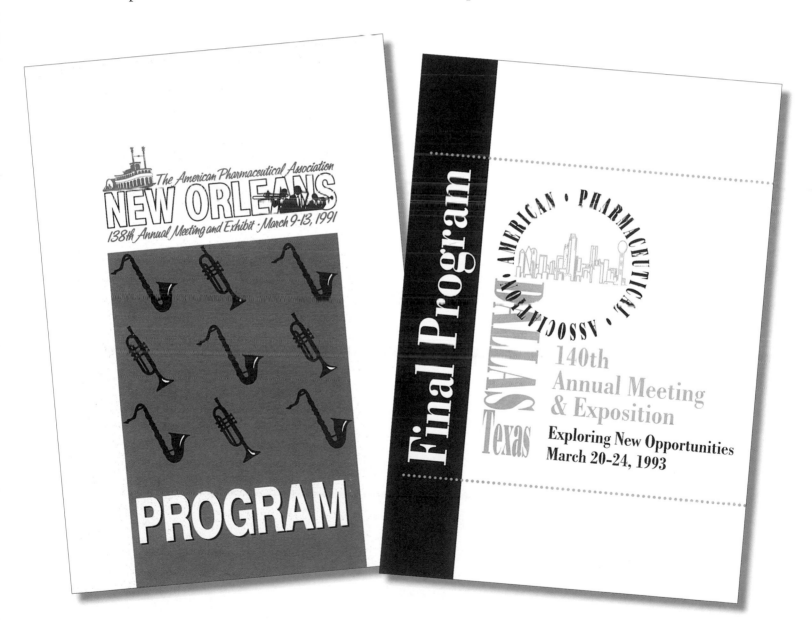

1957	April 28-May 3	New York, NY	1969	May 17-23	Montreal, Canada
1958	April 20-25	Los Angeles, CA	1970	April 12-17	Washington DC
1959	August 16-21	Cincinnati, OH	1971	March 27-April 2	San Francisco, CA
1960	August 14-19	Washington, DC	1972	April 22-28	Houston TX
1961	April 23-28	Chicago, IL	1973	July 21-27	Boston, MA
1962	March 25-30	Las Vegas, NV	1974	August 3-9	Chicago, IL
1963	May 12-17	Miami Beach	1975	April 19-25	San Francisco, CA
1964	August 2-7	New York, NY	1976	April 3-8	New Orleans, LA
1965	March 28-April 2	Detroit, MI	1977	May 14-19	New York, NY
1966	April 24-29	Dallas, TX	1978	May 13-18	Montreal, Canada
1967	April 9-14	Las Vegas, NV	1979	April 21-26	Anaheim, CA
1968	May 5-10	Miami Beach, FL	1980	April 19-24	Washington, DC

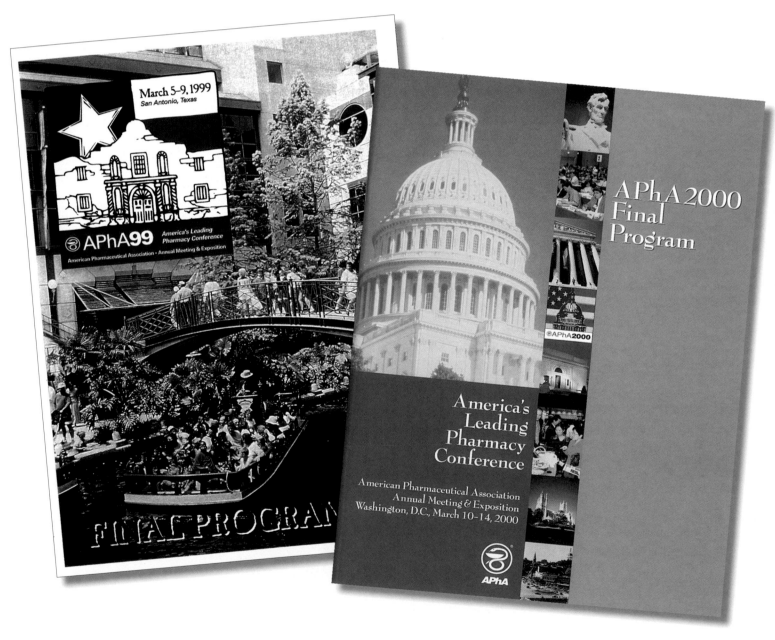

1981	March 28-April 2	St. Louis, MO	1992	March 14-19	San Diego, CA
1982	April 24-29	Las Vegas, NV	1993	March 20-24	Dallas, TX
1983	April 9-14	New Orleans, LA	1994	March 19-21	Seattle, WA
1984	May 5-10	Montreal, Canada	1995	March 18-22	Orlando, FL
1985	February 16-21	San Antonio, TX	1996	March 8-12	Nashville, TN
1986	March 16-20	San Francisco, CA	1997	March 7-12	Los Angeles, CA
1987	March 28-April 1	Chicago, IL	1998	March 21-25	Miami Beach, FL
1988	March 12-16	Atlanta, GA	1999	March 5-9	San Antonio, TX
1989	April 8-12	Anaheim, CA	2000	March 10-14	Washington, DC
1990	March 10-14	Washington, DC	2001	March 16-20	San Francisco, CA
1991	March 9-13	New Orleans, LA	2002	March 15-19	Philadelphia, PA

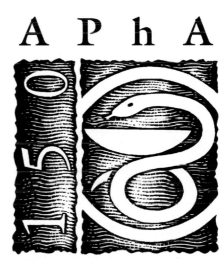

A P h A

1852 - 2002

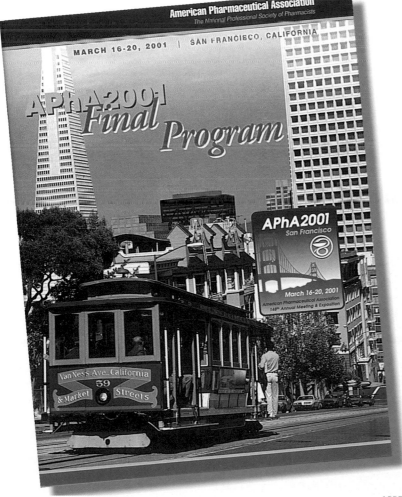

APhA Past President Trivia

How many APhA presidents served two terms?

Answer: Four (Henry Taylor Kiersted (1860-1862 because of the Civil War); George Allen Moulton (1944-1946 because of World War II); Mary Munson Runge (1979-1980 because of Bylaw amendments); and James Allen Main (1985-1986 because of Bylaw changes). Calvin Knowlton (1995-1997) served nearly two terms.

Which APhA president served the shortest term of office?

Answer: Alfred Robert Lewis Dohme thought he had served the shortest term of office. As 1917-1918 APhA first vice president, Dohme had ascended to president on the death of president Charles Holzhauer three months into Holzhauer's term of office; Dohme told APhA members accordingly in his 1918 presidential address:

> "For the first time in history, your duly elected president has not presided at the next annual meeting, and for the first time your duly elect-ed vice president has assumed the mantle of this high office."

Alfred Dohme was wrong; 28 years earlier, Karl Simmon of St. Paul, Minnesota, became APhA president when Emlen Painter died only six months into his term as APhA president.

Does this mean that Robert Earl Davis served the shortest term as APhA president when he resigned three months after assuming office at the 1995 APhA annual meeting?

Answer: Definitely not because there were six APhA presidents who only served for less than 24 hours. When the duly elected president failed to show up for the APhA annual meeting, they ascended to president in accordance with the APhA Bylaws until the new president was elected. They included:

- Henry Cummings in 1855 when retiring president William Chapman was unable to attend the annual meeting.
- Robert Battey in 1859 when retiring president John Kidwell failed to show at the annual meeting.
- Ferris Bringhurst in 1869 when retiring president Edward Parrish was unable to attend the annual meeting because Parrish was in Oklahoma as a U.S. Commissioner to manage the Indian tribes.

- George Schafer in 1881 when retiring president James Shinn was unable to attend the 1881 annual meeting because his pharmacy had burned down.
- Henry Menninger in 1887 in the absence of retiring president Charles Tufts who was too ill to attend the annual meeting.

But the shortest term of office was held by Charles Guthrie when William Brewer was unable to attend the 1854 annual meeting because of a cholera epidemic. Guthrie was president for only three hours since the convention assembled elected William Chapman on the same day as the 1854-1855 president.

Was any APhA president ever impeached?

Answer: Not during his term of office, but two years after Frederick Stearns completed his term of office in 1867, APhA expelled him as an APhA member for marketing "sweet quinine," which did not contain any quinine.

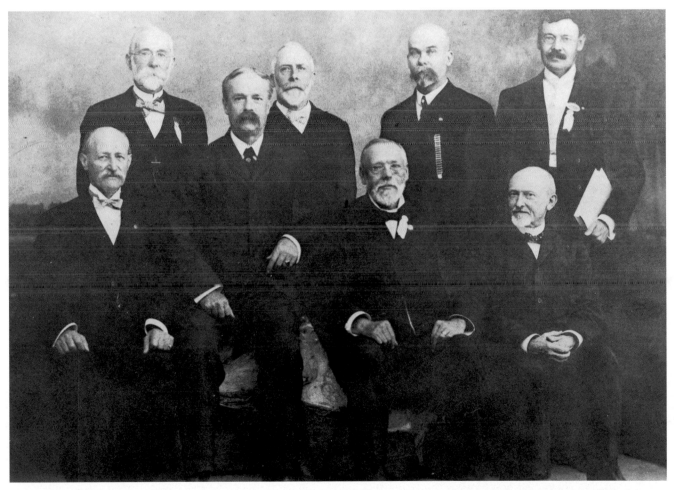

These eight APhA officers include (left to right with year of installation) top row: vice president Samuel Sheppard (1876); vice president Charles Caspari (1893); 1909 treasurer Henry Whelpley (1909); and general secretary James Beal (1911). Seated, president Joseph Lemberger (1905); president Joseph Remington (1892); president Conrad Lewis Diehl (1874); and president John Patton (1900).

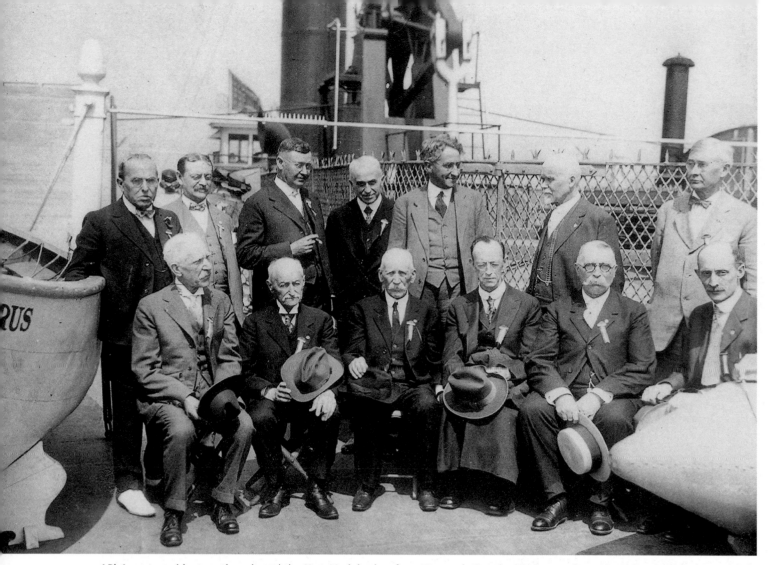

APhA past presidents gather aboard the New York harbor ferry *Taurus* during the 1919 annual meeting. They include (seated, left to right with year of installation) Lucius Sayre (1919); Joseph Lemberger (1905); John Hancock (1873); Edgar Patch (1893); John Godding (1911); and William Day (1912). Standing (left to right) are Caswell Mayo (1914); George Beringer (1913); James Beal (1904); Eugene Eberle (1910); Charles LaWall (1918); Henry Whelpley (1901); and Lewis Hopp (1903).

Were there any pairs of father and son who served as APhA president?

Answer: Yes, there were three. James Hartley Beal (1904-1905) and George Denton Beal (1936-1937); Charles Emile Dohme (1898-1899) and Alfred Robert Louis Dohme (1917-1918); and Charles Holzhauer (1917) and Charles William Holton (1924-1925) who had changed his name. (Holton married the daughter of Charles Dohme, thus bringing four APhA past presidents into a single family.)

Who was the youngest president when installed in office?

Answer: The youngest was German-born Albert Ethelbert Ebert (commemorated by the Ebert Prize) who was 32 years old when he became APhA president in 1872.

Who was the oldest when installed as APhA president?

Answer: Robert Gibson was nearly 75 years of age when he was installed as APhA presidnet in 2000.

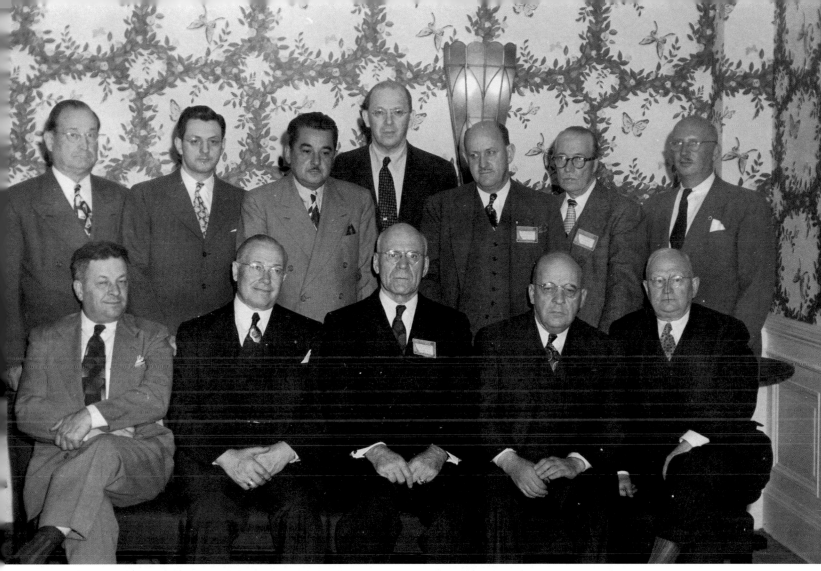

The APhA Council at the 1948 annual meeting in San Francisco includes seated (left to right) Glenn Jenkins, Martin Adamo, Ernest Little, George Beal, and Robert Swain. Standing (left to right) Bernard Christensen, Don Francke, Hugo Schaefer, Robert Fischelis, Mearl Pritchard, Hans Hansen, and Frederick Lascoff.

How many APhA presidents were not natives of the U.S.A.?

Answer: Ten APhA presidents were born in Germany, all serving in the 19th-century. This constituted 20 percent of all 19th century APhA presidents. Three others were born in Great Britain, and one each was born in Canada, in Chile, in Ireland, in Lithuania, and in Sweden. In most instances, each came to live in America during his youth.

What state claims to be the birth place of the most APhA presidents?

Answer: Twenty-one APhA presidents were born in Pennsylvania; eleven in New York; ten in Maryland; nine in Massachusetts; eight in New Jersey; seven in Wisconsin; five each in Illinois and Michigan; and four each in Delaware, Georgia, Ohio, Texas, Virginia, and West Virginia. The remaining were born in Alabama, California, Connecticut, Indiana, Iowa, Kansas, Kentucky, Louisiana, Minnesota, Mississippi, Misouri, Nebraska, New Hampshire, North Carolina, Oregon, South Dakota, Washington, and the District of Columbia.

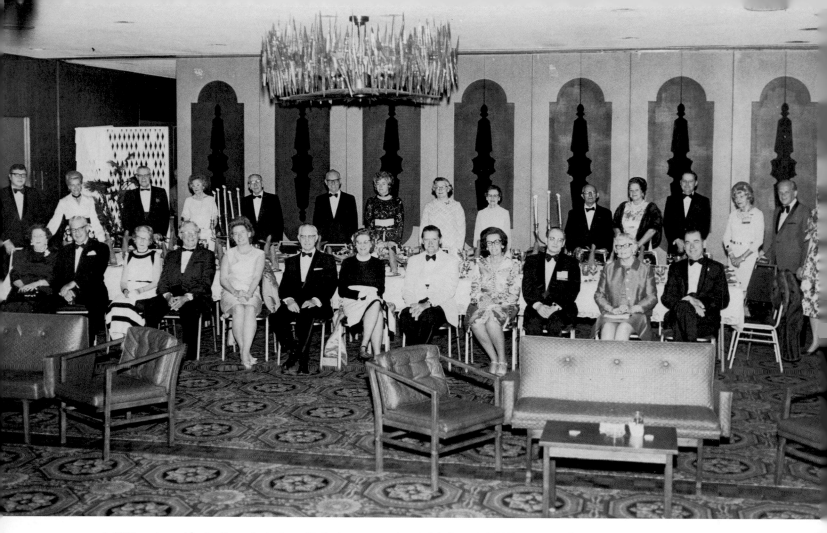

A 1971 past presidents dinner includes with their spouses, (seated, left to right) Warren Lansdowne; Louis Fischl; Linwood Tice; Curtis Nottingham; Don Francke; and George Grider. Standing (left to right) are Max Eggleston; Joseph Burt; Arthur Uhl (honorary president); William Whitten; Charles Rabe (staff); Grover Bowles; and William Hennessy.

What school of pharmacy graduated the most APhA presidents?

Answer: 32 APhA presidents were graduates of the Philadelphia College of Pharmacy. This is more than double the 15 graduates of the New York College of Pharmacy (Columbia University) and the 14 graduates of the Massachusetts College of Pharmacy. Nine graduated from the Chicago College of Pharmacy (University of Illinois); eight from the Maryland College of Pharmacy (University of Maryland); and five each from the University of Minnesota College of Pharmacy, the National College of Pharmacy (George Washington University), and the University of Wisconsin School of Pharmacy.

How many past presidents obtained additional degrees beyond those directly relating to pharmacy?

Answer: Seven went on to obtain an M.D. degree after qualifying as a pharmacist, but only two practiced medicine. Jefferson Medical College graduate Robert Battey, who served as APhA president *pro tem* in 1859, is noted for pioneering in gynecological surgical procedures. 1855 APhA president Henry Cummings graduated from Harvard Medical School, but gave up medical practice because of a hearing defect, and subsequently operated a Portland, Maine, pharmacy for nearly 50 years.

Four APhA past presidents obtained a law degree after obtaining their pharmacy degree. Three APhA past presidents were elected as a member of a state legislature, and more than a dozen APhA presidents served as mayor or as a member of their city council.

How many APhA presidents served in a similar capacity for other pharmacy associations?

Answer: Seventeen served as president of the American Association of Colleges of Pharmacy; fourteen served as president or executive officer of National Association of Boards of Pharmacy, and 47 were members of their state board of pharmacy. Six were president of the American College of Apothecaries; five were president of the American Society of Hospital Pharmacists; and three served as NARD vice presidents.

Sixty-four APhA past presidents were president of their state pharmaceutical association, and another nine served as executive officer. Seven APhA presidents were founding presidents or founding secretaries of the state pharmaceutical association in Iowa, Maine, New Hampshire, New York, Ohio, Pennsylvania, and South Carolina.

How many past presidents served in the military during various wars?

Answer: Veterans of the military service included one APhA president who served as a major general in the Mexican War of 1846-1848. Ten APhA presidents served in the Civil War — five with the Confederate Army, and five with the Union Army. Only one served during the Spanish-American War, while six served in France during World War One. Nine APhA presidents served in the military service during World War II.

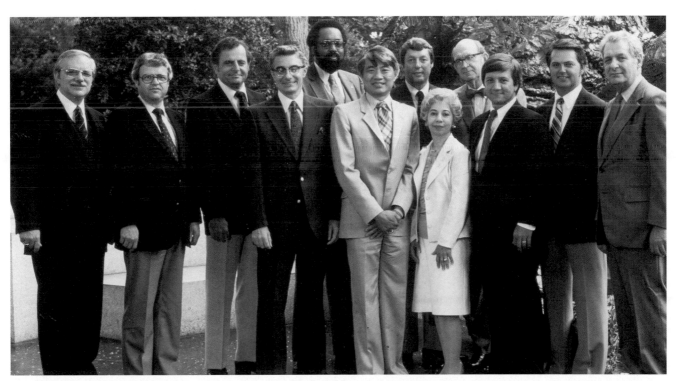

1982 APhA Board of Trustees gather at the Albert Einstein memorial at the National Academy of Sciences for this photograph. They are (left to right) Herbert Carlin; Donald Dee; Michael Schwartz; James Doluisio; Leonard Edloe; Chester Yee; Maurice Bectel; Natalie Certo; William Edwards; James Main; Stephen Crawford; and William Apple.

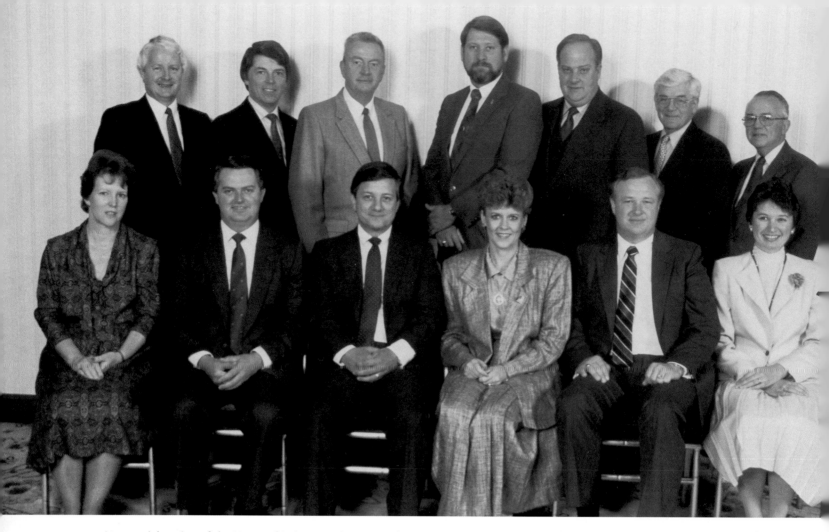

At a special session of the House of Delegates, the 1986 APhA Board of Trustees are (seated, left to right) Shirley McKee; Stephen Crawford; James Main; Marily Rhudy; John Schlegel; and Michelle Valentine. Standing (left to right) are John West; Charles Green; John Fay; David Cobb; Tim Vordenbaumen; August Lemberger; and Donald Gronewold.

Which APhA past presidents created the most controversy within the ranks of APhA?

Answer: Albert Benjamin Prescott was denied a seat at the 1871 APhA annual meeting because he was representing the University of Michigan School of Pharmacy. Unlike the Philadelphia, Massachusetts, Baltimore, and St. Louis Colleges of Pharmacy which were then basically local associations of pharmacists, the University of Michigan School of Pharmacy admittedly was not an organization of pharmacists. In belated tribute to his innovations in pharmaceutical education, Prescott was subsequently installed APhA president in 1899.

George Frederick Payne, who was installed in 1902 as APhA president, had been ousted as dean of the Atlanta College of Pharmacy, so he proceeded to purchase the college from the state of Georgia and operated it as a private institution.

The most controversial had to be William Charles Alpers who served as APhA president 1915-1916. Shocking all APhA members assembled at the 1916 annual meeting, Alpers attacked the establishment, claiming that the power of the APhA Council (now Board of Trustees) was "too autocratic." He denounced the APhA bookkeeping, which he asserted, "had for three years concealed an annual deficit," and he charged that the salaries of both the APhA *Journal* editor and the general secretary were excessive.

The following day, Joseph Remington exhibited to those assembled at the APhA annual meeting a copy of the Philadelphia *Public Ledger* with a blazing headline announcing that APhA was on the verge of bankruptcy. APhA members subsequently voted not to publish Alpers's presidential address until such time as Alpers would make suggested modifications,

but Alpers died six months later before any resolution was achieved.

Aside from Alpers's address, every APhA presidential address has been published by APhA from 1852 to 1990. However, the address of the APhA president was not published in any APhA journal from 1991 until 1998 when the publication of presidential addresses resumed in the *Journal of the American Pharmaceutical Association*.

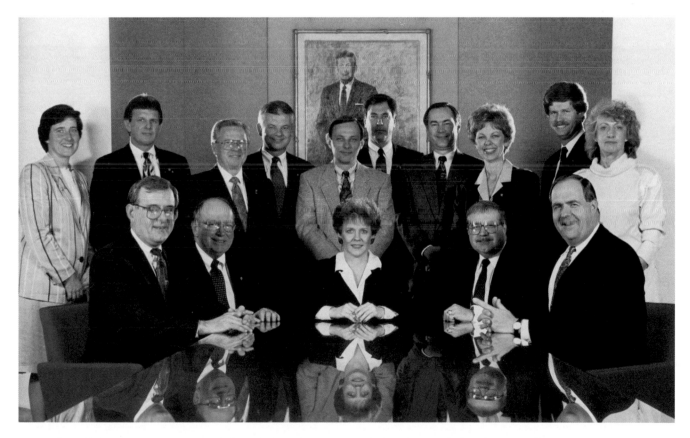

Shown here in the American Institute of Pharmacy are the 1992 Board of Trustees including (seated, left to right) Jean Paul Gagnon; Robert Osterhaus; Marily Rhudy: Philip Gerbino; and John Gans. Standing (left to right) are Lucinda Maine; Jerry Moore; John Hasty; Raymond Roberts; Timothy Burelle; Gary Schneider; Robert Davis; Susan Torrico; Tery Baskin; and Hazel Pipkin.

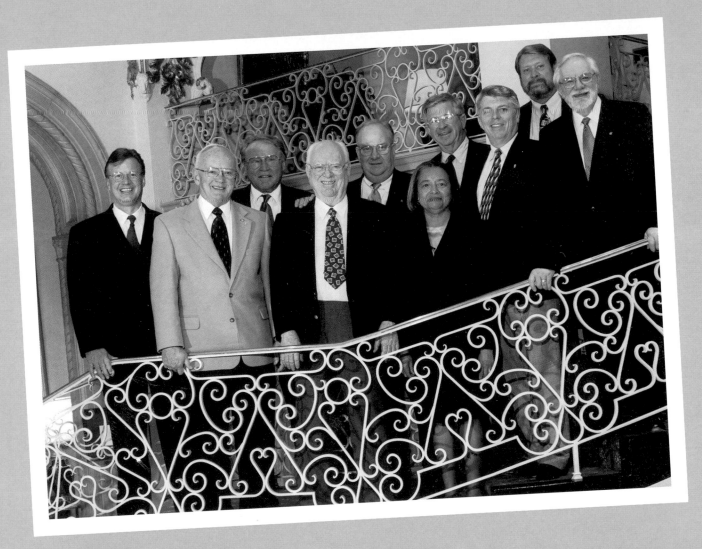

Ten APhA past presidents gather at the 1999 annual meeting in San Antonio, Texas. They are (left to right with year of installation) Gary Kadlec (1997), Jacob Miller (1978), Kenneth Tiemann (1975), William Whitten (1970), Tim Vordenbaumen (1994), Mary Munson Runge (1979), George Denmark (1973), Charles Green (1988), David Cobb (1989), and Herbert Carlin (1984).

Biographies of APhA Presidents 1852 – 2002

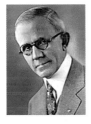

Walter Dickson Adams
(1871-1961)

APhA president 1931-1932, first vice president 1930-1931. Born in Kemp, Texas, December 31, 1871. Apprenticed pharmacy with his brother in Forney, Texas; subsequently became sole owner of the Adams Drug Co. which he operated for 60 years. Established the *Forney Tribune* 1887; *Texas Druggist* editor 1932-1942. Texas Pharmaceutical Association president 1914-1915, secretary 1921-1936. Died March 28, 1961, in Forney, Texas.

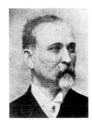

Maurice William Alexander
(1835-1898)

APhA president 1888-1889, first vice president 1887-1888, second vice president 1886-1887. Born in Philadelphia, Pennsylvania, in 1835. Philadelphia College of Pharmacy Ph.G. 1854. Bacon, Hyde & Co. St. Louis (drug wholesalers) clerk 1855; St. Louis community pharmacist 1855-1898. Missouri Board of Pharmacy founding president 1881-1890; Missouri Pharmaceutical Association president 1882-1883; National Retail Druggists Association vice president 1886-1887. Died June 6, 1898, in St. Louis, Missouri.

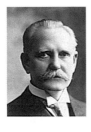

William Charles Alpers
(1851-1917)

APhA president 1915-1916, first vice president 1903-1904, Scientific Section chairman 1896-1897, Practical Pharmacy Section chairman 1905-1906, Historical Pharmacy Section chairman 1913-1914. Born in Hamburg, Germany, July 7, 1851; wounded as soldier during Franco-Prussian War; came to America in 1872; University of New York Sc.D. 1890. Bayonne, New Jersey community pharmacist 1879-1897, New York City 1898-1905; Western Reserve University School of Pharmacy professor and dean 1913-1917. New Jersey Pharmaceutical Association secretary 1892-1895, president 1899-1900; Manhattan (New York) Pharmaceutical Association president 1906-1907. Died February 20, 1917, in Cleveland, Ohio.

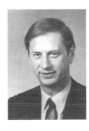

Lowell John Anderson
(1939-   )

APhA president 1993-1994, House of Delegates speaker 1983-1985, treasurer 1998-. Born in Hoodsport, Washington, February 14, 1939. University of Minnesota College of Pharmacy B.S. 1962; Philadelphia College of Pharmacy D.Sc. (hon) 1995. Northwestern Hospital (Minneapolis) pharmacist 1963-1965; St. Paul community pharmacist 1966-. Minnesota Pharmaceutical Association president 1978-1979; Minnesota State Board of Pharmacy president 1973-1974; American Council on Pharmaceutical Education 1974-1980. Minnesota Pharmacist Service Corporation director and president 1974-1980; Physicians Health Plan of Minnesota director and vice chairman 1981-1989; currently Watauga Corporation president. Presently resides in Ardon Hills, Minnesota.

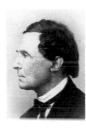

George Wansey Andrews
(1800-1877)

APhA president 1856-1857, first vice president at founding meeting 1852-1853. Born in Baltimore, Maryland, in 1800. Apprenticed pharmacy in Baltimore; operated community pharmacy first by himself and then in partnership with William S. Thompson 1829-1871. Maryland College of Pharmacy founder 1841, vice president 1852-1856, president 1856-1877; Maryland Academy of Sciences member 1822-1877. Died September 12, 1877, in Baltimore, Maryland.

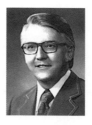

William Frank Appel
(1924-   )

APhA president 1976-1977, treasurer 1979-1981. Born in Minneapolis, Minnesota, October 8, 1924. University of Minnesota College of Pharmacy B.S. 1949; clinical instructor 1970-; Philadelphia College of Pharmacy D.Sc. (hon) 1978. U.S. Navy 1942-1945; Minneapolis community pharmacy 1949-. Twin City Retail Druggists Association director 1960; Minnesota Pharmaceutical Association vice president 1969-1970; Minnesota Board of Pharmacy member 1960-1965, president 1965-1966; USP Committee of Revision 1980-1989.

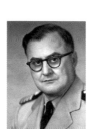

George Frances Archambault
(1909-2001)

APhA president 1962-1963, Council chairman 1960-1961, Pharmaceutical Economics Section secretary 1946-1947. Born in Springfield, Massachusetts, April 29, 1909. Massachusetts College of Pharmacy Ph.G. 1931, Ph.C. 1933, faculty 1931-1943; Northeastern University LL.B. Liggett Drug Company professional relations director 1945-1947; American Society of Hospital Pharmacists president 1954-1955; U.S. Public Health Service commissioned 1947, division of hospitals chief of pharmacy 1947-1965, liaison officer to the Surgeon General 1959-1967; Florida University College of Pharmacy dean 1968; United Mine Workers pharmacy consultant 1970-1976. Died January 1, 2001, in Bethesda, Maryland.

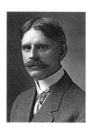

Henry Vincome Arny
(1868-1943)

APhA president 1923-1924, Reporter on Progress of Pharmacy 1916-1922, Scientific Section secretary 1898-1899, *APhA Year Book* editor 1916-1922. Born in Philadelphia, Pennsylvania, February 28, 1868. Philadelphia College of Pharmacy Ph.G. 1889; University of Goettingen, Germany Ph.D. 1896. New Orleans community pharmacist 1889-1892. Louisiana Pharmaceutical Association secretary 1897; Western Reserve University College of Pharmacy professor 1905-1911; Columbia University College of Pharmacy professor and dean 1912-1936; *Druggists Circular* editor 1914-1916; American Association of Colleges of Pharmacy president 1915-1916. Died November 3, 1943, in Montclair, New Jersey.

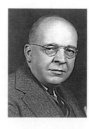

George Denton Beal
(1887-1972)

APhA president 1936-1937, first vice president 1934-1935, Historical Section chairman 1929-1930. Born in Scio, Ohio, August 12, 1887, son of James Hartley Beal. Columbia University Ph.D. 1911. University of Illinois professor 1911-1926; Mellon Institute research director 1926-1968; American Council on Pharmaceutical Education president 1948-1972; USP Committee of Revision first vice chairman 1940-1950; USP Board of Trustees chairman 1959-1968. Died June 4, 1972, in Cocoa, Florida.

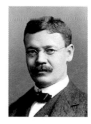

James Hartley Beal
(1861-1945)

APhA president 1904-1905, first vice president 1900-1901, second vice president 1898-1899, Council chairman 1902-1908, general secretary 1911-1914, and *APhA Journal* editor 1912-1914. Born in New Philadelphia, Ohio, September 23, 1861; Scio College Ph.G. 1884; Cincinnati School of Law LL.B. 1886. Scio College of Pharmacy dean 1887-1907; Ohio State Pharmaceutical Association president 1898-1899; Ohio State Legislature 1901-1903; American Association of Colleges of Pharmacy president 1907-1908; *Midland Druggist* editor 1908-1909; USP Board of Trustees chairman 1910-1940. National Drug Trade Conference president 1918-1919. Died September 20, 1945, in Fort Walton, Florida.

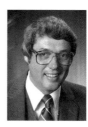

Maurice Quinn Bectel
(1935-   )

APhA president 1983, chief operating officer 1983-1984. Born in Muskegon, Michigan, July 9, 1935. Ferris State University School of Pharmacy B.S. 1960, D.Sc. (hon) 1994, Albany College of Pharmacy D.Sc. (hon) 1992. Owner Bectel Pharmacy, Muskegon 1963-1983; Western Michigan Pharmacists Association president 1963-1965; Michigan Pharmaceutical Association president 1971-1972; Pharmaceutical Research and Manufacturers of America Foundation president 1986-1997; Pharmaceutical Research and Manufacturers of America vice president for pharmacy affairs 1989-1997. Pan American Federation of Pharmacy treasurer 1992-1994.

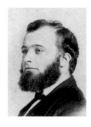

Peter Wendover Bedford
(1836-1892)

APhA president 1881-1882, secretary 1862-1866, Pharmaceutical Education Section chairman 1888-1890. Born in Johnsville, New York, August 1, 1836. New York College of Pharmacy Ph.G. 1858, secretary 1860-1870, trustee 1870-1873, professor 1873-1891. New York City community pharmacist 1859-1870; *Pharmaceutical Record* editor 1883-1892. New York Pharmaceutical Society founding president 1879-1881; USP Convention second vice president 1880-1890; *National Formulary* revision committee secretary 1888-1892. Died July 20, 1892, in White Mountain, New Hampshire.

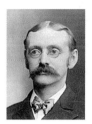

George Mahlon Beringer
(1860-1928)

APhA president 1913-1914, Practical Pharmacy Section chairman 1902-1903. Born in Philadelphia, Pennsylvania, February 3, 1860. Philadelphia College of Pharmacy Ph.G. 1880, trustee 1893-1921, board of trustees chairman 1910-1921, *American Journal of Pharmacy* editor 1917-1921. Bullock and Crenshaw department manager 1880-1892; Camden, New Jersey, community pharmacist. New Jersey Pharmaceutical Association president 1904-1905. Died June 23, 1928, in Collingswood, New Jersey.

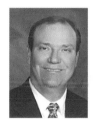

J. Lyle Bootman
(1950-   )

APhA president 1999-2000, trustee 1987-1989, 1998-2001. Born in Upland, California, on May 15, 1950. University of Arizona B.S. 1974, M.S. 1976, University of Minnesota Ph.D. 1978. U.S. Public Health Service (active duty) 1973-1975; clinical pharmacy residency 1975; GEMCO community pharmacist 1979-1983; Hennepin County Medical Center, Minneapolis, Minnesota, clinical pharmacist 1976-1978, University of Arizona College of Pharmacy dean and professor 1990-; Center for PharmacoEconomic Research, Tucson, Arizona, founding director. Elected member National Academy of Sciences Institute of Medicine, 1998.

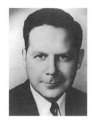

Grover Cleveland Bowles, Jr.
(1920-   )

APhA president 1965-1966, treasurer 1967-1978, House of Delegates speaker 1960-1962, Board of Trustees chairman 1963-1964. Born in Piedmont, Missouri, February 15, 1920. University of Tennessee College of Pharmacy B.S. 1942, professor emeritus 1992, Philadelphia College of Pharmacy D.Sc. (hon) 1968. U.S. Navy Hospital Corps 1942-1946; Strong Memorial Hospital (Rochester, New York) chief pharmacist 1948-1955; Memorial Hospital Association of Kentucky associate administrator 1955-1956; Baptist Memorial Hospital (Memphis, Tennessee) department of pharmacy director 1956-1984. Tennessee Society of Hospital Pharmacists president 1956; American Society of Hospital Pharmacists president 1952-1953; American Council on Pharmaceutical Education president 1982-1986.

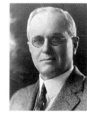

Theodore James Bradley
(1874-1936)

APhA president 1926-1927, first vice president 1919-1920, second vice president 1918-1919, third vice president 1917-1918. Born in Albany, New York, August 8, 1874. Union University Department of Pharmacy Ph.G. 1895; Rensselaer Polytechnic Institute B.S. 1904. New York Department of Health and Agriculture chemist 1895-1905; Albany College of Pharmacy professor 1895-1912; Massachusetts College of Pharmacy dean 1912-1935. Boston Druggists' Association president 1921-1922; American Association of Colleges of Pharmacy secretary-treasurer 1917-1922. Died December 11, 1936, in Brookline, Massachusetts.

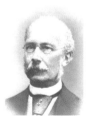

William A. Brewer
(1807-1890)

APhA president 1853-1854. Born in Boston, Massachusetts in 1807. Initially worked for Bortlett and Brewer, and then employed until his retirement in 1884 by the wholesale and manufacturing firm of William H. Schieffelin & Company in New York City; responsible for reviving the Massachusetts College of Pharmacy in 1850. Died April 11, 1890, in South Orange, New Jersey.

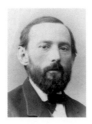

Charles Bullock
(1826-1900)

APhA president 1876-1877, secretary
1859-1860. Born in Wilmington,
Delaware, February 25, 1826. Philadelphia
College of Pharmacy Ph.G. 1847, secretary
1864-1873, first vice president 1874-1885,
president 1886-1900. Apprenticed with APhA's first president,
Daniel B. Smith, 1844-1848; joined in partnership (1849) with
Edmund A. Crenshaw to establish the firm of Bullock &
Crenshaw. Franklin Institute president and curator 1874-
1900; Died March 21, 1900, in Philadelphia, Pennsylvania.

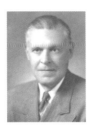

Joseph B. Burt
(1895-1974)

APhA president 1957-1958, first vice president 1951-1952, Scientific Section chairman 1939-1940. Born in Woodland,
Illinois, September 8, 1895. Purdue
University School of Pharmacy B.S. 1920;
University of Wisconsin Ph.D. 1935. World War I veteran;
University of Nebraska College of Pharmacy professor 1920-
1961, dean 1946-1961; War Production Board 1943-1946;
American Association of Colleges of Pharmacy president
1974-1975; Pan American Federation of Pharmacy president
1957-1960; Rho Chi national president. Died December 12,
1974, in Lincoln, Nebraska.

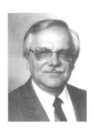

Herbert Sylvester Carlin
(1932-   )

APhA president 1984, House of Delegates
vice speaker 1978-1979, trustee 1978-
1984. Born in Providence, Rhode Island,
December 5, 1932. University of Rhode
Island College of Pharmacy B.Sc. 1954;
Philadelphia College of Pharmacy M.Sc. 1958; D.Sc. (hon)
1984. Warwick, Rhode Island, community pharmacist 1954-
1956; Jefferson Medical College Hospital assistant director of
pharmacy 1958-1959; University of Colorado pharmacy director 1959-1962; University of Illinois pharmacy director 1962-
1972; New York Hospital apothecary-in-chief 1972-1986;
Schein Pharmaceutical vice president 1987-2000;
Pharmaceutical Management Insight president 2000-.
American Society of Hospital Pharmacists president 1970-
1971, speaker 1972, director 1962-1972; USP drug nomenclature and labeling committee chairman 1985-.

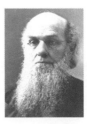

William Barker Chapman
(1813-1874)

APhA president 1854-1855, founding
member, secretary 1853-1854. Born in
Philadelphia, Pennsylvania, June 5, 1813.
Philadelphia College of Pharmacy Ph.G.
1834; Ohio Medical College M.D. 1839.
Cincinnati, Ohio, community pharmacist 1835-1874; Civil
War surgeon; Cincinnati College of Pharmacy professor 1872-
1874; Cincinnati Board of Pharmacy member 1873-1874.
Died October 10, 1874, in Cincinnati, Ohio.

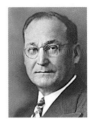

Bernard Victor Christensen
(1885-1956)

APhA president 1941-1942,
Pharmaceutical Education Section chair-
man 1930-1931, Scientific Section chair-
man 1937-1938. Born in Westfield,
Wisconsin, April 15, 1885. University of
Wisconsin School of Pharmacy Ph.B. 1917, Ph.D. 1927,
instructor 1924-1927. University of Florida College of
Pharmacy professor 1927-1939; Ohio State University College
of Pharmacy dean 1939-1955; Plant Science Seminar presi-
dent 1931-1932; American Association of Colleges of
Pharmacy president 1949-1950. Died September 13, 1956, in
Columbus, Ohio.

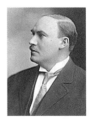

Henry C. Christensen
(1865-1947)

APhA president 1930-1931, Council vice
chairman 1935-1937. Born in Union
Grove, Wisconsin, December 10, 1865.
Northwestern University College of
Pharmacy Ph.G. 1893. Apprenticed phar-
macy in Minden, Nebraska; Chicago, Illinois, community
pharmacist 1893-1911. Illinois Board of Pharmacy member
1907-1921; National Association of Boards of Pharmacy secretary 1914-1942, honorary president 1942-1943. Died January
20, 1947, in Chicago, Illinois.

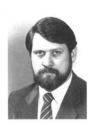

Ronald David Cobb
(1945-   )

APhA president 1989-1990, Academy of
Pharmacy Practice president 1983-1984.
Born in Louisville, Kentucky, May 10,
1945. University of Kentucky College of
Pharmacy B.S. 1968, Pharm.D. 1973, asso-
ciate professor of pharmacy 1970-2000. Kentucky Pharmacists
Association president 1976-1977.

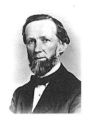

Samuel Marshall Colcord

(1817-1895)

APhA president 1859-1860, president *pro tem* 1853, second vice president 1852-1853, treasurer 1854-1859. Born in Somersworth, New Hampshire, May 8, 1817. New York College of Pharmacy, attended lectures 1837; moved to New Orleans for health reasons 1838-1842. Apprenticed pharmacy in Portsmouth 1834-1837; Boston community pharmacist 1843-1877; Massachusetts College of Pharmacy first vice president 1854-1860, president 1871-1887. Died March 5, 1895, in Dover, Massachusetts.

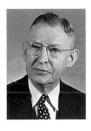

Roy Bird Cook

(1886-1961)

APhA president 1942-1943, House of Delegates chairman 1935-1936, Historical Pharmacy Section chairman 1959-1960. Born in Weston, West Virginia, April 1, 1886. Apprenticed pharmacy in Weston, registered 1905; Huntington, West Virginia, community pharmacist 1907-1919, Charleston 1919-1932; Independent Publishing Co. president 1933-1941; West Virginia Newspaper Council president 1939-1940; *Virginia History Magazine* editor 1939-1941. West Virginia Pharmaceutical Association president 1918-1919; West Virginia Board of Pharmacy secretary 1932-1961; National Association of Boards of Pharmacy president 1938-1939; Died November 23, 1961, in Charleston, West Virginia.

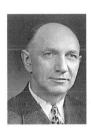

Patrick Henry Costello

(1897-1971)

APhA president 1935-1936, House of Delegates chairman 1933-1934. Born in Sauk Center, Minnesota, January 17, 1897. North Dakota Agricultural College School of Pharmacy, Ph.G. 1917. World War I veteran; Cooperstown, North Dakota, community pharmacist 1919-1942; Cooperstown mayor 1938-1942; North Dakota Pharmaceutical Association president 1924-1925, treasurer 1927-1942; North Dakota Board of Pharmacy secretary 1927-1942; National Association of Boards of Pharmacy president 1939-1940, secretary 1942-1962. Died May 23, 1971, in Lakefield, Michigan.

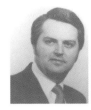

David Stephen Crawford

(1945-   )

APhA president 1987, House of Delegates speaker 1981-1983, Academy of Pharmacy Practice president 1979-1980. Born in Parkersburg, West Virginia, October 23, 1945. West Virginia University School of Pharmacy B.S. 1968. Elkins, West Virginia, community pharmacist 1968-. West Virginia Pharmaceutical Association president 1975-1976; International Pharmaceutical Federation community pharmacy section executive committee member.

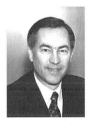

Robert Earl Davis

(1951-   )

APhA president 1995, trustee 1989-1995, Section on Clinical Pharmacy chairman 1980-1981. Born in Danville, Virginia, May 18, 1951. Medical University of South Carolina College of Pharmacy B.S. 1974; Pharm.D. 1975; clinical associate professor 1977-1986. Lexington, South Carolina, community pharmacist 1976-1986; FoxMeyer Health Corporation director 1986-1991; Health Mart general manager 1991-1993; ScriptCard president 1993-1996, senior vice president 1994-1907; Clinical Affairs VHA Inc. vice president 1997-. South Carolina Pharmaceutical Association president 1986-1987.

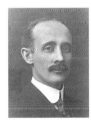

William Baker Day

(1871-1938)

APhA president 1912-1913, first vice president 1910-1911, second vice president 1909-1910, general secretary 1914-1925. Born in Peru, Illinois, February 15, 1871. Chicago College of Pharmacy Ph.G. 1892. University of Illinois School of Pharmacy professor and dean 1913-1938. Illinois Pharmaceutical Association secretary 1906-1936; USP Board of Trustees secretary 1930-1938. Died December 10, 1938, in Oak Park, Illinois.

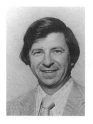

George David Denmark
(1934-)

APhA president 1973-1974, first vice president 1967-1968. Born in Quincy, Massachusetts, May 13, 1934. Massachusetts College of Pharmacy B.S. 1957, trustee 1975-. Pocasset, Massachusetts, community pharmacist 1960-1994; Barnstable County Hospital pharmacist 1962-1982. Cape Cod Pharmaceutical Association president 1963-1964; Massachusetts Pharmaceutical Association recording secretary 1965; Denmark's Home Medical Equipment owner 1973-.

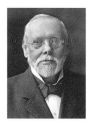

Conrad Lewis Diehl
(1840-1917)

APhA president 1874-1875, first vice president 1871-1872, *Progress of Pharmacy* reporter 1873-1891, 1894-1915, *National Formulary* committee of revision chairman 1896 1917. Born in Neustadt (Bavaria), Germany, August 3, 1840; came to America 1851. Philadelphia College of Pharmacy Ph.G. 1862. Apprenticed pharmacy in Philadelphia 1854-1858; John Wyeth & Co. laboratory director 1858-1862; Civil War veteran, wounded at Stone River; U.S. Army Laboratory chemist 1863-1865; Louisville Chemical Company manager 1865-1869; Louisville community pharmacist 1869-1903. Louisville College of Pharmacy founding president 1870-1881, professor 1871-1916; Kentucky Pharmaceutical Association president 1900-1901; Kentucky Board of Pharmacy president 1885-1886. Died March 25, 1917, in Louisville, Kentucky.

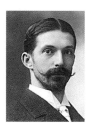

Alfred Robert Louis Dohme
(1867-1952)

APhA president 1917-1918 succeeding presidency on the death of Charles Holzhauer, advancing from first vice president 1917, Scientific Section chairman 1894-1895. Born in Baltimore, Maryland, February 15, 1867, son of APhA president Charles Emile Dohme. Johns Hopkins University A.B. 1886, Ph.D. 1889, instructor 1900-1912. Sharp & Dohme chief chemist 1891-1910, vice president 1908-1911, president 1911-1929; Maryland Pharmaceutical Association president 1899-1900. Died June 11, 1952, in Baltimore, Maryland.

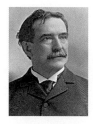

Charles Emile Dohme
(1843-1911)

APhA president 1898-1899, first vice president 1895-1896, second vice president 1890-1891. Born in Obernkirchen, Germany, March 12, 1843. Came to America in 1851. Maryland College of Pharmacy Ph.G. 1862. Apprenticed in the Baltimore pharmacy of Alpheus P. Sharp; obtained a position with APhA past president John Kidwell of Georgetown, District of Columbia; joined the firm of [Alpheus] Sharp & [Louis] Dohme as laboratory director 1866-1892; Sharp & Dohme vice president 1892-1910, president 1910-1911; USP Board of Trustees chairman 1901-1910. Died December 9, 1911, in Baltimore, Maryland.

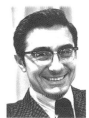

James Thomas Doluisio
(1935-)

APhA president 1982; Basic Pharmaceutics section chairman 1973-1974. Born in Bethlehem, Pennsylvania, September 28, 1935; Temple University School of Pharmacy B.S. 1957; Purdue University Ph.D. 1962. Philadelphia College of Pharmacy professor 1961-1967; University of Kentucky professor 1967-1973; University of Texas College of Pharmacy dean 1973-1998; USP Board of Trustees chairman 1990-1995; American Association of Pharmaceutical Scientists president 1988; International Pharmaceutical Federation vice president 1995-1998.

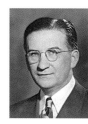

Sylvester H. Dretzka
(1894-1980)

APhA president 1947-1948, House of Delegates chairman 1944-1946. Born in Cudahy, Wisconsin, December 5, 1894. Marquette University School of Pharmacy Ph.G. 1914. World War I veteran; Milwaukee community pharmacist 1920-1937. Wisconsin Pharmaceutical Association president 1934-1935; Wisconsin Board of Pharmacy secretary 1937-1958; National Association of Boards of Pharmacy president 1941-1942; American Institute of the History of Pharmacy treasurer 1942-1968, honorary president 1962. Died January 12, 1980, in Milwaukee, Wisconsin.

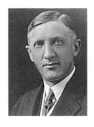

Andrew Grover DuMez

(1885-1948)

APhA president 1939-1940, Scientific Section chairman 1920-1921, *Year Book* editor 1922-1926, *APhA Journal, Scientific Edition* editor 1940-1942. Born in Horicon, Wisconsin, April 26, 1885. University of Wisconsin School of Pharmacy B.S. 1907, Ph.D. 1917, instructor 1905-1910. Pacific University (Oregon) professor 1910-1911; Oklahoma Agricultural and Mechanical College professor 1911-1912; University of the Philippines School of Pharmacy director 1912-1916; U.S. Public Health Service pharmacologist 1917-1926; University of Maryland School of Pharmacy dean 1926-1948. American Association of Colleges of Pharmacy president 1929-1930. Died September 27, 1948, in the District of Columbia.

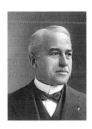

Henry Armitt Brown Dunning

(1877-1962)

APhA president 1929-1930, APhA Foundation president 1953-1961, Practical Pharmacy Section chairman 1906-1907. Born in Denton, Maryland, October 24, 1877. Maryland College of Pharmacy Ph.G. 1897, Pharm.D. 1908, associate professor 1903-1913. Apprenticed as pharmacist in Denton 1895; Spanish-American War veteran; purchased part ownership in Hynson, Wescott & Company, manufacturing pharmacists in Baltimore 1901; Hynson, Wescott & Dunning president 1930-1962. Maryland Pharmaceutical Association president 1926-1927. Died July 26, 1962, in Baltimore, Maryland.

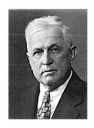

Eugene Gustave Eberle

(1863-1942)

APhA president 1910-1911, first vice president 1908-1909, second vice president 1902-1903, Council chairman 1911-1916, Historical Section secretary 1906-1909, chairman 1909-1911; *APhA Journal* editor 1915-1940. Born in Watertown, Wisconsin, June 3, 1863. Philadelphia College of Pharmacy Ph.G. 1884. Texas Drug Company (Dallas) manager 1894-1900; Dallas University Department of Pharmacy professor 1900-1915, dean 1903-1915; *Southern Pharmaceutical Journal* editor 1908-1915. Texas Pharmaceutical Association president 1901-1903, secretary 1909-1914. Died May 2, 1942, in the District of Columbia.

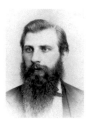

Albert Ethelbert Ebert

(1840-1906)

APhA president 1872-1873, third vice president 1868-1869, Historical Section chairman 1904-1905. Born in Bavaria, Germany, December 23, 1840, Came to America 1841. Philadelphia College of Pharmacy Ph.G. 1864; Munich (Germany) University Ph.D. 1868. Apprenticed as pharmacist in Chicago, Illinois, 1853-1861; Chicago community pharmacist 1868-1877; Chicago College of Pharmacy professor 1871-1876; *The Pharmacist* editor 1868-1876. Died November 20, 1906, in Chicago, Illinois.

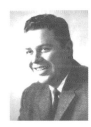

Max Ward Eggleston

(1922-1997)

APhA president 1968-1969; Board of Trustee chairman 1969-1970, member 1965-1970. Born in Waverly, Iowa, August 4, 1922. University of Iowa College of Pharmacy B.S. 1947. Waverly community pharmacist 1948-1984; Pharmacy Sales and Management Co. 1984-1997. Iowa Pharmacists Association president 1960-1961, House of Delegates chairman 1965-1966; Iowa Interprofessional Society president 1966; Iowa Pharmacy Foundation president 1990-1992; American Council on Pharmaceutical Education president 1978-1982. Died November 6, 1997, in Waverly, Iowa.

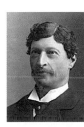

Leo Eliel

(1845-1911)

APhA president 1906-1907, first vice president 1893-1894, Commercial Interests Section chairman 1889-1890. Born in Germany, October 26, 1845. Came to America in 1856; South Bend, Indiana, community pharmacist 1873-1911. Indiana Pharmaceutical Association president 1886-1887; USP fourth vice president 1910-1911. Died February 11, 1911, in South Bend, Indiana.

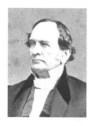

Charles Ellis
(1800-1874)

APhA president 1857-1858, founding member 1852, second vice president 1855-1856. Born in Muncy, Pennsylvania, January 31, 1800. Apprenticed pharmacy with Elizabeth Marshall in Philadelphia 1817-1820; Philadelphia community pharmacist 1825-1874. Philadelphia College of Pharmacy founding member 1821, secretary 1828-1842, first vice president 1842-1854, president 1854-1869. Died May 16, 1874, in Philadelphia, Pennsylvania.

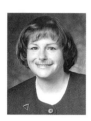

Janet P. Engle (Donnelly)
(1959 -   )

APhA president 2002-2003, trustee 1995-2001, Academy of Pharmacy Practice and Management president 1994-1995, section of clinical/pharmacotherapeutic practice chairman 1990-1991. Born in Summit, New Jersey, August 25, 1959. Rutgers University College of Pharmacy BS in Pharmacy 1982; University of Illinois College of Pharmacy Pharm.D. 1985. Illinois Pharmacy Foundation treasurer 1991-1993; Illinois Pharmacists Association secretary 1994; American Association of Colleges of Pharmacy teachers of pharmacy practice awards committee chairman 1989-1990, professional affairs committee chairman 1990-1991, bylaws and policy development committee chairman 1992-1993. University of Illinois at Chicago College of Pharmacy clinical professor of pharmacy practice 1992-1999 and associate dean for academic affairs 1993-.

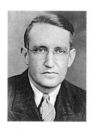

Charles Hall Evans
(1895-1983)

APhA president 1940-1941, House of Delegates chairman 1947-1948. Born in Norwood, Georgia, December 15, 1895. Mercer University Southern School of Pharmacy Ph.G. 1915. Warrenton, Georgia, community pharmacist 1915-1947. Georgia Board of Pharmacy 1929-1934; National Association of Boards of Pharmacy president 1934-1935, vice president 1932-1934; Georgia Pharmaceutical Association president 1946-1947, first vice president 1945-1946. Died March 5, 1983, in Warrenton, Georgia.

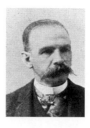

Alexander Kirkwood Finlay
(1843-1911)

APhA president 1891-1892, second vice president 1887-1889. Born in Ireland in 1843. Came to America 1858. Louisiana University Medical Department Ph.G. 1874. Apprenticed pharmacy with his brother in New Orleans 1867-1872; New Orleans community pharmacist 1874-1901. Orleans Pharmaceutical Association president 1886-1888; Louisiana Pharmaceutical Association founding first vice president 1882-1884, president 1885-1886; National Retail Druggists Association founding executive committee member 1883; New Orleans city councilor 1888-1890. Died October 20, 1911, in New Orleans, Louisiana.

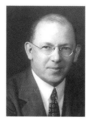

Robert Phillip Fischelis
(1891-1981)

APhA president 1934-1935, first vice president 1933-1934, Council chairman 1941-1945, secretary and general manager 1945-1959, Foundation secretary 1953-1959, editor *APhA Journal* 1949-1951. Born in Philadelphia, Pennsylvania, August 16, 1891. Medico-Chirurgical College Department of Pharmacy Ph.G. 1911, Pharm.D. 1913, faculty 1916-1921. H. K. Mulford Company scientific staff 1916-1918; Drug Trade Bureau of Public Information editor 1920-1932; War Production Board division of chemicals, drugs, and health supplies director 1943-1945. Pennsylvania Pharmaceutical Association secretary 1916-1919, president 1919-1920; New Jersey College of Pharmacy dean 1921-1925; New Jersey Pharmaceutical Association secretary 1926-1929; and president 1942-1945; *New Jersey Journal of Pharmacy* founding editor 1928-1935; New Jersey Board of Pharmacy executive secretary 1926-1944; National Drug Trade Conference president 1958-1960; Ohio Northern University College of Pharmacy dean 1962-1965. Died October 14, 1981, in Ada, Ohio.

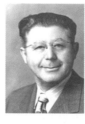

Louis James Fischl, Sr.
(1894-1979)

APhA president 1958-1959, Council chairman 1961-1962, House of Delegates chairman 1951-1952, second vice president 1950-1951, Foundation president 1958-1959. Born in Chicago, Illinois, March 4, 1894. Montana University School of Pharmacy Ph.C. 1914. Helena, Montana community pharmacist 1914-1925, Oakland, California 1926-1979. Alameda County Pharmaceutical Association president; Berkeley Retail Druggists Association president; California Pharmaceutical Association president 1937-1938; American College of Apothecaries president 1954-1955; Died October 28, 1979, in Oakland, California.

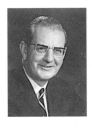

Don Eugene Francke
(1910-1978)

APhA president 1951-1952. Born in Athens, Pennsylvania, August 28, 1910. University of Michigan College of Pharmacy B.S. 1936, M.S. 1948, faculty 1948-1963. University of Michigan Medical Center chief pharmacist 1944-1963; *American Journal of Hospital Pharmacy* editor 1944-1966; *Drug Intelligence* editor 1972-1978; Michigan Academy of Pharmacy director 1947-1957; University of Cincinnati College of Pharmacy faculty and Cincinnati General Hospital director of pharmacy 1967-1971. Michigan Board of Pharmacy member 1950-1952; American Society of Hospital Pharmacy president 1943-1946, International Pharmaceutical Federation vice president 1958-1966, press and documentation section president 1964-1978. Drug Information Association president 1969; Died November 6, 1978, in the District of Columbia.

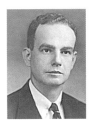

Fred Royce Franzoni, Jr.
(1913-1965)

APhA president 1953-1954. Born in Washington, District of Columbia, March 15, 1913. George Washington University College of Pharmacy B.Sc. 1936, instructor 1936-1937, U.S. Army 1931-1948 including World War II veteran. District of Columbia community pharmacist 1936-1965, Z. D. Gilman president 1946-1965. District of Columbia Pharmaceutical Association president 1951-1952; District of Columbia Board of Pharmacy president 1953-1955; National Association of Boards of Pharmacy president 1951-1952. Died August 22, 1965, in the District of Columbia.

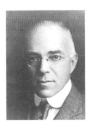

Edmund Norris Gathercoal
(1874-1954)

APhA president 1937-1938, first vice president 1922-1923, Scientific Section chairman 1918-1919, Committee of Revision for the *National Formulary* revision committee chairman 1929-1940; Scientific Section chairman 1918-1919. Born in Sycamore, Illinois, in 1874. Chicago College of Pharmacy Ph.G. 1895; Rush Medical College two years of study. Apprenticed in Chicago pharmacy 1891-1893; Wilmette, Illinois, community pharmacist 1897-1907; University of Illinois College of Pharmacy faculty 1907-1944; National Conference on Pharmaceutical Research president 1929-1930; Died December 27, 1954, in Pentwater, Michigan.

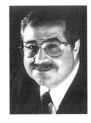

Philip Paul Gerbino
(1947-   )

APhA president 1990-1991, Academy of Pharmacy Practice president 1986-1987, Clinical Practice Section chairman 1978-1979. Born in Jersey City, New Jersey, March 11, 1947. Philadelphia College of Pharmacy B.S. 1969, Pharm.D. 1970, assistant professor 1971-1973, 1975-1976, associate professor 1976-1983, professor 1983-1987, vice president and dean 1992-1994, president 1994-, Linwood F. Tice professor 1999. St. John's University College of Pharmacy professor 1973-1975; New York Hospital drug information director 1973-1975; West Windsor Township, New Jersey, deputy mayor 1979-1981.

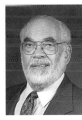

Robert Daniel Gibson
(1925-   )

APhA president 2000-2001, Trustee 1992-2002. Born in Tacoma, Washington, on July 2, 1925. University of Oregon B.A. 1949; B.S. 1954, Pharm.D. 1958. U.S. Army Medical Corp, 1944-1946; University of California hospital pharmacist 1954-1964; San Francisco community pharmacist 1964-1966; pharmaceutical technology laboratory director 1970-1982; school of pharmacy associate dean, 1970-1982, 1995-1998; University of California - San Francisco associate vice chancellor 1982-1995. Northern California Hospital Pharmacists Association president 1964-1965; American Association of Colleges of Pharmacy president 1984-1985.

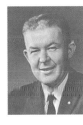

Robert John Gillespie
(1917-1995)

APhA president 1963-1964, first vice president 1959-1960. Born in St. Joseph, Michigan, June 11, 1917. Philadelphia College of Pharmacy B.S. 1941. World War II veteran; St. Joseph and Benton Harbor, Michigan, community pharmacist 1945-1990. Michigan Pharmaceutical Association president 1973-1974; Michigan Board of Pharmacy president 1957; National Association of Boards of Pharmacy president 1959-1960. Died January 7, 1995, in St. Joseph, Michigan.

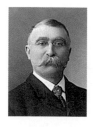

John Granville Godding
(1853-1929)

APhA president 1911-1912, Council vice chairman 1913-1916, Historical Section chairman 1912-1913. Born in Gardiner, Maine, March 28, 1853. Massachusetts College of Pharmacy Ph.G. 1874, trustee 1886-1890, treasurer 1890-1929. Apprenticed pharmacy in Brandon and Rutland, Vermont; Philadelphia community pharmacist 1875-1878; Boston, Massachusetts, community pharmacist 1879-1929; Boston Druggists Association treasurer; Died April 7, 1929, in Newton, Massachusetts.

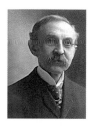

James Michener Good
(1842-1919)

APhA president 1895-1896, Council chairman 1884-1894, Education Section chairman 1894-1895. Born in Birmingham, Pennsylvania, January 12, 1842. Philadelphia College of Pharmacy course 1867-1868. St. Louis, Missouri, community pharmacist 1869-1918; St. Louis College of Pharmacy professor 1875-1912, dean 1880-1904. Missouri Pharmaceutical Association treasurer 1883-1887, president 1888-1889; St. Louis Retail Druggists Association president 1912-1913; National Association of Retail Druggists founding member 1898. Died May 15, 1919, in St. Louis, Missouri.

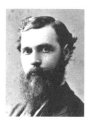

William John Maclester Gordon
(1825-1909)

APhA president 1864-1865, first vice president 1860-1862, secretary 1855-1859, Council vice chairman 1881-1883. Born in Somerset County, Maryland, December 25, 1825. Maryland University Medical College chemistry courses 1847. Apprenticed pharmacy in Baltimore 1844-1846; Cincinnati, Ohio, community pharmacist 1848-1865; manufacturing pharmacist 1867-1900; Cincinnati College of Pharmacy president; Cincinnati Board of Trade president. Died July 7, 1909, in Cincinnati, Ohio.

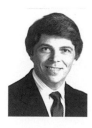

Charles Rowand Green
(1943-   )

APhA president 1988. Born in Stockton, California, July 30, 1943. University of the Pacific School of Pharmacy B.S. 1968, assistant clinical professor 1969-1971, associate professor 1971-1985. Stockton, California, community pharmacist 1968-; California Pharmacy Inc. president 1984-1993; Pacific Pharmacy Associates president 1987; *Pharmacist Letter* senior editorial advisor for 13 years. California Pharmaceutical Association president 1983-1984, long-range planning committee chairman 1981, pharmacy law revision task force 1991-1995, committee to restructure 2000. San Joaquin Pharmacists Association president.

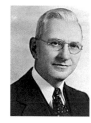

Henry Hamilton Gregg III
(1899-1982)

APhA president 1950-1951, second vice president 1940-1941, House of Delegates chairman 1941-1942, Council vice chairman 1955-1958. Born in Purceville, Virginia, May 24, 1899. Philadelphia College of Pharmacy Ph.G. 1899. World War I veteran; Minneapolis community pharmacist 1929-1975. Minneapolis Retail Druggists Association president and secretary; APhA Northwestern Branch president 1945-1946; American College of Apothecaries president 1960-1961. Died August 24, 1982, in Edina, Minnesota.

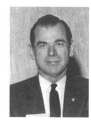

George W. Grider
(1914-   )

APhA president 1967-1968. Born in Albany, Kentucky, August 20, 1914. Louisville College of Pharmacy B.S. 1940, associate clinical professor 1971-1989. Danville, Kentucky, community pharmacist 1940-; Ephraim McDowell Memorial Hospital consultant pharmacist 1956-1975; Northpoint Training Center (Prison) chief pharmacist 1984-1990. Kentucky Board of Pharmacy president 1959 and 1963; Kentucky Council on Pharmaceutical Education vice president 1960-1967; American Institute of the History of Pharmacy president 1964-1965; Pan American Federation of Pharmacy professional pharmacy section chairman 1969-1973; McDowell Apothecary Museum curator.

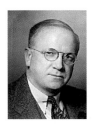

Ivor Griffith
(1891-1961)

APhA president 1943-1944, Practical Pharmacy Section chairman 1920-1922, Historical Section chairman 1940-1941. Born in Rhiwlas, North Wales, Great Britain, January 3, 1891. Came to America 1907. Philadelphia College of Pharmacy P.D. 1912, instructor 1916-1922, associate professor 1922-1936, professor 1936-1940, dean 1936-1959, president 1941-1961. Stetson Hospital pharmacist 1913-1915; *American Journal of Pharmacy* editor 1921-1941; World War II National Quinine Pool creator; Welsh Society president; *To the Lilacs* [poems and essays] author. Died May 16, 1961, in Philadelphia, Pennsylvania.

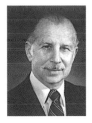

Leonard Grossman
(1917-   )

APhA president 1981, Academy of Pharmacy Practice president 1977-1978, Foundation vice president 1985-1990. Born in Cambridge, Massachusetts, February 1, 1917. Northeastern University School of Pharmacy Ph.G. 1939; Massachusetts College of Pharmacy D.Sc. (hon) 1981. Jamaica Plains, Massachusetts, community pharmacist 1939-; Massachusetts Association of Durable Medical Equipment Companies founder and board chairman 1974, Massachusetts Health Council director 1968-1970. Massachusetts Pharmaceutical Association first vice president 1970, second vice president 1969.

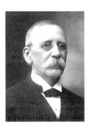

John Francis Hancock
(1834-1923)

APhA president 1873-1874, honorary president 1920-1921, Historical Section chairman 1905-1906. Born in Anne Arundel County, Maryland, September 9, 1834. Maryland College of Pharmacy Ph.G. 1860, president 1872-1874. Apprenticed pharmacy in Baltimore 1854-1858. Maryland Pharmaceutical Association president 1894-1895, secretary 1895-1986; Baltimore Board of Pharmacy 1890-1902. Died November 12, 1923, in Baltimore, Maryland.

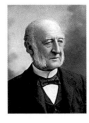

Charles Augustus Heinitsh
(1822-1898)

APhA president 1882-1883, third vice president 1865-1866. Born in Lancaster, Pennsylvania, July 31, 1822. Apprenticed in father's Lancaster pharmacy 1838-1841; Lancaster community pharmacist 1841-1891. Pennsylvania Pharmaceutical Association founding president 1878-1880; Lancaster Pharmaceutical Association president 1882-1883; National Retail Druggists Association vice president 1884-1885; Linnean Society of Lancaster founding member 1860, president, treasurer, curator. Died December 29, 1898, in Lancaster, Pennsylvania.

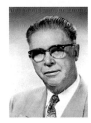

John B. Heinz
(1890-1965)

APhA president 1955-1956, first vice president 1954-1955, Council chairman 1956-1958. Born in Raeville, Nebraska, September 25, 1890. Creighton University School of Pharmacy Ph.G. 1912. Laurel, Montana, community pharmacist 1912-1929, Salt Lake City, Utah, 1930-1960. Utah Pharmaceutical Association president 1944-1945; Utah Board of Pharmacy president, American College of Apothecaries president 1952-1953; Died April 29, 1965, in Salt Lake City, Utah.

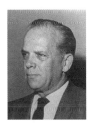

William B. Hennessy
(1911-1989)

APhA president 1969-1970. Born in London, Ontario, Canada, March 25, 1911. Detroit Institute of Technology B.S. 1947. Detroit, Michigan, community pharmacist, Grosse Pointe, Michigan, 1947-1989; Saratoga General Hospital chief pharmacist 1960-1989. Metropolitan Detroit Pharmaceutical Association president, Michigan Pharmaceutical Association president 1962-1963; American College of Apothecaries president 1966-1967. Died August 18, 1989, in St. Clair Shores, Michigan.

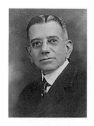

Samuel Louis Hilton
(1866-1944)

APhA president 1921-1922, House of Delegates chairman 1919-1920, Council chairman 1925-1940. Born in District of Columbia, March 18, 1866. National College of Pharmacy Ph.G. 1888. Apprenticed pharmacy in District of Columbia 1844-1846; District of Columbia community pharmacist 1889-1936. City of Washington Retail Druggists Association president; District of Columbia Board of Pharmacy secretary 1906-1908; USP treasurer 1910-1940. Died January 30, 1944, in the District of Columbia.

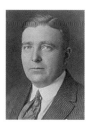

Charles William Holton
(1882-1970)

APhA president 1924-1925, treasurer 1925-1941, Commercial Interests Section chairman 1921-1922. Born in Newark, New Jersey, November 6, 1882, son of APhA president Charles Holzhauer. Princeton University B.A. 1904; New York College of Pharmacy Ph.B. 1907, secretary 1917-1930. Newark, New Jersey, community pharmacist 1906-1928. New Jersey Pharmaceutical Association president 1913-1914; Essex Falls, New Jersey, mayor 1930-1952; Died January 26, 1970, in Essex Falls, New Jersey.

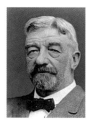

Charles Holzhauer
(1848-1917)

APhA president 1917, first vice president 1905-1906, Historical Section chairman 1915-1916. Born in Kassel, Germany in 1848. Came to America 1851. New York College of Pharmacy Ph.G. 1873, trustee 1892-1897, vice president 1891. Apprenticed pharmacy in Newark, New Jersey, 1862-1866; Newark community pharmacist 1880-1917. New Jersey Pharmaceutical Association president 1881-1882; New Jersey Board of Pharmacy founding member 1877-1880, president 1880-1890; National Retail Druggists Association executive committee member 1885-1886. Died November 19, 1917, in Newark, New Jersey, while serving as APhA president.

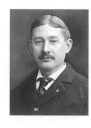

Lewis Christopher Hopp
(1856-1925)

APhA president 1903-1904, first vice president 1899-1900, Council chairman 1916-1920, Commercial Interests Section chairman 1896-1897. Born in Cleveland, Ohio, in 1856. Philadelphia College of Pharmacy Ph.G. 1875. Cleveland, Ohio, community pharmacist 1882-1925. Ohio Pharmaceutical Association founding secretary 1879-1903, president 1903-1904; Cleveland School of Pharmacy president 1903-1919; National Retail Druggists Association founding executive committee member 1883-1884; National Association of Retail Druggists first vice president 1902-1903. Died May 7, 1925, in Cleveland, Ohio.

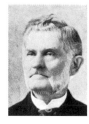

John Ingalls
(1829-1898)

APhA president 1884-1885, first vice president 1882-1883, second vice president 1877-1878. Born in New Bern, North Carolina, in 1829. Apprenticed pharmacy in New Bern 1848-1850; Columbia, South Carolina, community pharmacist 1851-1859, Macon, Georgia, 1860-1898. Georgia Pharmaceutical Association president 1879-1880, first vice president 1875-1876, treasurer 1876-1879; Georgia Board of Pharmacy founding member 1881-1887. Died November 12, 1898, in Macon, Georgia.

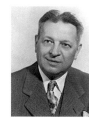

Glenn Llewellyn Jenkins
(1898-1979)

APhA president 1949-1950, second vice president 1937-1938, House of Delegates chairman 1943-1944, Council chairman 1940-1941, Scientific Section chairman 1936-1937, Education Section chairman 1929-1930. Born in Sparta, Wisconsin, March 25, 1898. University of Wisconsin School of Pharmacy B.S. 1922, Ph.D. 1926, instructor 1926-1927. University of Maryland professor 1927-1936; University of Minnesota professor 1936-1941; Purdue University School of Pharmacy dean 1941-1965; Indiana State Board of Health chairman 1958-1960; Indiana Interprofessional Health Council chairman 1941-1956. American Association of Colleges of Pharmacy president 1944-1946; Rho Chi president 1930-1934. Died January 12, 1979, in Lafayette, Indiana.

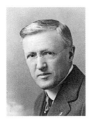

Charles Willis Johnson
(1873-1949)

APhA president 1927-1928, second vice president 1909-1910, Education Section chairman 1910-1911. Born in Concord, Indiana, September 23, 1873. University of Michigan College of Pharmacy Ph.C. 1896, B.S. 1900, Ph.D. 1903. Ann Arbor and Detroit, Michigan, community pharmacist 1896-1898; Iowa State University professor 1900-1902; University of Washington College of Pharmacy dean 1903-1939. Washington State Pharmaceutical Association president 1915-1917; American Association of Colleges of Pharmacy president 1923-1924. Died January 9, 1949, in Seattle, Washington.

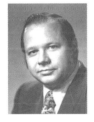

Robert Charles Johnson
(1935-   )

APhA president 1974-1975, vice president 1972-1973, trustee 1963-1976. Born in Detroit, Michigan, August 24, 1935. Wayne State University College of Pharmacy B.Sc. 1958, M.Sc. 1962; University of the Pacific D.Sc. (hon). Trenton, Michigan, community pharmacist 1958-1960; Michigan Pharmaceutical Association field director 1959-1962, executive director 1961-1969; *Michigan Pharmacist* editor 1963-1969; California Pharmaceutical Association executive vice president 1969-1990; *California Pharmacist* editor 1969-1990; Nevada Pharmaceutical Association executive officer 1980-1985; PCS Health Systems chief executive officer 1990-1995; Midwestern University College of Pharmacy Center for the Advancement of Pharmacy Practice executive director 1998-. National Council of State Pharmaceutical Association Executives president 1976-1977; American Council on Pharmaceutical Education vice president 1982-1988; Medic-Alert Foundation International Board chairman 1990-1992.

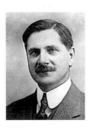

David Franklin Jones
(1869-1944)

APhA president 1928-1929, second vice president 1921-1922. Born in Sparta, Wisconsin, October 26, 1867. Northwestern University Pharmacy Department Ph.G. 1894. Apprenticed pharmacy in Barrow, Wisconsin, 1888-1891; Watertown, North Dakota, community pharmacist 1894-1933; South Dakota College Pharmacy Department professor 1896-1897. South Dakota Pharmaceutical Association president; South Dakota Board of Pharmacy member 15 years; National Association of Boards of Pharmacy vice president 1910-1911, honorary president 1941; Watertown, South Dakota councilor 1903-1908. Died February 10, 1944, in Watertown, South Dakota.

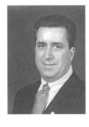

Ronald Philip Jordan
(1952-   )

APhA president 1998-1999, trustee 1994-1999. Born in Hartford, Connecticut, December 25, 1952. University of Rhode Island B.S. 1976. Blue Cross & Blue Shield of Rhode Island assistant vice president 1980-1989; Drug Benefit Management Systems president 1989-1995; HCaliber Consulting Corporation president 1995-; Hospice Pharmacia/excelleRx senior vice president 1994-2000; PharmasMarket.com senior vice president 2000-2001. Rhode Island Institute for Pharmaceutical Care president and founder 1999-. Rhode Island Pharmaceutical Association president 1981-1982.

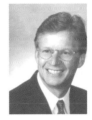

Gary William Kadlec
(1948-   )

APhA president 1997-1998, trustee 1993-1999. Born in Pontiac, Michigan, on June 29, 1948. Ferris State University B.S. 1971, Michigan State University M.B.A. 1991. Specialized Pharmacy Services, Livonia, Michigan, president 1976-1996; Omnicare Regional vice president 1980-1996; Americare senior vice president 2000-. Oakland County Pharmacists Association president 1985-1986; Michigan Pharmacists Association president 1991-1992.

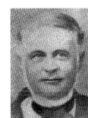

John Lawrence Kidwell
(1819-1885)

APhA president 1858-1859, first vice president 1856-1857. Born in Rockville, Maryland, in 1819. Apprenticed pharmacy in Georgetown, District of Columbia 1836-1840; District of Columbia community pharmacist 1840-1878; known as "Quinine King" because of profitable quinine contracts with the Union Army during the Civil War; acquired marshlands in 1869 (called Kidwell Meadows or Potomac Flats where Lincoln Memorial is presently located) leading to 12-year legal battle before the U.S. government took it back. Died February 16, 1885, in his home (Halcyon House) in Georgetown, District of Columbia.

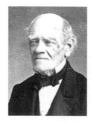

Henry Taylor Kiersted
(1793-1882)

APhA president 1860-1862, third vice president 1856-1857. Born in New York City, March 13, 1793. War of 1812 veteran; Mexican War major general 1846-1848; apprenticed pharmacy in New York City 1814-1818; New York City community pharmacist 1820-1870; New York College of Pharmacy founding trustee 1829-1832, vice president 1859-1861, president 1861-1866; St. Nicholas Society president 1844. Died September 13, 1882, in New York City.

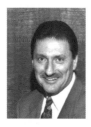

Calvin Haines Knowlton
(1949-)

APhA president 1995-1997, trustee 1992-1997, Academy of Pharmacy Practice and Management president 1991. Born in Audubon, New Jersey, October 5, 1949. Temple University School of Pharmacy B.S. 1972; Princeton Theological Seminary M.Div. 1984; University of Maryland Ph.D. 1992. Lumberton, New Jersey community pharmacist 1975-1996; Philadelphia College of Pharmacy and Science associate professor of pharmacy, 1983-1996; CEO ExcelleRx Inc., Philadelphia 1996-. American College of Apothecaries president, 1991.

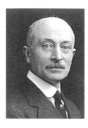

Julius Arnold Koch
(1865-1956)

APhA president 1922-1923, third vice president 1904-1905, Education Section secretary 1899-1901, *APhA Year Book* editor 1915-1916. Born in Bremen, Germany, August 15, 1864. Came to America in infancy. Pittsburgh College of Pharmacy Ph.G. 1884, Pharm.D. 1895, professor and dean 1891-1932. Apprenticed pharmacy in Pittsburgh, Pennsylvania, 1880-1884; Pittsburgh community pharmacist 1885-1891. Pennsylvania Pharmaceutical Association president 1904-1905; American Association of Colleges of Pharmacy executive committee chairman 1908-1920. Died February 10, 1956, in Ocala, Florida.

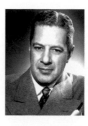

J. Warren Lansdowne
(1902-1972)

APhA president 1961-1962, first vice president 1957-1958, House of Delegates chairman 1958-1960, Foundation president 1964-1966. Born in Adrian, Missouri, August 14, 1902. St. Louis College of Pharmacy Ph.G. 1924. Missouri community pharmacist 1926-1933; Eli Lilly & Company salesman 1935-1943, trade relations assistant manager 1944-1955, professional relations manager 1956-1965; *Tile and Till* editor 1956-1965. Died February 13, 1972, in Cassville, Missouri.

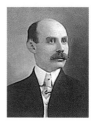

J. Leon Lascoff
(1867-1943)

APhA president 1938-1939, first vice president 1936-1937, Practical Pharmacy Section chairman 1912-1913. Born in Vilna, Lithuania (then part of Russia), August 28, 1867. Came to America 1892. Apprenticed pharmacy in New York City 1892-1898; Merck & Co. tablet department manager 1896; New York City community pharmacist 1899-1943. New York Board of Pharmacy president 1914, 1921, 1929; New York County Pharmaceutical Association founding president 1911-1913; Columbia University College of Pharmacy trustee 1916-1943; American College of Apothecaries founder 1940; National Association of Boards of Pharmacy honorary president 1940. Died May 4, 1943, in New York City.

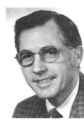

Clifton Joseph Latiolais
(1926-1995)

APhA president 1972-1973, second vice president 1969-1970, House of Delegates speaker 1970-1971. Born in Breaux Bridge, Louisiana, January 13, 1926. Loyola University (New Orleans) College of Pharmacy B.S. 1949; University of Michigan College of Pharmacy M.S. 1952. World War II veteran; Ohio State University Hospitals director of pharmacy 1958-1983. Ohio Society of Hospital Pharmacists president 1965-1966; American Society of Hospital Pharmacists president 1960-1961; American Managed Care Pharmacy Association president 1989-1993; Baxter-Travenol Laboratories consultant. Died May 30, 1995, in Granville, Ohio.

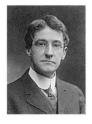

Charles Herbert LaWall
(1871-1937)

APhA president 1918-1919, first vice president 1915-1916, Council chairman 1920-1922, Education Section chairman 1909-1910. Born in Allentown, Pennsylvania, May 7, 1871. Philadelphia College of Pharmacy Ph.G. 1893, lecturer 1900-1905, professor 1906-1918, dean 1918-1937. Apprenticed pharmacy in Bloomsburg, Pennsylvania, 1888-1891; Smith Kline & French Laboratories chemist 1891-1893; Pennsylvania Board of Pharmacy chemist 1905-1912; Pennsylvania state chemist 1909-1915. Pennsylvania Pharmaceutical Association president 1910-1911; USP Committee of Revision secretary 1900-1937, chairman 1918-1930. Died December 7, 1937, in Philadelphia, Pennsylvania.

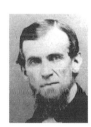

Joseph Lyon Lemberger
(1834-1927)

APhA president 1905-1906, second vice president 1879-1880, Historical Pharmacy Section chairman 1910-1911. Born in Myerstown, Pennsylvania, December 7, 1834. Philadelphia College of Pharmacy Ph.G. 1854. Apprenticed pharmacy in Philadelphia 1850; Lebanon, Pennsylvania, community pharmacist 1857-1922; Civil War hospital steward 1862-1863. Pennsylvania Pharmaceutical Association founding treasurer 1878-1911, president 1911-1912; Pennsylvania Asylum for Chronic Insane secretary 1892-1922. Died September 29, 1927, in Lebanon, Pennsylvania.

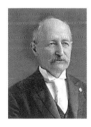

Henry Ware Lincoln
(1822-1887)

APhA president 1865-1866. Born in Highland, Massachusetts in 1822; Massachusetts College of Pharmacy Ph.G., secretary 1851-1874, trustee 1875-1878. Boston, Massachusetts, community pharmacist; compiled outstanding library on botany. Died September 12, 1887, in Boston, Massachusetts.

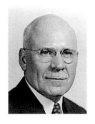

Ernest Little
(1888-1973)

APhA president 1948-1949, Council chairman 1952-1953, House of Delegates vice speaker 1937-1938. Born in Johnstown, New York, June 9, 1888. Rochester University B.S. 1911, instructor 1911-1914; Columbia University Ph.D. 1924. New Jersey College of Pharmacy professor 1924-1953, dean 1926-1946; Pratt Institute instructor 1914-1918. American Association of Colleges of Pharmacy president 1934-1935; American Foundation for Pharmaceutical Education founding president 1942-1943, director 1943-1950, acting secretary 1950. Died October 30, 1973, in Saint Johnsbury, Vermont.

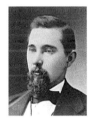

John Uri Lloyd
(1849-1936)

APhA president 1887-1888. Born in West Bloomfield, New York, April 19, 1849. Moved to Kentucky 1853; apprenticed pharmacy in Cincinnati, Ohio; Cincinnati College of Pharmacy professor 1883-1887; Eclectic Medical Institute president 1896-1904; *Pharmaceutical Review* and *Eclectic Medical Journal* associate editor; H. M. Merrell Company laboratory manager 1871-1877; Lloyd Brothers president 1885-1936; author of numerous popular novels including *Springtown on the Pike* (1900), *Warwick of the Knobs* (1901), *Red Head* (1903), and *Scroggins* (1904). Died April 9, 1936, in Los Angeles, California.

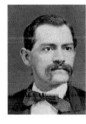

Gustavus Johann Luhn
(1839-1888)

APhA president 1878-1879, second vice president 1876-1877. Born in Genthin, Saxony, Germany, June 7, 1839. Came to America in 1847. Apprenticed pharmacy in Baltimore, Maryland, and in Richmond, Virginia; Civil War cavalryman veteran; Charleston, South Carolina, community pharmacist 1868-1888. South Carolina Pharmaceutical Association founding president 1876-1877; South Carolina Board of Pharmacy founding president 1876. Died April 4, 1888, in Charleston, South Carolina.

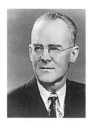

John A. MacCartney
(1905-1989)

APhA president 1956-1957, first vice president 1953-1954, second vice president 1951-1952, Pharmaceutical Economics Section chairman 1950-1951. Born in Claysville, Pennsylvania, June 8, 1905. Pittsburgh University College of Pharmacy Ph.G. 1928. World War II Okinawa campaign veteran 1943-1944; U.S. Military Government in Korea chief medical supply officer 1945-1946; Parke Davis and Company salesman 1928-1942, professional relations manager 1946-to retirement. Died July 23, 1989, in Upper Arlington, Franklin County, Ohio.

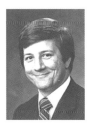

James Allen Main
(1945-   )

APhA president 1985-1986. Born in Troy, Alabama, April 8, 1945. Auburn University School of Pharmacy B.S. 1968; Alabama University J.D. 1972. Anniston, Alabama, practicing attorney 1973-. Alabama Pharmaceutical Association president 1977-1978.

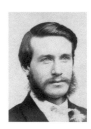

George Frederic Holmes Markoe
(1840-1896)

APhA president 1875-1876, second vice president 1871-1872. Born in Valparaiso, Chile, January 10, 1840. Came to America 1850. Apprenticed pharmacy in Boston, Massachusetts, 1855-1860; Boston and Roxbury community pharmacist 1861-1890; Massachusetts College of Pharmacy professor 1867-1896, alumni association founding president 1870-1871; Harvard Medical School materia medica instructor 1872-1879; Burnett Company (Boston) product formulation director 1890-1896. Boston Druggists Association president 1883-1884. Died September 25, 1896, in Boston, Massachusetts.

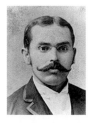

Caswell Armstrong Mayo
(1862-1928)

APhA president 1914-1915, second vice president 1912-1913, Historical Pharmacy Section secretary 1904-1905 and 1911-1912. Born in Columbus, Mississippi, July 5, 1862. Philadelphia College of Pharmacy Ph.G. 1887. *Druggists Circular* associate editor 1887-1891; *American Druggist* editor 1892-1919; William S. Merrell publications director and *Merrell Messenger* editor 1919-1925; New York College of Pharmacy trustee 1910-1921; New Jersey (Rutgers) College of Pharmacy dean 1925-1926. Died January 13, 1928, in Cincinnati, Ohio.

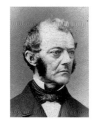

John Meakim
(1812-1863)

APhA president 1855-1856, second vice president 1854-1855. Born in New York City in 1812. New York College of Pharmacy Ph.G. 1836, secretary 1842-1850, vice president 1851-1863, president 1854-1861. Apprenticed pharmacy at New York City Dispensary 1828-1830; New York City community pharmacist 1837-1863. Died October 17, 1863, at his New York City pharmacy.

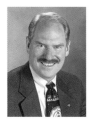

Thomas Edward Menighan
(1952-   )

APhA president 2001-2002, trustee 1995-1998; 2000-2003. Born in Sistersville, West Virginia, on January 14, 1952. West Virginia University B.S. 1974; Averett College M.B.A. 1990. Huntington, West Virginia, community pharmacist 1978-1998; Pharmacy Associates partner 1981-; APhA senior director of external affairs 1987-1992; PharMark vice president 1992-1993; Comprecare Home Health CEO 1997-1999. West Virginia Pharmacists Association president 1985.

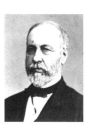

John [Tiburce Gregoire Francis de] Milhau
(1795-1874)

APhA president 1867-1868, first vice president 1862-1863. Born in Baltimore, Maryland, August 11, 1795, son of displaced French nobleman. Attended Parisian School of Pharmacy 1828-1829. Baltimore, Maryland, community pharmacist 1813-1819; New York City 1830-1869; New York College of Pharmacy vice president 1836-1846, president 1846-1851 and 1866-1869. Died December 23, 1874, in New York City.

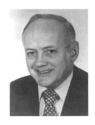

Jacob Willis Miller
(1927-   )

APhA president 1978-1979, vice president 1971-1972, House of Delegates speaker 1972-1974, Foundation president 1993-2000. Born in Louisville, Kentucky, September 5, 1927. University of Kentucky College of Pharmacy B.S. 1951; Washburn University School of Law J.D. 1964. Merck Sharp & Dohme professional service representative 1951-1961; Topeka, Kansas, community pharmacist 1961-1979. A.H. Robins assistant vice president for professional relations director 1979-1990; Wyeth-Ayerst Laboratories assistant vice president for professional affairs 1990-1993. Kansas Pharmaceutical Association president 1970-1971; Kansas Board of Pharmacy member 1974-1977.

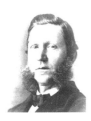

Jacob Faris Moore
(1826-1888)

APhA president 1863-1864 and 1871, third vice president 1862-1863. Born in Port Penn, Delaware, February 20, 1826. Maryland College of Pharmacy Ph.G. 1847, professor 1861-1879, president 1872-1875; Jefferson Medical College M.D. 1849. Apprenticed pharmacy in Baltimore, Maryland, 1842-1846; Baltimore, Maryland, community pharmacist 1850-1858. Died February 3, 1888, in Baltimore, Maryland.

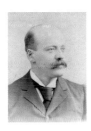

Joseph Edward Morrison
(1862-1913)

APhA president 1896-1897, third vice president 1894-1895. Born in Waterford, Ireland, January 15, 1862. Montreal College of Pharmacy Ph.G. 1882, professor 1894-1912, dean 1907-1912. Quebec Board of Pharmacy Examiners 1887-1893; Lyman Sons & Co. (manufacturing chemists of Montreal) laboratory supervisor; *Philatelic Gazette* editor 1896; *Canadian Pharmaceutical Journal* editor 1897-1900; Died September 2, 1913, in Montreal, Canada.

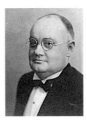

George Allen Moulton
(1890-1981)

APhA president 1944-1946, second vice president 1938-1939, Council vice chairman 1947-1950 and 1953-1955, Education Section chairman 1937-1938. Born in Lewiston, Maine, September 29, 1890. Massachusetts College of Pharmacy Ph.C. 1913, Pharm.D. 1914. Peterborough, New Hampshire, community pharmacist 1917-1949. New Hampshire Pharmaceutical Association vice president 1933-1935, president 1935-1940, executive secretary 1940-1949; New Hampshire Board of Pharmacy president 1946; National Association of Boards of Pharmacy president 1936-1937. Moved to Fort Myers, Florida, 1949, where he died in July 1981.

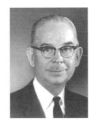

Howard Chamberlain Newton
(1892-1964)

APhA president 1959-1960, Practical Pharmacy Section chairman 1925-1926 and 1929-1930, APhA Foundation president 1961-1964. Born in Southborough, Massachusetts, September 16, 1892. Massachusetts College of Pharmacy Ph.G. 1914, dean 1936-1964. Creighton University School of Pharmacy professor 1914-1916, dean 1916-1935. Boston Druggists Association president 1939-1940; American Association of Colleges of Pharmacy president 1942-1943; Died January 5, 1964, in Wellesley Hills, Massachusetts.

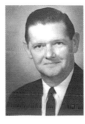

John Curtis Nottingham
(1912-   )

APhA president 1964-1965, first vice president 1961-1962, Council chairman 1965-1966, Foundation treasurer 1968-1994. Born in Cape Charles, Virginia, September 15, 1912. Medical College of Virginia School of Pharmacy B.S. 1935, D.Sc. (hon); Philadelphia College of Pharmacy M.Ph. (hon). Williamsburg, Virginia, community pharmacist 1955-1977; Virginia Pharmaceutical Association executive director 1948-1955, president 1961-1962; *Virginia Pharmacist* editor 1948-1955; National Conference of State Pharmaceutical Association Executives president; Williamsburg Chamber of Commerce president 1957-1958; Virginia Yacht Club past commander; Williamsburg National Bank past director.

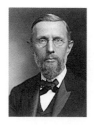

Oscar Oldberg

(1846-1913)

APhA president 1908-1909, first vice president 1907-1908, Scientific Section chairman 1900-1901, Education Section chairman 1905-1907. Born in Helsingland, Sweden, January 22, 1846. Apprenticed pharmacy in Uppsala, Sweden, 1861-1864; came to America 1864; Swedish vice consul in Memphis, Tennessee, 1872; U.S. Marine Hospital Service (Washington, D.C.) medical purveyor 1874-1881; National College of Pharmacy professor 1874-1880; St. Louis, Missouri, pharmaceutical manufacturer 1881-1884; Chicago College of Pharmacy professor 1884-1886; Northwestern University College of Pharmacy dean 1886-1911; International Pharmaceutical Congress (Chicago) secretary 1893; *Bulletin of Pharmacy* editor 1895-1898. Died February 27, 1913, in Pasadena, California.

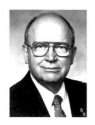

Robert Joseph Osterhaus

(1931-   )

APhA president 1992-1993. Born in Dyersville, Iowa, January 30, 1931. Iowa University College of Pharmacy B.S. 1952. U.S. Army 1952-1954; Anamosa, Iowa, community pharmacist 1954-1965, Maquoketa 1965-. Iowa Pharmaceutical Association House of Delegates speaker 1980-1981, president 1983-1984; Iowa Board of Pharmacy member 1972-1977, chairman 1974-1976; International Pharmaceutical Federation community pharmacists section executive committee 1990-1996; American Council on Pharmaceutical Education president 2000-; Iowa state legislator (34th District House of Representatives) 1996-.

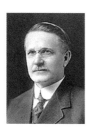

Charles Herbert Packard

(1863-1937)

APhA president 1920-1921, second vice president 1914-1915, third vice president 1912-1913. Born in Amherst, Massachusetts, in 1863. Massachusetts College of Pharmacy Ph.G. 1892, president 1909-1922. Apprenticed pharmacy in Boston 1880-1884; Boston community pharmacist 1885-1937; Massachusetts Pharmaceutical Association president 1907-1908; Boston Druggists' Association treasurer 1917-1937. Died October 3, 1937, in Boston, Massachusetts.

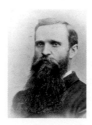

Emlen Painter

(1844-1890)

APhA president 1889-1890, first vice president 1881-1882, third vice president 1877-1878, Scientific Section chairman 1888-1889. Born in Concord, Pennsylvania, September 8, 1844. Philadelphia College of Pharmacy Ph.G. 1866. Apprenticed pharmacy in Philadelphia 1860-1864; San Francisco, California, community pharmacist 1867-1883, New York City 1883-1889; California College of Pharmacy professor 1876-1883; New York College of Pharmacy trustee 1885-1888. Died January 15, 1890, in Spuyten Duyvil, New York, while serving as APhA president.

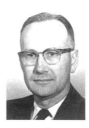

Lloyd McClain Parks

(1912-   )

APhA president 1971-1972, vice president 1970-1971, Council chairman 1967-1969, Foundation president 1976-1979, task force on pharmacy education vice chairman 1982-1984. Born in Scottsburg, Indiana, March 21, 1912. Purdue University School of Pharmacy B.S. 1933, M.S. 1936; University of Wisconsin Ph.D. 1938, instructor 1938-1940, professor 1946-1956. World War II veteran 1941-1945; Mishawaka, Indiana, community pharmacist 1933-1934; Ohio State University College of Pharmacy dean 1956-1977. American Association of Colleges of Pharmacy president 1961-1962; Rho Chi president 1961-1963.

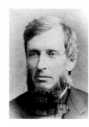

Edward Parrish

(1822-1872)

APhA president 1868-1869, first vice president 1866-1867, recording secretary 1853-1854, corresponding secretary 1857-1858. Born in Philadelphia, Pennsylvania, May 31, 1822. Philadelphia College of Pharmacy Ph.G. 1842, secretary 1854-1864, professor 1864-1872. Apprenticed pharmacy in Philadelphia 1838-1840; Philadelphia community pharmacist 1843-1872; Died September 19, 1872, in Fort Sill, Indian Territory (Oklahoma), where he was serving as a U.S. Government commissioner to manage the Indian tribes.

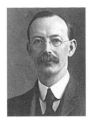

Edgar Leonard Patch
(1851-1924)

APhA president 1893-1894, Scientific Section chairman 1890-1891. Born in Spencer, Massachusetts, December 2, 1851. Massachusetts College of Pharmacy Ph.G. 1872, treasurer 1874-1878, professor 1879-1892. Apprenticed pharmacy in Boston 1869-1870; Boston community pharmacist 1870-1888; E. L. Patch Company (Stoneham, Massachusetts) president 1888-1924. Boston Druggists' Association president 1917-1918; Stoneham, Massachusetts, YMCA president. Died February 27, 1924, in Stoneham, Massachusetts.

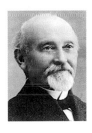

John Franklin Patton
(1839-1919)

APhA president 1900-1901. Born in Lower Windsor, Pennsylvania. Apprenticed pharmacy in York, Pennsylvania, 1856-1859; Baltimore, Maryland, community pharmacist 1859-1866, York, Pennsylvania, 1869-1919. Pennsylvania Pharmaceutical Association president 1891-1892; National Retail Druggists Association executive committee member 1884-1885. Died March 17, 1919, in York, Pennsylvania.

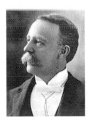

George Frederick Payne
(1853-1923)

APhA president 1902-1903, first vice president 1896-1897 and 1898-1899, second vice president 1901-1902. Born in Macon, Georgia, April 7, 1853. New York College of Pharmacy Ph.G. 1876; Atlanta Medical College M.D. 1891. Apprenticed in father's Macon pharmacy; Macon, Georgia, community pharmacist 1877-1890; Atlanta College of Pharmacy professor 1891-1899, dean 1899-1910, president 1910-1922. Georgia Pharmaceutical Association vice president 1893-1894; Georgia Board of Pharmacy secretary 1899-1906; National Association of Boards of Pharmacy first vice president 1904-1905. Died April 18, 1923, in Atlanta, Georgia.

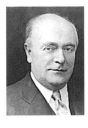

Waldemar Bruce Philip
(1878-1936)

APhA president 1932-1933, third vice president 1923-1924, House of Delegates chairman 1924-1925, Commercial Interests Section chairman 1924-1925. Born in Sacramento, California, July 19, 1878. University of California College of Pharmacy Ph.G. 1903; New York College of Pharmacy Pharm.D. 1904; University of California LL.B. 1923. Apprenticed pharmacy in Sacramento and Fresno, California; Fruitvale, California, community pharmacist 1905-1920. National Association of Retail Druggists vice president and counsel; Kappa Psi grand regent 1925-1932. Died July 13, 1936 in Oakland, California.

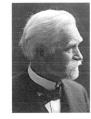

Albert Benjamin Prescott
(1832-1905)

APhA president 1899-1900, second vice president 1885-1886, Council chairman 1901-1902. Born in Hastings, New York, December 12, 1832. University of Michigan M.D. 1864, professor 1865-1876; Civil War U.S. Army assistant surgeon; University of Michigan School of Pharmacy dean 1876-1905. American Chemical Society president 1886; American Association for the Advancement of Science president 1891. Died February 25, 1905, in Ann Arbor, Michigan.

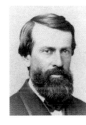

William Procter, Jr.
(1817-1874)

APhA president 1862-1863, first vice president 1859-1860, corresponding secretary 1852-1857. Born in Baltimore, Maryland, May 3, 1817. Philadelphia College of Pharmacy Ph.G. 1837, professor 1846-1866 and 1872-1874, secretary 1855-1867, president 1867-1868 and 1869-1874. Apprenticed pharmacy in Philadelphia, Pennsylvania, 1831-1836; Philadelphia community pharmacist 1844-1874; *American Journal of Pharmacy* editor 1850-1871; International Pharmaceutical Conference (Paris) vice president 1867. Died February 10, 1874, in Philadelphia, Pennsylvania.

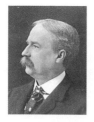

Joseph Price Remington
(1847-1918)

APhA president 1892-1893, general secretary 1893-1894. Born in Philadelphia, Pennsylvania, March 26, 1847. Philadelphia College of Pharmacy Ph.G. 1866, professor 1874-1918, dean 1893-1918. Edward R. Squibb & Co. pharmacist 1867-1869; Powers & Weightman pharmacist 1870-1872; Philadelphia community pharmacist 1872-1885. Pennsylvania Pharmaceutical Association president 1896-1897; USP Committee of Revision first vice chairman 1880-1890, chairman 1901-1918; International Pharmaceutical Congress (Chicago) president 1893. Died January 1, 1918, in Philadelphia, Pennsylvania.

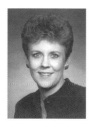

Marily Harper Rhudy
(1948-   )

APhA president 1991-1992, treasurer 1985-1988. Born in Colby, Kansas, February 15, 1948. University of Kansas School of Pharmacy B.S. 1972. Topeka, Kansas, community pharmacist 1975-1993; Wyeth-Ayerst Laboratories public affairs vice president 1993-1997; American Home Products global vice president, public affairs 1997-. Kansas Pharmaceutical Association president 1978-1979.

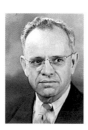

Richard Quintus Richards
(1892-1968)

APhA president 1952-1953, House of Delegates chairman 1949-1950, Council chairman 1955-1956, Foundation vice president 1953-1958. Born in Sandersville, Georgia, December 1, 1892. Emory University Medical School attended 1912-1914. Lakeland, Florida, community pharmacist 1915-1919, Fort Myers, Florida 1920-1965; Florida Pharmaceutical Association secretary 1940-1965; *Florida Pharmacist* editor 1937-1965. Florida Board of Pharmacy secretary 1940-1950; National Association of Boards of Pharmacy president 1946-1947. Died June 1, 1968, in Fort Myers, Florida.

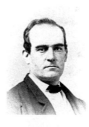

Joseph Roberts
(1824-1888)

APhA president 1885-1886, first vice president 1874-1875, second vice president 1859-1860. Born in Baltimore, Maryland, February 15, 1824. New York College of Pharmacy Ph.G. 1845. Apprenticed pharmacy in New York City, 1841-1843; Baltimore community pharmacist 1846-1888; Maryland College of Pharmacy president 1878-1888; Baltimore City Council serving two terms. Died January 31, 1888, in Baltimore, Maryland.

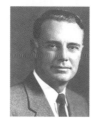

Ronald V. Robertson
(1903-1962)

APhA president 1960-1961, first vice president 1956-1957, second vice president 1954-1955. Born in La Grande, Oregon, August 5, 1903. Washington State University College of Pharmacy Ph.C., B.S.. Spokane, Washington, community pharmacist 1925-1962. American College of Apothecaries president 1949-1950; Washington State Society for Crippled Children president; Spokane Kiwanis Club president. Died June 3, 1962, in Spokane, Washington.

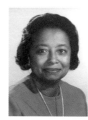

Mary Munson Runge
(1928-   )

APhA president 1979-1980, House of Delegates speaker 1977-1978. Born in Donaldsonville, Louisiana, July 25, 1928. Xavier University College of Pharmacy B.S. 1948. Richmond, California, community pharmacist 1949-1951, Oakland 1971-1991; Martinez, California, hospital pharmacist 1951-1965, San Pablo 1965-1971. California Society of Hospital Pharmacists president 1967-1968; California Pharmaceutical Association president 1974-1975, Education Foundation president 1978-1992; California Board of Pharmacy member 1983-1991, vice president 1986-1988. National Pharmaceutical Association Chauncey I. Cooper award (first recipient) 1997.

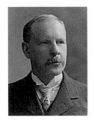

Henry Hurd Rusby
(1855-1940)

APhA president 1909-1910, second vice president 1907-1908, Scientific Section chairman 1898-1899. Born in Franklin, New Jersey, April 26, 1855. New York University Medical College M.D. 1884. Smithsonian Institution botanical expedition 1880; Parke-Davis & Co. expeditions 1885-1887; H. K. Mulford & Co. expedition 1921-1922; New York College of Pharmacy professor 1888-1930, dean 1905-1930. Died November 18, 1940, in Sarasota, Florida.

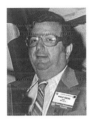

Philip Sacks
(1919-1997)

APhA president 1977-1978, House of Delegates speaker 1971-1972, Foundation vice president 1979-1985. Born in Wilmette, Illinois, July 18, 1919. University of Illinois College of Pharmacy B.S. 1940. World War II combat medic veteran; Illinois community pharmacist 1951-1978. Chicago Retail Druggists Association president 1965-1966; Illinois Pharmaceutical Association president 1969-1970; Illinois Board of Pharmacy member 1968-1976, chairman 1972-1974; Retired to Fort Lauderdale, Florida in 1979 where he died January 22, 1997.

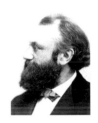

Enno Sander
(1822-1912)

APhA president 1871-1872, second vice president 1864-1865, honorary president 1909-1910. Born in Trinum, Germany, February 27, 1822. Baden (Germany) assistant secretary of war 1849, taken prisoner during Baden Revolution, exiled to America 1850; St. Louis community pharmacist 1853-1861; Civil War veteran 1862-1865; St. Louis analytical laboratory manager 1865-1894; St. Louis College of Pharmacy president 1859-1860, professor 1871-1874; Enno Sander Mineral Water Company president 1894-1912; St. Louis Academy of Science treasurer 1862-1890. Died February 12, 1912, in St. Louis, Missouri.

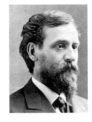

Eziekiel Henry Sargent
(1830-1904)

APhA president 1869-1870, second vice president 1866-1867. Born in Dover, New Hampshire, November 13, 1830. Apprenticed pharmacy in Lowell, Massachusetts, 1844-1851; Chicago community pharmacist 1852-1904. Chicago College of Pharmacy charter member 1859; Illinois Pharmaceutical Association founding member 1880. Died April 24, 1904, in Chicago, Illinois.

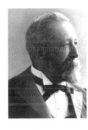

William Saunders
(1836-1914)

APhA president 1877-1878, first vice president 1873-1874, played role in bringing 1877 annual meeting to Toronto. Born in Devonshire, England, June 16, 1836. Came to Canada 1848. Ontario College of Pharmacy president 1879-1881; Canadian Pharmaceutical Association founding member 1867; Dominion Experimental Farms (Ottawa) director 1886-1911. Died September 13, 1914, in London, Ontario, Canada.

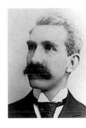

Lucius Elmer Sayre
(1846-1925)

APhA president 1919-1920, second vice president 1916-1917, Scientific Section chairman 1893-1894, Historical Section chairman 1917-1918. Born in Bridgeton, New Jersey, November 2, 1846. Philadelphia College of Pharmacy Ph.G. 1866. Apprenticed pharmacy in Bridgeton 1862-1865; Frederick Brown Manufacturing Chemist Laboratory director 1866-1869; Philadelphia community pharmacist 1869-1884; Women's Medical College of Philadelphia lecturer on pharmacy 1880-1885; University of Kansas School of Pharmacy dean 1885-1925; Kansas Board of Health director of drug analysis 1907-1925. Died July 21, 1925, in Lawrence, Kansas.

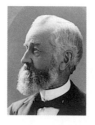

William Martin Searby
(1835-1909)

APhA president 1907-1908, first vice president 1901-1902, second vice president 1889-1890, Council chairman 1908-1909. Born in Croft, Lincolnshire, England, January 21, 1835. Pharmaceutical Society of Great Britain qualified 1855. Apprenticed pharmacy in Guilford, England, 1849-1854; Norwich, England, community pharmacist 1857-1859; Victoria, British Columbia, Canada, 1860-1865; San Francisco, California, 1866-1906; California College of Pharmacy professor 1873-1881, dean 1891-1909; California Board of Pharmacy president 1897-1905; *Pacific Drug Review* editor 1892-1894; *Pacific Pharmacist* editor 1907-1909. Died October 7, 1909, in San Francisco, California.

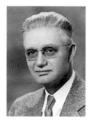

Earl Roy Serles
(1890-1957)

APhA president 1946-1948, House of Delegates chairman 1937-1938. Born in Salem, South Dakota, November 18, 1890. South Dakota State School of Pharmacy Ph.G. 1911, B.S. 1915, faculty member 1913-1923, dean 1923-1940; University of Minnesota Ph.D. 1934. World War I U.S. Army chemical warfare service veteran 1917-1918; University of Illinois College of Pharmacy dean 1940-1957. American Association of Colleges of Pharmacy president 1938-1939. Died March 13, 1957, in River Forest, Illinois.

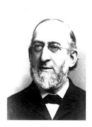

James Thornton Shinn
(1834-1907)

APhA president 1880-1881. Born in Philadelphia, Pennsylvania, January 9, 1834. Philadelphia College of Pharmacy Ph.G. 1854, treasurer 1894-1907. Apprenticed pharmacy with Charles Ellis & Co.; Philadelphia community pharmacist 1855-1907; Working Home of Blind Men manager 1876-1884; Pennsylvania Hospital secretary 1890-1907; Pennsylvania Board of Pharmacy founding secretary 1872-1887; Association Center of University Extension Teaching president 1896-1907. Died October 4, 1907, in Bryn Mawr, Pennsylvania.

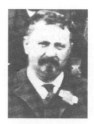

Karl Simmon
(1854-1911)

APhA president 1890, first vice president 1889-1890, third vice president 1887-1888. Born in New York City, December 1854. Apprenticed pharmacy in St. Paul, Minnesota, 1871-1874; St. Paul, Minnesota, community pharmacist (as owner) 1875-1889, (as employee) 1890-1895. Minnesota Pharmaceutical Association secretary 1888-1890; Northern Pacific Railway sales solicitor in Helena, Montana, 1895-1905. Died June 19, 1911, in St. Paul, Minnesota.

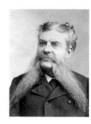

William Simpson
(1839-1905)

APhA president 1894-1895, third vice president 1880-1881. Born in New York City, May 21, 1839. Apprenticed pharmacy in New York City, Warrenton, North Carolina, and Richmond, Virginia 1855-1860; Civil War Confederate Army veteran 1862-1865; Raleigh, North Carolina, community pharmacist 1867-1905. North Carolina Pharmaceutical Association president 1882-1883; North Carolina Board of Pharmacy secretary 1881-1902; Shaw University (a Raleigh, North Carolina, institution for Negro students) Leonard School of Pharmacy dean 1893-1905. Died June 23, 1905, in Raleigh, North Carolina.

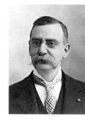

George White Sloan
(1835-1903)

APhA president 1879-1880. Born in Harrisburg, Pennsylvania, June 28, 1835. Apprenticed pharmacy in Indianapolis, Indiana, 1848-1850. Indianapolis, Indiana, community pharmacist 1850-1903; Civil War veteran 1862-1865. Indianapolis Pharmaceutical Association founding vice president 1874-1875; Indiana Board of Pharmacy founding president 1901-1902, secretary 1902-1903; Interstate Retail Druggists' League founding treasurer 1891-1893; Indianapolis School Board president. Died February 15, 1903, in Indianapolis, Indiana.

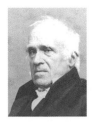

Daniel B. Smith
(1792-1883)

APhA founding president 1852-1853, honorary president 1856. Born in Philadelphia, Pennsylvania, July 14, 1792. Apprenticed pharmacy in Philadelphia 1812-1818. Philadelphia community pharmacist 1819-1853; Philadelphia College of Pharmacy founding secretary 1821-1828, first vice president 1828-1829, president 1829-1854. Society for the Prevention of Pauperism founding secretary 1817-1823; Philadelphia Savings Fund manager 1819-1835; Franklin Institute founding member 1824-1874; Pennsylvania Historical Society founding corresponding secretary 1825-1826; Haverford College professor 1834-1846. Died March 29, 1883, in Germantown, Pennsylvania.

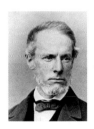

Richard Hartshorn Stabler
(1820-1878)

APhA president 1870-1871, first vice president 1864-1865. Born in Alexandria, Virginia, December 1, 1820. University of Pennsylvania M.D. 1843. Apprenticed pharmacy in Alexandria, Virginia, with his father Edward Stabler 1836-1840; Alexandria community pharmacist 1844-1878; National College of Pharmacy professor 1872-1878. Died November 18, 1878, in Alexandria, Virginia.

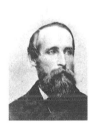

Frederick Stearns
(1831-1907)

APhA president 1866-1867, first vice president 1864-1865. Born in Lockport, New York, April 8, 1831. Apprenticed pharmacy in Buffalo, New York, 1845-1853. Detroit, Michigan, community pharmacist 1854-1881; Frederick Stearns & Company president 1871-1887; established branches in Australia, Canada, and Great Britain; among first to use steam power in pharmaceutical laboratory; devoted remainder of life to collecting objects of historical and scientific interest. Died January 13, 1907, in Savannah, Georgia.

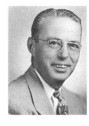

Newell W. Stewart
(1900-1989)

APhA president 1954-1955, House of Delegates chairman 1950-1951. Born in Sistersville, West Virginia. University of West Virginia School of Pharmacy Ph.G. 1923. World War I veteran 1918-1919; Moundsville, West Virginia community pharmacist 1923-1926; Phoenix, Arizona, 1926-1952; Phoenix mayor 1942-1944; Arizona Pharmaceutical Association secretary 1947-1954; Arizona Board of Pharmacy secretary 1942-1953; National Pharmaceutical Council executive vice president 1954-1965. National Association of Boards of Pharmacy president 1948-1949. Died March 12, 1989, in Phoenix, Arizona.

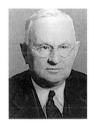

Robert Lee Swain
(1887-1963)

APhA president 1933-1934, House of Delegates chairman 1929-1930, Council chairman 1958-1959. Born in Redden, Delaware, September 29, 1887. University of Maryland Pharm.D. 1909, LL.B. 1932. Sykesville, Maryland, community pharmacist 1909-1927; *Maryland Pharmacist* editor 1925-1939; Maryland Board of Pharmacy secretary 1925-1940; Temple University School of Pharmacy professor 1938-1948; *Drug Topics* editor 1939-1960. Maryland Pharmaceutical Association president 1937-1938; National Association of Boards of Pharmacy president 1928-1929, treasurer 1940-1957; USP Board of Trustees chairman 1944-1959. Died February 4, 1963, in Jackson Heights, New York.

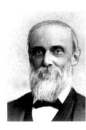

Alfred Bower Taylor
(1824-1898)

APhA president 1890-1891, founding member 1852, treasurer 1852-1854. Born in Philadelphia, Pennsylvania, January 6, 1824. Philadelphia College of Pharmacy Ph.G. 1844, corresponding secretary 1867-1886. Apprenticed pharmacy in Philadelphia 1841-1843; New York City community pharmacist 1845-1847, Philadelphia 1847-1887; Philadelphia Inspector of Drugs 1848. USP Committee of Revision secretary 1860-1880. Died February 28, 1898, in Philadelphia, Pennsylvania.

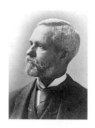

William Scott Thompson
(1838-1901)

APhA president 1883-1884, second vice president 1880-1881 and 1897-1898, Council chairman 1886-1887 and 1894-1901. Born in Frederick County, Maryland, February 14, 1838. Apprenticed pharmacy in District of Columbia 1850-1854; community pharmacist 1854-1901. District of Columbia Board of Pharmacy founding president 1878-1888; National College of Pharmacy founder 1871; USP Convention first vice president 1890-1900; USP Board of Trustees chairman 1900-1901. Died September 26, 1901, in the District of Columbia.

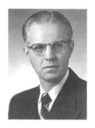

Linwood Franklin Tice
(1909-1996)

APhA president 1966-1967, House of Delegates chairman 1964-1965. Born in Salem, New Jersey, February 17, 1909. Philadelphia College of Pharmacy Ph.C. 1929, B.Sc. 1933, M.Sc. 1935, professor 1938-1956, dean 1959-1975; *American Journal of Pharmacy* editor 1941-1977. Baylor University professor 1930-1931; U.S. Coast Guard during World War II. American Association of Colleges of Pharmacy president 1955-1956; American Council on Pharmaceutical Education vice president 1964-1966; American Association for the Advancement of Science vice president 1972-1973. Died August 18, 1996, in Salem, New Jersey.

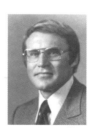

Kenneth Edward Tiemann
(1929-   )

APhA president 1975-1976. Born in Seguin, Texas, July 12, 1929. University of Texas College of Pharmacy B.S. 1952, M.S. 1958, Ph.D. 1983, adjunct associate professor 1980-1988. Austin, Texas, community pharmacist 1961-1994; American Pharmaceutical Services consultant 1994-. Capitol Area (Texas) Pharmaceutical Association president 1963-1964; Texas Society of Hospital Pharmacists secretary 1958-1959; Texas Pharmaceutical Association vice president 1966-1967, president 1968-1969.

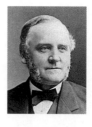

Charles Augustus Tufts
(1822-1899)

APhA president 1886-1887, second vice president 1863-1864, treasurer 1865-1886. Born in New Hampshire 1822. Massachusetts College of Pharmacy Ph.G.; Dartmouth Medical College M.D. Dover, New Hampshire, community pharmacist 1849-1899. New Hampshire Pharmaceutical Association president 1874-1875; New Hamphire Board of Pharmacy president 1875-1899; Dover City Council member 1868-1870, alderman 1872-1874, chairman 1892-1894; Dover School Board member 1874-1881; New Hampshire state senator 1861-1862. Died February 12, 1899, in Dover, New Hampshire.

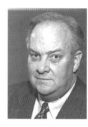

Timothy Lee Vordenbaumen, Sr.
(1939-   )

APhA president 1994-1995, APhA-PAC founding chairman/treasurer 1986-1991. Born in San Antonio, Texas, December 20, 1939. University of Texas College of Pharmacy B.S. 1964; ex-students association president. San Antonio, Texas, community pharmacist 1964-1993, T. L. Vordenbaumen & Associates (data processing) president 1979-1991; American Pharmaceutical Services regulatory affairs vice president 1993-. Bexar County Pharmaceutical Association secretary 1965-1969, president 1972-1973; Texas Pharmaceutical Association president 1978-1979, secretary 1970-1971, House of Delegates chairman 1974-1975, treasurer 1981-1983. Good Samaritan board of directors.

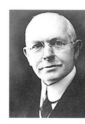

Lucius Leedom Walton
(1865-1935)

APhA president 1925-1926, House of Delegates chairman 1923-1924. Born in Clinton, New Jersey, July 8, 1865. Philadelphia College of Pharmacy Ph.G. 1888. Danbury, Connecticut, community pharmacist 1888-1892, Williamsport, Pennsylvania 1892-1935. Pennsylvania Pharmaceutical Association president 1908-1909; Pennsylvania Board of Pharmacy secretary 1909-1926; National Association of Boards of Pharmacy president 1921-1922. Died December 26, 1935, in Clifton Springs, New York.

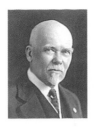

Henry Milton Whelpley
(1861-1926)

APhA president 1901-1902, treasurer 1908-1921, acting general secretary 1893, Scientific Section chairman 1889-1890. Born in Harmonia, Michigan, May 24, 1861. St. Louis College of Pharmacy Ph.G. 1883, dean 1904-1926; Missouri Medical College M.D. 1890. Apprenticed pharmacy in Otsego, Michigan, and Cobden, Illinois; *National Druggist* editor 1884-1887; *Meyer Brothers Druggist* editor 1888-1926. Missouri Pharmaceutical Association secretary 1892-1922; American Association of Colleges of Pharmacy president 1905-1906; USP Convention secretary 1900-1910; USP Board of Trustees secretary 1910-1926; St. Louis Anthropology Society president 1921-1925. Died June 26, 1926, in Argentine, Kansas.

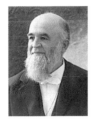

Henry Martin Whitney
(1827-1903)

APhA president 1897-1898, Council vice chairman 1892-1895. Born in Winchendon, Massachusetts, August 21, 1827. Apprenticed pharmacy in Boston, Massachusetts, 1844-1849; Boston community pharmacist 1849-1899. Massachusetts Pharmaceutical Association president 1891-1892; Massachusetts Board of Pharmacy president 1885-1899; Edison Electric Light Company treasurer 1892-1899. Died December 2, 1903, in North Andover, Massachusetts.

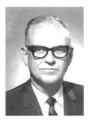

William Ray Whitten
(1921-   )

APhA president 1970-1971, House of Delegates speaker 1966-1967, North Texas APhA Chapter president. Born in Bogata, Texas, August 25, 1921. University of Texas College of Pharmacy B.S. 1947. Fort Worth, Texas, community pharmacist 1953-1977; realtor 1978-. Texas Board of Pharmacy president 1967-1968.

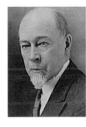

Frederick John Wulling
(1866-1947)

APhA president 1916-1917. Born in Brooklyn, New York, December 24, 1866. New York College of Pharmacy Ph.G. 1888. *Pharmaceutical Record* associate editor 1887-1891; Brooklyn College of Pharmacy professor 1891-1892; University of Minnesota College of Pharmacy founding dean 1892-1947. American Association of Colleges of Pharmacy president 1914-1915; Minnesota Academy of Sciences chairman 1910. Died October 21, 1947, in Minneapolis, Minnesota.

APhA Presidents (*Pro Tem*)

Nine 19th-century presidents failed to attend the meeting at which their term expired; in each case, a President Pro Tem was seated at the opening of the convention, serving only until the new president was elected within 24 hours. Three of the Presidents Pro Tem also served a full term as elected APhA presidents (Colcord, Moore, and Stearns) and are therefore covered in the preceding biographies.

Robert Battey
(1828-1895)

APhA president *pro tem* 1850, third vice president 1858-1859. Born in Augusta, Georgia, November 26, 1828. Philadelphia College of Pharmacy Ph.G. 1856; Jefferson Medical College M.D. 1857. Served four years in Confederate Army as surgeon during Civil War; Atlanta Medical College professor 1872-1875; Georgia Medical Association president; developed gynecological procedure for surgical removal of ovaries; established first hospital in Rome, Georgia. Died November 8, 1895, in Rome, Georgia.

Ferris Bringhurst
(1837-1871)

APhA president *pro tem* 1869, first vice president 1868-1869. Born in Wilmington, Delaware, in 1837. Philadelphia College of Pharmacy Ph.G. 1857. Operated Wilmington pharmacy established by his father, Edward Bringhurst, Sr. Died from an accidental explosion in his laboratory, March 16, 1871, in Wilmington, Delaware.

Henry Thornton Cummings
(1822-1901)

APhA president *pro tem* 1855, first vice president 1854-1855. Born in Yarmouth, Maine, November 12, 1822. Bowdoin College graduate 1841; Harvard Medical School M.D. 1843. Deafness caused him to give up medical practice and open a pharmacy in Portland, Maine, 1845-1892. Maine Pharmaceutical Association founding president 1867-1873; Maine Board of Pharmacy founding president 1877-1892; moved to Tacoma, Washington, in 1892 where he died December 15, 1901.

Charles B. Guthrie
(1815-1875?)

APhA president *pro tem* 1854, first vice president 1855-1856, third vice president 1853-1854, New York City 1851 convention (precursor to founding of APhA) president. Born in Logan, Ohio, 1815. Memphis Medical College M.D. 1853, faculty 1853-1855. New York City community pharmacist 1848-1852, Memphis, Tennessee, 1853-1855; New York College of Pharmacy trustee 1850-1852; Memphis City Dispensary for the Poor director 1853-1855; New York City drug broker 1855-1870; Orange, New Jersey, contractor 1870-1874. Probably died in Orange, New Jersey, in 1875.

Henry Joseph Menninger
(1838-1890)

APhA president *pro tem* 1887, first vice president 1886-1887. Born in Metz, Germany, 1838. Came to America 1850. New York College of Pharmacy Ph.G. 1861, vice president 1877-1890. Apprenticed pharmacy in New York City 1858-1860; Civil War medical staff veteran; appointed North Carolina military secretary by President Andrew Johnson; New Bern and Raleigh, North Carolina, community pharmacist 1865-1873; Brooklyn, New York, community pharmacist 1873-1890; elected Brooklyn alderman for three terms. Died September 8, 1890, in Brooklyn, New York.

George Henry Schafer
(1847-1923)

APhA president *pro tem* 1881, first vice president 1880-1881, honorary president 1914-1915. Born in Fort Madison, Iowa, July 15, 1847. Apprenticed pharmacy in Fort Madison 1862-1867; Fort Madison community pharmacist 1868-1872; manufacturing pharmacist 1872-1923. Iowa Pharmaceutical Association founding president 1880-1881; Iowa Board of Pharmacy founding secretary 1880-1888. Died April 8, 1923, in Fort Madison, Iowa.

APhA Chief Executive Officers

In 1852, the Association elected both a Recording Secretary who "kept the Association's minutes," and a Corresponding Secretary who "attended to the official correspondence of the Association." In 1865, the two secretaries were merged into a single office called "permanent secretary," creating the first chief executive officer. In 1895 the title of the office was changed to "general secretary," and in 1945 the title became "secretary and general manager." The title of APhA's chief executive officer changed to "executive director" in 1959, and then in 1989 the title was converted to "executive vice president."

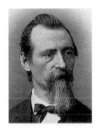

John Michael Maisch
permanent secretary 1866-1893

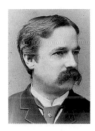

Joseph Price Remington
permanent secretary 1893-1894

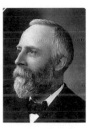

Charles Caspari, Jr.
general secretary 1894-1911

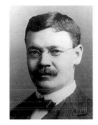

James Hartley Beal
general secretary 1911-1914

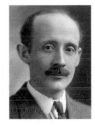

William Baker Day
general secretary 1914-1925

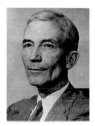

Evander Frank Kelly
general secretary 1925-1944

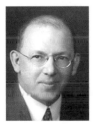

Robert Phillip Fischelis
secretary and general manager
1944-1959

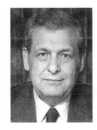

William Shoulden Apple
executive director 1959-1983

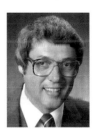

Maurice Quinn Bectel
acting executive director
1983-1984

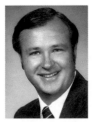

John F. Schlegel
executive director 1984-1989

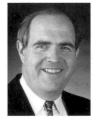

John A. Gans
executive vice president 1989-

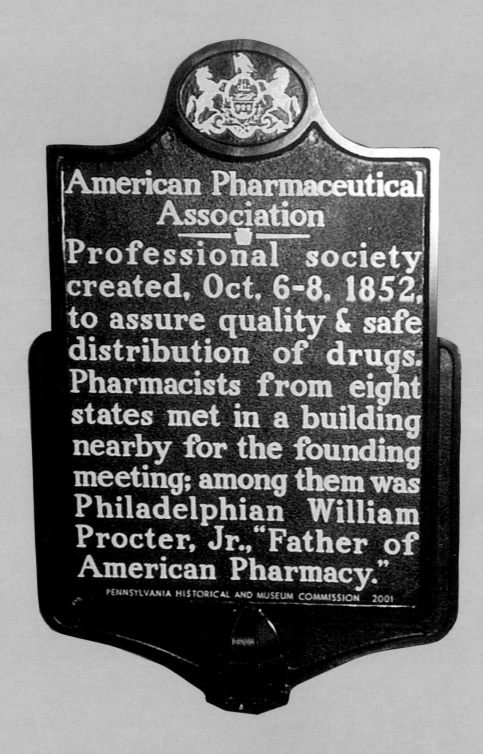

Official Commonwealth of Pennsylvania historical marker commemorating the founding on October 6-8, 1852, of the American Pharmaceitical Association. The marker was installed October 24, 2001, on Seventh Street near Market Street in Philadelphia, near the building where APhA was founded.

The Leadership of APhA 1852-2002

APhA Presidents

Two presidents died in office (identified by +) and the first vice president assumed the presidency (identified by ++). Nine 19th-century presidents failed to attend the meeting at which their term expired; in each case, a vice president was elevated to president at the opening of the convention, serving only until the new president was elected (identified by °). A resignation is identified by @. Three pairs are father and son indentified by #. [NOTE: Holton was the son of 1917 president Charles Holzhauer, but Holton changed his last name.]

Term	President	Birth-Death	Term	President	Birth-Death
1852-1853	Daniel B. Smith	(1792-1883)	1875-1876	George Frederic Holmes Markoe	(1840-1896)
1853	Samuel Marshall Colcord *	(1817-1895)	1876-1877	Charles Bullock	(1826-1900)
1853-1854	William A. Brewer	(1807-1890)	1877-1878	William Saunders	(1836-1914)
1854	Charles B. Guthrie °	(1815-1875)	1878-1879	Gustavus Johann Luhn	(1839-1888)
1854-1855	William Barker Chapman	(1813-1874)	1879-1880	George White Sloan	(1835-1903)
1855	Henry Thornton Cummings °	(1822-1902)	1880-1881	James Thornton Shinn	(1834-1907)
1855-1856	John Meakim	(1812-1863)	1881	George Henry Schafer °	(1847-1919)
1856-1857	George Wansey Andrews	(1800-1877)	1881-1882	Peter Wendover Bedford	(1836-1892)
1857	Frederick Stearns °	(1831-1907)	1882-1883	Charles Augustus Heinitsh	(1822-1898)
1857-1858	Charles Ellis	(1800-1874)	1883-1884	William Scott Thompson	(1838-1901)
1858-1859	John Lawrence Kidwell	(1819-1885)	1884-1885	John Ingalls	(1829-1898)
1859	Robert Battey *	(1828-1895)	1885-1886	Joseph Roberts	(1824-1888)
1859-1860	Samuel Marshall Colcord	(1817-1895)	1886-1887	Charles Augustus Tufts	(1822-1899)
1860-1862	Henry Taylor Kiersted	(1793-1882)	1887	Henry Joseph Menninger °	(1838-1890)
1862-1863	William Procter, Jr.	(1817-1874)	1887-1888	John Uri Lloyd	(1849-1936)
1863-1864	Jacob Faris Moore	(1826-1888)	1888-1889	Maurice William Alexander	(1835-1898)
1864-1865	William John Maclester Gordon	(1825-1909)	1889-1890	Emlen Painter +	(1844-1890)
1865-1866	Henry Ware Lincoln	(1822-1887)	1890	Karl Simmon ++	(1854-1911)
1866-1867	Frederick Stearns	(1831-1907)	1890-1891	Alfred Bower Taylor	(1824-1898)
1867-1868	John Milhau	(1795-1874)	1891-1892	Alexander Kirkwood Finlay	(1843-1911)
1868-1869	Edward Parrish	(1822-1872)	1892-1893	Joseph Price Remington	(1847-1918)
1869	Ferris Bringhurst °	(1837-1871)	1893-1894	Edgar Leonard Patch	(1851-1924)
1869-1870	Ezekial Henry Sargent	(1830-1904)	1894-1895	William Simpson	(1839-1905)
1870-1871	Richard Hartshorn Stabler	(1820-1878)	1895-1896	James Michener Good	(1842-1919)
1871	Jacob Faris Moore °	(1826-1888)	1896-1897	Joseph Edward Morrison	(1862-1913)
1871-1872	Enno Sander	(1822-1912)	1897-1898	Henry Martin Whitney	(1827-1903)
1872-1873	Albert Ethelbert Ebert	(1840-1906)	1898-1899	Charles Emile Dohme #	(1834-1911)
1873-1874	John Francis Hancock	(1834-1923)	1899-1900	Albert Benjamin Prescott	(1832-1905)
1874-1875	Conrad Lewis Diehl	(1840-1917)	1900-1901	John Franklin Patton	(1839-1919)

Term	President	Birth-Death
1901-1902	Henry Milton Whelpley	(1861-1926)
1902-1903	George Frederick Payne	(1853-1923)
1903-1904	Lewis Christopher Hopp	(1856-1925)
1904-1905	James Hartley Beal #	(1861-1945)
1905-1906	Joseph Lyon Lemberger	(1834-1927)
1906-1907	Leo Eliel	(1845-1911)
1907-1908	William Martin Searby	(1835-1909)
1908-1909	Oscar Oldberg	(1846-1913)
1909-1910	Henry Hurd Rusby	(1855-1940)
1910-1911	Eugene Gustave Eberle	(1863-1942)
1911-1912	John Granville Godding	(1853-1929)
1912-1913	William Baker Day	(1871-1938)
1913-1914	George Mahlon Beringer	(1860-1928)
1914-1915	Caswell Armstrong Mayo	(1862-1928)
1915-1916	William Charles Alpers	(1851-1917)
1916-1917	Frederick John Wulling	(1866-1947)
1917	Charles Holzhauer + #	(1848-1917)
1917-1918	Alfred Robert Louis Dohme ++ #	(1867-1952)
1918-1919	Charles Herbert LaWall	(1871-1937)
1919-1920	Lucius Elmer Sayre	(1847-1925)
1920-1921	Charles Herbert Packard	(1863-1937)
1921-1922	Samuel Louis Hilton	(1866-1944)
1922-1923	Julius Arnold Koch	(1865-1956)
1923-1924	Henry Vincome Arny	(1868-1943)
1924-1925	Charles William Holton #	(1882-1970)
1925-1926	Lucius Leedom Walton	(1865-1935)
1926-1927	Theodore James Bradley	(1874-1935)
1927-1928	Charles Willis Johnson	(1873-1949)
1928-1929	David Franklin Jones	(1869-1944)
1929-1930	Henry Armitt Brown Dunning	(1877-1962)
1930-1931	Henry C. Christensen	(1865-1947)
1931-1932	Walter Dickson Adams	(1871-1961)
1932-1933	Waldemar Bruce Philip	(1878-1936)
1933-1934	Robert Lee Swain	(1887-1963)
1934-1935	Robert Phillip Fischelis	(1891-1981)
1935-1936	Patrick Henry Costello	(1896-1971)
1936-1937	George Denton Beal #	(1887-1972)
1937-1938	Edmund Norris Gathercoal	(1874-1954)
1938-1939	J. Leon Lascoff	(1867-1943)
1939-1940	Andrew Grover DuMez	(1885-1948)
1940-1941	Charles Hall Evans	(1895-1983)
1941-1942	Bernard Victor Christensen	(1885-1956)
1942-1943	Roy Bird Cook	(1886-1961)
1943-1944	Ivor Griffith	(1891-1961)
1944-1946	George Allen Moulton	(1890-1981)
1946-1947	Earl Roy Serles	(1890-1957)
1947-1948	Sylvester Dretzka	(1892-1980)
1948-1949	Ernest Little	(1888-1973)
1949-1950	Glenn Llewellyn Jenkins	(1898-1979)
1950-1951	Henry Hamilton Gregg III	(1899-1982)

Term	President	Birth-Death
1951-1952	Don Eugene Francke	(1910-1978)
1952-1953	Richard Quintus Richards	(1892-1968)
1953-1954	Fred Royce Franzoni, Jr.	(1913-1965)
1954-1955	Newell W. Stewart	(1900-1989)
1955-1956	John B. Heinz	(1890-1965)
1956-1957	John A. MacCartney	(1905-1989)
1957-1958	Joseph B. Burt	(1895-1974)
1958-1959	Louis James Fischl, Jr.	(1894-1979)
1959-1960	Howard Chamberlain Newton	(1892-1964)
1960-1961	Ronald V. Robertson	(1903-1962)
1961-1962	James Warren Lansdowne	(1902-1972)
1962-1963	George Frances Archambault	(1909-2001)
1963-1964	Robert John Gillespie	(1917-1995)
1964-1965	John Curtis Nottingham	(1912-)
1965-1066	Grover Cleveland Bowles, Jr.	(1920-)
1966-1967	Linwood Franklin Tice	(1909-1996)
1967-1968	George W. Grider	(1914-)
1968-1969	Max Ward Eggleston	(1922-1997)
1969-1970	William B. Hennessy	(1911-1989)
1970-1971	William Ray Whitten	(1921-)
1971-1972	Lloyd McClain Parks	(1912-)
1972-1973	Clifton Joseph Latiolais	(1916-1995)
1973-1974	George David Denmark	(1934-)
1974-1975	Robert Charles Johnson	(1935-)
1975-1976	Kenneth Edward Tiemann	(1929-)
1976-1977	William Frank Appel	(1924-)
1977-1978	Philip Sacks	(1919-1997)
1978-1979	Jacob Willis Miller	(1927-)
1979-1980	Mary Munson Runge	(1928-)
1981	Leonard Grossman	(1917-)
1982	James Thomas Doluisio	(1935-)
1983	Maurice Quinn Bectel	(1935-)
1984	Herbert Sylvester Carlin	(1932-)
1985-1986	James Allen Main	(1945-)
1987	David Stephen Crawford	(1945-)
1988	Charles Rowand Green	(1943-)
1989-1990	Ronald David Cobb	(1945-)
1990-1991	Philip Paul Gerbino	(1947-)
1991-1992	Marily Harper Rhudy	(1948-)
1992-1993	Robert Joseph Osterhaus	(1931-)
1993-1994	Lowell John Anderson	(1939-)
1994-1995	Tim Lee Vordenbaumen, Sr.	(1939-)
1995	Robert Earl Davis @	(1951-)
1995-1997	Calvin Haines Knowlton	(1949-)
1997-1998	Gary William Kadlec	(1948-)
1998-1999	Ronald Philip Jordan	(1952-)
1999-2000	J. Lyle Bootman	(1950-)
2000-2001	Robert Daniel Gibson	(1925-)
2001-2002	Thomas Edward Menighan	(1952-)
2002-2003	Janet P. Engle	(1959-)

First Vice Presidents

Those who subsequently became APhA president are identified by °.

1852-1853	George Wansey Andrews °	Maryland	1906-1907	William Mittelbach	Missouri
1853-1854	George D. Coggeshall	New York	1907-1908	Oscar Oldberg °	Illinois
1854-1855	Henry Thornton Cummings °	Maine	1908-1909	Eugene Gustavus Eberle °	Texas
1855-1856	Charles B. Guthrie °	Tennessee	1909-1910	Clement Belton Lowe	Pennsylvania
1856-1857	John Lawrence Kidwell °	Washington, DC	1910-1911	William Baker Day °	Illinois
1857-1858	James Cooke	Virginia	1911-1912	Wilhelm Bodemann	Illinois
1858-1859	Edward Robinson Squibb	New York	1912-1913	Charles Mangan Ford	Colorado
1859-1860	William Procter, Jr. °	Pennsylvania	1913-1914	Franklin Muhlenberg Apple	Pennsylvania
1860-1862	William John M. Gordon °	Ohio	1914-1915	L. D. Havenhill	Kansas
1862-1863	John Milhau °	New York	1915-1916	Charles Herbert LaWall °	Pennsylvania
1863-1864	John Michael Maisch	Pennsylvania	1916-1917	Leonard Adams Seltzer	Michigan
1864-1865	Richard Hartshorn Stabler °	Virginia	1917-1918	Alfred Robert Louis Dohme °	Maryland
1865-1866	George C. Close	New York	1918-1919	Ferd Wilhelm Nitardy	New York
1866-1867	Edward Parrish °	Pennsylvania	1919-1920	Theodore James Bradley °	Massachusetts
1867-1868	Robert J. Brown	Kansas	1920-1921	Ernest Fullerton Cook	Pennsylvania
1868-1869	Ferris Bringhurst °	Delaware	1921-1922	Charles Edward Caspari	Missouri
1869-1870	Ferdinand W. Sennewald	Missouri	1922-1923	Edmund Norris Gathercoal °	Illinois
1870-1871	Fleming G. Grieve	Georgia	1923-1924	Lyman Frederic Kebler	Washington, DC
1871-1872	Conrad Lewis Diehl °	Kentucky	1924-1925	Paul Stewart Pittinger	Pennsylvania
1872-1873	Samuel S. Garrigues	Michigan	1925-1926	William Christine Anderson °	New York
1873-1874	William Saunders °	Ontario, Canada	1926-1927	George Judisch	Iowa
1874-1875	Joseph Roberts °	Maryland	1927-1928	Ambrose Hunsberger	Pennsylvania
1875-1876	Frederick Hoffmann	New York	1928-1929	Alfred Washington Pauley	Missouri
1876-1877	Samuel A. D. Sheppard	Massachusetts	1929-1930	Arthur L. I. Winne	Virginia
1877-1878	Ewen McIntyre	New York	1930-1931	Walter Dickson Adams °	Texas
1878-1879	Frederick T. Whiting	Massachusetts	1931-1932	John G. Beard	North Carolina
1879-1880	Thomas Roberts Baker	Virginia	1932-1933	Rowland Jones	South Dakota
1880-1881	George Henry Schafer °	Iowa	1933-1934	Robert Phillip Fischelis °	New Jersey
1881-1882	Emlen Painter °	California	1934-1935	George Denton Beal °	Pennsylvania
1882-1883	John Ingalls °	Georgia	1935-1936	Frank Anthony Delgado	Washington, DC
1883-1884	Charles Rice	New York	1936-1937	J. Leon Lascoff °	New York
1884-1885	John Alfred Dadd	Wisconsin	1937-1938	W. MacChilds	Kansas
1885-1886	Albert H. Hollister	Wisconsin	1938-1939	A. O. Michelsen	Oregon
1886-1887	Henry Joseph Menninger	New York	1939-1940	Francis Owen Taylor	Michigan
1887-1888	Maurice William Alexander °	Missouri	1940-1941	Harvey A. K. Whitney	Michigan
1888-1889	James Vernor	Michigan	1941-1942	J. K. Attwood	Florida
1889-1890	Karl Simmon °	Minnesota	1942-1943	Donald A. Clarke	New York
1890-1891	Alviso Burdett Stevens	Michigan	1943-1944	Paul G. Stodghill	Colorado
1891-1892	George John Seabury	New York	1944-1946	Charles E. Wilson	Mississippi
1892-1893	Andrew Peabody Preston	New Hampshire	1946-1947	A. Lee Adams	Illinois
1893-1894	Leo Eliel °	Indiana	1947-1948	Augustus J. Affleck	California
1894-1895	Charles Mangan Ford	Colorado	1948-1949	Mearl D. Pritchard	New York
1895-1896	Charles Emile Dohme °	Maryland	1949-1950	Harold C. Kinner	Washington, DC
1896-1897	George Frederick Payne °	Georgia	1950-1951	Roy A. Bowers	New Jersey
1897-1898	George Case Bartells	Illinois	1951-1952	Joseph B. Burt °	Nebraska
1898-1899	George Frederick Payne °	Georgia	1952-1953	Thomas D. Rowe	Michigan
1899-1900	Lewis Christopher Hopp °	Ohio	1953-1954	John A. MacCartney °	Michigan
1900-1901	James Hartley Beal °	Ohio	1954-1955	John B. Heinz °	Utah
1901-1902	William Martin Searby °	California	1955-1956	Troy C. Daniels	California
1902-1903	William Lincoln Cliffe	Pennsylvania	1956-1957	Ronald V. Robertson °	Washington
1903-1904	William Charles Alpers °	New York	1957-1958	James Warren Lansdowne °	Indiana
1904-1905	Philip Charles Candidus	Alabama	1958-1959	Stephen Wilson	Michigan
1905-1906	Charles Holzhauer °	New Jersey	1959-1960	Leo F. Godley	Texas

1960-1961	Robert John Gillespie °	Michigan		1970-1971	Lloyd McClain Parks °	Ohio
1961-1962	Rudolph H. Blythe	Pennsylvania		1971-1972	Jacob Willis Miller °	Kansas
1962-1963	John Curtis Nottingham °	Virginia		1972-1973	Robert Charles Johnson °	California
1963-1964	John Stadnik	Florida		1973-1974	Joe D. Taylor	Kentucky
1964-1965	Thomas J. Macek	Pennsylvania		1974-1975	Joseph E. McSoley	Indiana
1965-1966	Mike Harris	Arizona		1975-1976	M. Donald Pritchard	New York
1966-1967	Robert G. Gibbs	Iowa		1976-1977	Thomas H. Holland	Virginia
1967-1968	George David Denmark °	Massachusetts		1977-1978	Angele C. D'Angelo	New York
1968-1969	Victor M. Morganroth	Maryland		1978-1979	Charles C. Rabe	Missouri
1969-1970	Clifton Joseph Latiolais °	Ohio		1979-1980	Bernard J. Cimino	Florida
					Position abolished	

Second Vice Presidents

1852-1853	Samuel Marshall Colcord °	Massachusetts		1891-1892	Willard Horatio Torbert	Iowa
1853-1854	Alexander Duval	Virginia		1892-1893	Sidney Powell Watson	Georgia
1854-1855	John Meakim °	New York		1893-1894	Wiley Rogers	Kentucky
1855-1856	Charles Ellis °	Pennsylvania		1894-1895	John Newell Hurty	Indiana
1856-1857	Frederick Stearns °	Michigan		1895-1896	Adolph Brandenberger	Missouri
1857-1858	Samuel P. Peck	Vermont		1896-1897	William Arthur Frost	Minnesota
1858-1859	James O'Gallagher	Missouri		1897-1898	William Scott Thompson °	Washington, DC
1859-1860	Joseph Roberts °	Maryland		1898-1899	James Hartley Beal °	Ohio
1860-1862	William Silver Thompson °	Maryland		1899-1900	William Lawrene Dewoody	Arkansas
1862-1863	Eugene L. Massot	Missouri		1900-1901	John William Gayle	Kentucky
1863-1864	Charles Augustus Tufts °	New Hampshire		1901-1902	George Frederick Payne °	Georgia
1864-1865	Enno Sander °	Missouri		1902-1903	Eugene Gustave Eberle °	Texas
1865-1866	Elijah W. Sackrider	Ohio		1903-1904	Albert Michael Roehrig	New York
1866-1867	Ezekial Henry Sargent °	Illinois		1904-1905	William Mittelbach	Missouri
1867-1868	N. Hynson Jennings	Maryland		1905-1906	Charles Andrew Rapelye	Connecticut
1868-1869	Edward S. Wayne	Ohio		1906-1907	Carl S. N. Hallberg	Illinois
1869-1870	John H. Pope	Louisiana		1907-1908	Oscar Oldberg °	Illinois
1870-1871	James G. Steele	California		1908-1909	William Mittelbach	Missouri
1871-1872	George Frederic H. Markoe °	Massachusetts		1909-1910	Charles Willis Johnson °	Washington
1872-1873	Edward P. Nichols	New Jersey		1910-1911	Otto Ferdinand Claus	Missouri
1873-1874	John T. Buck	Mississippi		1911-1912	Charles Mangan Ford	Colorado
1874-1875	William T. Wenzell	California		1912-1913	Caswell Armstrong Mayo °	New York
1875-1876	Thomas Roberts Baker °	Virginia		1913-1914	Franklin Muhlenberg Apple	Pennsylvania
1876-1877	Gustavus Johann Luhn °	South Carolina		1914-1915	Charles Herbert Packard °	Massachusetts
1877-1878	John Ingalls °	Georgia		1915-1916	Edsel Alexander Ruddiman	Tennessee
1878-1879	Henry J. Rose	Ontario, Canada		1916-1917	Lucius Elmer Sayre °	Kansas
1879-1880	Joseph Lyon Lemberger °	Pennsylvania		1917-1918	Leonard Adams Seltzer	Michigan
1880-1881	William Scott Thompson °	Washington, DC		1918-1919	Theodore James Bradley °	Massachusetts
1881-1882	George Leis	Kansas		1919-1920	Harry Whitehouse	Tennessee
1882-1883	Louis Dohme	Maryland		1920-1921	Charles Edward Caspari	Missouri
1883-1884	Frederick H. Masi	Virginia		1921-1922	David Franklin Jones °	South Dakota
1884-1885	Henry Canning	Massachusetts		1922-1923	Lyman Frederic Kebler	Washington, DC
1885-1886	Albert Benjamin Prescott °	Michigan		1923-1924	Francis Eugene Bibbins	Indiana
1886-1887	Maurice William Alexander °	Missouri		1924-1925	William Mansfield	New York
1887-1888	Alexander Kirkwood Finlay °	Louisiana		1925-1926	Clyde L. Eddy	New York
1888-1889	Frederick Wilcox	Connecticut		1926-1927	Arthur G. Hulett	Arizona
1889-1890	William Martin Searby °	California		1927-1928	Joseph Jacobs	Georgia
1890-1891	Charles Emile Dohme °	Maryland		1928-1929	Washington Hayne Ziegler	South Carolina

1929-1930	Wilbur B. Goodyear	Pennsylvania		1949-1950	Leib L. Riggs	Oregon
1930-1931	David B. Ray Johnson	Oklahoma		1950-1951	Louis James Fischl °	California
1931-1932	John W. Dargavel	Minnesota		1951-1952	John A. MacCartney °	Michigan
1932-1933	G. H. Grommet	Florida		1952-1953	Charles F. Lanwermeyer	Illinois
1933-1934	John Christian Krantz, Jr.	Maryland		1953-1955	Ronald V. Robertson °	Washington
1934-1935	Oscar Rennebohm	Wisconsin		1955-1956	George C. Roberts	Mississippi
1935-1936	Joseph Lester Hayman	West Virginia		1956-1957	John J. Dugan	Connecticut
1936-1937	James Clyde Munch	Pennsylvania		1957-1958	Leroy A. Weidle, Sr.	Missouri
1937-1938	Glenn Llewellyn Jenkins °	Minnesota		1958-1959	Howell R. Jordan	Texas
1938-1939	George Allen Moulton °	New Hampshire		1959-1960	Paul W. Wilcox	Pennsylvania
1939-1940	Frederick Jefferson Cermak	Ohio		1960-1961	John J. Dugan	Connecticut
1940-1941	Henry Hamilton Gregg °	Minnesota		1961-1962	Noel E. Foss	Maryland
1941-1942	Lewis William Rowe	Michigan		1962-1963	Lee E. Eiler	Ohio
1942-1943	Charles O. Lee	Indiana		1963-1964	Mike Harris	Arizona
1943-1944	John Grover Beard	North Carolina		1964-1965	James W. Alexander	Minnesota
1944-1946	R. S. Lehman (deceased)	New York		1965-1966	Marc F. Laventurier	California
1946-1947	Harold V. Darnell	Indiana		1966-1967	Benjamin J. Kingwell	California
1947-1948	Roy L. Sanford	Oklahoma		1967-1968	Mary Louise Andersen	Delaware
1948-1949	Frederick D. Lascoff	New York		1968-1969	Arnold Albert	Florida
					Position abolished	

Third Vice Presidents

1852-1853	Charles Augustus Smith	Ohio		1882-1883	William B. Blanding	Rhode Island
1853-1854	Charles B. Guthrie °	Tennessee		1883-1884	Edward Wheelock Runyon	California
1854-1855	Joseph Laidley	Virginia		1884-1885	Charles F. Goodman	Nebraska
1855-1856	Henry F. Fish	Connecticut		1885-1886	Joseph Spragg Evans	Pennsylvania
1856-1857	Henry Taylor Kiersted °	New York		1886-1887	Norman Archibald Kuhn	Nebraska
1857-1858	A. E. Richards	Louisiana		1887-1888	Karl Simmon °	Minnesota
1858-1859	Robert Battey °	Georgia		1888-1889	Alvin A. Yeager	Tennessee
1859-1860	Edwin O. Gale	Illinois		1889-1890	Joseph William Eckford	Mississippi
1860-1862	Theodore Metcalf	Massachusetts		1890-1891	James Michener Good °	Missouri
1862-1863	Jacob Faris Moore °	Maryland		1891-1892	Lyman T. Dunning	South Dakota
1863-1864	George W. Weyman	Pennsylvania		1892-1893	William Henry Averill	Kentucky
1864-1865	Thomas Hollis	Massachusetts		1893-1894	Charles Caspari, Jr	Maryland
1865-1866	Charles A. Heinitsch °	Pennsylvania		1894-1895	Joseph Edward Morrison °	Quebec, Canada
1866-1867	John W. Shedden	New York		1895-1896	Mary Olds Miner	Kansas
1867-1868	Daniel Henchman	Massachusetts		1896-1897	George Warren Parisen	New Jersey
1868-1869	Albert Ethelbert Ebert °	Illinois		1897-1898	Jacob Augustus Miller	Pennsylvania
1869-1870	Joel S. Orne	Massachusetts		1898-1899	Josephine Anna Wanous	Minnesota
1870-1871	Eugene L. Massot	Missouri		1899-1900	Henry Robert Grey	Quebec, Canada
1871-1872	Matthew F. Ash	Mississippi		1900-1901	Edsel Alexander Ruddiman	Tennessee
1872-1873	Henry C. Gaylord	Ohio		1901-1902	William Scott Thompson °	Washington, DC
1873-1874	Paul Balluff	New York		1902-1903	Henry Willis	Quebec, Canada
1874-1875	Augustus R. Bayley	Massachusetts		1903-1904	Otto Ferdinand Claus	Missouri
1875-1876	Christian F. G. Meyer	Missouri		1904-1905	Julius Arnold Koch °	Pennsylvania
1876-1877	Jacob D. Wells	Ohio		1905-1906	Fabius Chapman Godbold	Louisiana
1877-1878	Emlen Painter °	California		1906-1907	Thomas Penrose Cook	New York
1878-1879	William H. Crawford	Missouri		1907-1908	Oscar Walter Bethea	Mississippi
1879-1880	Philip Charles Candidus	Alabama		1908-1909	James Hartley Beal °	Ohio
1880-1881	William Simpson °	North Carolina		1909-1910	William Baker Day °	Illinois
1881-1882	John F. Judge	Ohio		1910-1911	Leonard Adams Seltzer	Michigan

1911-1912	Ernest Berger	Florida
1912-1913	Charles Herbert Packard °	Massachusetts
1913-1914	William Stowell Richardson	Washington, DC
1914-1915	Charles Gietner	Missouri
1915-1916	Linwood Arnold Brown	Kentucky
1916-1917	Philip Asher	Louisiana
1917-1918	Theodore James Bradley °	Massachusetts
1918-1919	Francis Hemm	Missouri
1919-1920	Ernest Fullerton Cook	Pennsylvania
1920-1921	William Perry Porterfield	North Dakota
1921-1922	Hugo Herman Schaefer	New York
1922-1923	Clyde L. Eddy	New York
1923-1924	Waldemar Bruce Philip °	California
	Position abolished	

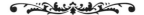

Secretary/Executive Director

1852-1853	George D. Coggeshall	Recording Secy
1852-1853	William Procter, Jr. °	Corresponding Secy
1853-1854	Edward Parrish °	Recording Secy
1853-1854	William B. Chapman °	Corresponding Secy
1854-1855	Edward S. Wayne	Recording Secy
1854-1857	William Procter, Jr. °	Corresponding Secy
1855-1859	William John M. Gordon °	Recording Secy
1857-1858	Edward Parrish °	Corresponding Secy
1858-1859	Ambrose Smith	Corresponding Secy
1859-1860	Charles Bullock °	Recording Secy
1859-1860	William Hegeman	Corresponding Secy
1860-1862	James Thornton Shinn °	Recording Secy
1860-1862	Peter Wendover Bedford °	Corresponding Secy
1862-1863	Peter Wendover Bedford °	Recording Secy
1862-1863	John Michael Maisch	Corresponding Secy
1863-1864	William Evans, Jr.	Recording Secy
1863-1866	Peter Wendover Bedford °	Corresponding Secy
1864-1865	Henry N. Rittenhouse	Recording Secy
1865-1866	John Michael Maisch	Recording Secy
1866-1893	John Michael Maisch	General Secretary
1893-1894	Joseph Price Remington °	General Secretary
1894-1911	Charles Caspari, Jr.	General Secretary
1911-1914	James Hartley Beal °	General Secretary
1914	Ernest C. Marshall	Acting Secretary
1914-1925	William Baker Day °	General Secretary
1925-1944	Evander Frank Kelly	General Secretary
1944-1959	Robert Phillip Fischelis °	General Secretary
1959-1983	William Shoulden Apple	Executive Director
1983-1984	Maurice Q. Bectel °	Acting Director
1984-1988	John F. Schlegel	Executive Director
1989-	John A. Gans	Exec. Vice President

Local Secretaries

(Local Secretaries were responsible for annual meeting arrangements)

1866-1867	Peter Wendover Bedford °		1879-1880	Charles F. Fish
1867-1868	Alfred Bower Taylor °		1880-1881	William T. Ford
1868-1869	Henry W. Fuller		1881-1882	Hiram E. Griffith
1869-1870	Jacob Faris Moore °		1882-1883	Charles Becker
1870-1871	William H. Crawford		1883-1884	Henry C. Schranck
1871-1872	Henry C. Gaylord		1884-1885	George A. Kelly
1872-1873	Thomas H. Hazard		1885-1886	William B. Blanding
1873-1874	Emil Scheffer		1886-1887	George W. Voss
1874-1875	Samuel A. D. Sheppard		1887-1888	James Vernor
1875-1876	Adolphus W. Miller		1888-1889	Edward W. Runyon
1876-1877	Henry J. Rose		1889-1890	Charles Emile Dohme °
1877-1878	Jesse W. Rankin		1890-1891	Alexander Kirkwood Finlay °
1878-1879	Eli Lilly		1891-1892	Henry Martin Whitney °

Local Secretaries *(continued)*

1892-1893	Henry Biroth
1893-1894	Whiteford Gamewell Smith
1894-1895	Edmund Louis Scholtz
1895-1896	James Edward Morrison °
1896-1897	Edward Shumpik
1897-1898	Henry Parr Hynson
1898-1899	Lewis Christopher Hopp °
1899-1900	Turner Ashby Miller
1900-1901	Henry Milton Whelpley °
1901-1902	William Lincoln Cliffe
1902-1903	Frederick W. R. Perry
1903-1904	Joseph Charles Wirthman
1904-1905	William Carter Wescott
1905-1906	Frank Henry Carter
1906-1907	Thomas Penrose Cook
1907-1908	Martin Augustine Eisele
1908-1909	Thomas William Jones

1909-1910	Turner Ashby Miller
1910-1911	Charles Herbert Packard °
1911-1912	Charles Mangan Ford
1912-1913	James Oscar Burge
1913-1914	Leonard Adams Seltzer
1914-1915	Albert Schneider
1915-1916	Charles Holzhauer °
1916-1917	Francis Eugene Bibbins
1917-1918	Edmund Norris Gathercoal °
1918-1919	Hugo Herman Schaefer
1919-1920	Samuel Louis Hilton °
1920-1921	George W. McDuff
1921-1922	Edward Spease
1922-1923	John G. Beard
1923-1924	Willis George Gregory
1924-1925	Elbert O. Kagy
	Position abolished

Treasurer

1852-1854	Alfred Bower Taylor °	Pennsylvania
1854-1855	Samuel Marshall Colcord °	Massachusetts
1856-1857	James S. Aspinwall	New York
1857-1859	Samuel Marshall Colcord °	Massachusetts
1859-1860	Ashel Boyden	Massachusetts
1860-1863	Henry C. Haviland	New York
1863-1865	J. Brown Baxley	Maryland
1865-1886	Charles Augustus Tufts °	New Hampshire
1886-1908	Samuel A. D. Sheppard	Massachusetts
1909-1921	Henry Milton Whelpley °	Missouri

1921-1925	Evander Frank Kelly	Maryland
1925-1941	Charles William Holton °	New Jersey
1941-1967	Hugo Herman Schaefer	New York
1967-1978	Grover Cleveland Bowles °	Tennessee
1979-1981	William Frank Appel °	Minnesota
1982-1984	William J. Edwards	Texas
1985-1988	Marily H. Rhudy °	Kansas
1988-1991	August P. Lemberger	Wisconsin
1991-1998	Jean Paul Gagnon	Missouri
1998-	Lowell J. Anderson °	Minnesota

Editor, Progress of Pharmacy

1873-1891	Conrad Lewis Diehl °
1891-1892	Charles Rice
1892-1895	Henry Kraemer
1896-1915	Conrad Lewis Diehl °

1915-1916	Julius Arnold Koch °
1916-1922	Henry Vincome Arny °
1922-1926	Andrew Grover DuMez °

House of Delegates

Year	Chairman/Speaker	Vice Chairman/Vice Speaker
1912-1913	William Christine Anderson	Clyde Mason Snow
1913-1914	Clyde Mason Snow	Willard Stowell Richardson
1914-1915	Willard Stowell Richardson	Charles Bernard Jordan
1915-1916	Henry Parr Hynson	Ferd Wilhelm Nitardy
1916-1917	James Hartley Beal °	Samuel Clements Henry
1917-1918	Samuel Clements Henry	Otto Ferdinand Claus
1918-1919	Otto Ferdinand Claus	Samuel Louis Hilton °
1919-1920	Samuel Louis Hilton °	Evander Frank Kelly
1920-1921	Evander Frank Kelly	John G. Beard
1921-1923	Evander Frank Kelly	Edwin Leigh Newcomb
1923-1924	Lucius Leedom Walton °	Waldemar Bruce Philip °
1924-1925	Waldemar Bruce Philip °	William D. Jones
1925-1926	William D. Jones	Jacob Diner
1926-1927	Jacob Diner	Leonard Adams Seltzer
1927-1928	Leonard Adams Seltzer	Ambroise Hunsberger
1928-1929	Ambroise Hunsberger	Robert Lee Swain °
1929-1930	Robert Lee Swain °	Charles Bernard Jordan
1930-1931	Charles Bernard Jordan	Thomas Roach
1931-1932	Thomas Roach	J. W. Slocum
1932-1933	J. W. Slocum	Patrick H. Costello °
1933-1934	Patrick H. Costello °	Sam A. Williams
1934-1935	Rowland Jones, Jr.	Sam A. Williams
1935-1936	Roy Bird Cook °	C. Thurston Gilbert
1936-1937	Robert Cumming Wilson	Andrew F. Ludwig
1937-1938	Arthur L. I. Winne	Ernest Little °
1938-1939	Charles Herbert Rogers	Rudolph A. Kuever
1939-1940	Myron Nile Ford	Edwin Clair Severin
1940-1941	Hugo Herman Schaefer	C. L. Guthrie
1941-1942	Henry Hamilton Gregg °	C. Leonard O'Connell
1942-1943	J. K. Attwood	Glenn Llewellyn Jenkins °
1943-1944	Glenn Llewellyn Jenkins °	Sylvester H. Dretzka °
1944-1946	Sylvester H. Dretzka °	E. L. Hammond
1946-1947	Hugh Cornelius Muldoon	E. M. Josey
1947-1948	Charles Hall Evans °	Emil C. Horn
1948-1949	Bert R. Mull	Louis James Fischl °
1949-1950	Richard Quintus Richards °	Newell W. Stewart °
1950-1951	Newell W. Stewart °	Thomas D. Wyatt
1951-1952	Louis James Fischl °	D. Mearl Pritchard
1952-1953	E. M. Josey	Paul Wilcox
1953-1954	Leib L. Riggs	Louis C. Zopf
1954-1955	Thomas D. Wyatt	James J. Lynch
1955-1956	James J. Lynch	William B. Shangraw
1956-1957	Troy C. Daniels	John Butts
1957-1958	Nicholas Gesoalde	Ewart A. Swinyard
1958-1959	James Warren Lansdowne °	Calvin Berger
1959-1960	James Warren Lansdowne °	Wilbur Powers
1960-1961	Grover Cleveland Bowles °	John G. Adams
1961-1962	Grover Cleveland Bowles °	Donald Brodie

Year	Chairman/Speaker	Vice Chairman/Vice Speaker
1962-1963	H. C. McAllister	David Stewart
1963-1964	Calvin Berger	Robert Charles Johnson °
1964-1965	Linwood Franklin Tice °	Robert G. Gibbs
1965-1966	William Ray Whitten °	Jack Karlin
1966-1967	Charles A. Schreiber	W. Byron Rumford
1967-1968	W. Byron Rumford	W. J. Smith
1968-1970	Mary Louise Andersen	Merritt Skinner
1970-1971	Clifton Joseph Latiolais °	Philip Sacks °
1971-1972	Philip Sacks °	George Inman
1972-1973	Jacob Willis Miller °	Joseph McSoley
1973-1974	Jacob Willis Miller °	James Wagner
1974-1975	David J. Krigstein	Louis Jeffrey
1975-1976	David J. Krigstein	Mark J. Sullivan
1076-1977	Merritt L. Skinner	Herbert Sylvester Carlin°
1977-1078	Mary Munson Runge °	Herbert Sylvester Carlin°
1978-1979	Ralph S. Levi	Earl Giacolini
1979-1980	William J. Edwards	Earl Giacolini
1980-1981	William J. Edwards	David Stephen Crawford *
1981-1982	David Stephen Crawford °	Stephen W. Schondelmeyer
1982-1983	David Stephen Crawford °	E. Michelle Valentine
1983-1984	Lowell John Anderson °	Joseph Fink III
1984-1985	Lowell John Anderson °	Shirley McKee
1985-1986	Raymond W. Roberts	Lucinda L. Maine
1986-1987	Shirley P. McKee	Lucinda L. Maine
1987-1988	Shirley P. McKee	Position Abolished
1988-1990	Lucinda L. Maine	
1990-1991	E. Michelle Valentine	
1991-1993	Hazel M. Pipkin	
1993-1994	Leonard N. "Red" Camp	
1994-1996	Wilma K. Wong	
1996-1997	Susan Bartlemay	
1997-1998	Timothy L. Tucker	
1998-1999	Betty Jean Harris	
1999-2000	Pamela W. Tribble	
2000-2001	Bethany J. Boyd	

Judicial Board

	Chairman			Chairman	
1972-1973	Kenneth S. Griswold	New York	1975-1978	W. Allen Daniels	Wisconsin

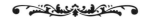

APhA Foundation Presidents

1953-1958	Henry Armitt Brown Dunning °	1970-1976	Merritt L. Skinner
1958-1959	Louis James Fischl, Jr. °	1976-1979	Lloyd McClain Parks °
1959-1961	Henry Armitt Brown Dunning °	1979-1990	Joseph E. McSoley
1961-1964	Howard Chamberlain Newton °	1990-1991	Leonard Grossman °
1964-1966	James Warren Lansdowne °	1991-2000	Jacob Willis Miller °
1966-1968	Rudolph H. Blythe	2000-	Brian Isetts
1968-1970	Robert G. Gibbs		

APhA Council/Board of Trustees

The executive body of the Association was known as the executive committee from 1852 until 1879. The APhA Council was formed in 1880, and remained as such until 1966, except for a single year (1923) when it was known as the Board of Directors. The current designation as Board of Trustees was adopted in 1966. From 1907 to 1921, each APhA Branch could elected a member of the Council. Since 1995, Academy presidents (APPM, APRS, and ASP) were *ex-officio* members of the Board of Trustees. Elected and *ex-officio* members are listed in alphabetical order, except for APhA presidents who usually served many terms on the Council/Board of Trustees, and whose biographical sketches appear in Appendix C.

Member	Term of Service	Member	Term of Service
Martin E. Adamo	1948-1954	Tery Baskin	1991-1997
A. Lee Adams	1946-1947	John G. Beard	1931-1932
Walter D. Adams	1931-1935	John G. Beard	1943-1945
Augustus J. Affleck	1947-1948	Joshua S. Benner	1997 (ASP)
Arnold Albert	1967-1971	Calvin Berger	1963-1964
James W. Alexander	1964-1965	Ernest Berger	1911-1912
Loyd V. Allen, Jr.	2000 (APRS)	Oscar W. Bethea	1907-1908
Mary Louise Andersen	1967-1970	Francis E. Bibbins	1921-1924
William C. Anderson	1912-1913	Francis E. Bibbins	1941-1945
William C. Anderson	1925-1926	W. James Bicket	1971-1974
Franklin M. Apple	1913-1918	W. James Bicket	1978-1980
William S. Apple	1959-1983	William B. Blanding	1882-1883
Roberta M. Armstrong	1998 (APPM)	Rudolph H. Blythe	1961-1962
Philip Asher	1909-1914	Roy A. Bowers	1950-1951
Philip Asher	1916-1917	Roy A. Bowers	1958-1963
J. K. Attwood	1941-1943	Bethany J. Boyd	1999-2001
Nick M. Avellone	1974-1977	Adolph Brandenberger	1895-1896
William H. Averill	1892-1893	Linwood A. Brown	1915-1916
Edward L. Baker, Jr.	1971-1972	Rinaldo A. Brusadin	1975-1977
Thomas Roberts Baker	1900-1903	Rinaldo A. Brusadin	1983-1985
George C. Bartells	1897-1898	Carol A. Bugdalski	1999-2001
Susan Bartlemay	1996-1997	Timothy N. Burelle	1991-1993

Academies

(in alphabetical order)

ACADEMY OF GENERAL PRACTICE OF PHARMACY
ACADEMY OF PHARMACY PRACTICE

	Chairman	Secretary
1965-1966	Raymond L. Dunn	John T. Fay, Jr.
1966-1967	Martin Golden	Richard P. Penna
1967-1968	Thurman H. Miller	Richard P. Penna
1968-1969	Thomas H. Holland	Richard P. Penna
1969-1970	Byron C. Spoon, Jr.	Richard P. Penna
1970-1971	C. Albert Olson	Richard P. Penna
1971-1972	W. James Bicket	Richard P. Penna
1972-1973	William R. Bacon	Ronald L. Williams
1973-1974	Donald O. Fedder	Ronald L. Williams
1974-1975	William J. Edwards	Ronald L. Williams
1975-1976	James R. Ramseth	Ronald L. Williams
1976-1977	Gary R. Cornell	Ronald L. Williams
1977-1978	Leonard Grossman °	Ronald L. Williams
1978-1979	George B. Browning	Ronald L. Williams
1979-1980	David Stephen Crawford °	Ronald L. Williams
1980-1981	Susan E. Torrico	Ronald L. Williams
1981-1982	James J. Bensel	Ronald L. Williams
1982-1983	Rinaldo J. Brusadin	Ronald L. Williams
1983-1984	Ronald David Cobb °	Ronald L. Williams
1984-1985	Dennis A. Smith	Ronald L. Williams
1985-1986	Ron Gieser	Maude A. Babington
1986-1987	Philip Paul Gerbino °	Maude A. Babington

ACADEMY OF PHARMACEUTICAL MANAGEMENT

	Chairman
1985-1986	Terry D. Grant
1986-1987	Terry D. Grant
1987-1988	Donald L. Beck

ACADEMY OF PHARMACEUTICAL SCIENCES

	Chairman/President	Secretary
1965-1967	Takeru Higuchi	Samuel W. Goldstein
1967-1968	Joseph V. Swintosky	Samuel W. Goldstein
1968-1969	George P. Hager	Samuel W. Goldstein
1969-1970	Leon Lachman	William C. Roemer
1970-1971	Thomas J. Macek	William C. Roemer
1971-1972	Harry B. Kostenbauder	William C. Roemer
1972-1973	Chester J. Cavallito	William C. Roemer
1973-1974	George H. Schneller	William F. McGhan
1974-1975	Louis W. Busse	William F. McGhan
1975-1976	Dale E. Wurster	William F. McGhan
1976-1977	Roy Kuramoto	Lloyd Kennon
1977-1978	George Zografi	Lloyd Kennon
1978-1979	James C. Boylan	Ronald L. Williams

1979-1980	Patrick P. DeLuca	Ronald L. Williams
1980-1981	Klaus G. Florey	Ronald L. Williams
1981-1982	Lawrene C. Weaver	Ronald L. Williams
1982-1983	Kenneth R. Heimlich	Ronald L. Williams
1983-1984	August P. Lemberger	Ronald L. Williams
1984-1985	Arthur R. Mlodozeniec	Edward G. Feldmann
1985-1986	Leslie Z. Benet	Arthur M. Horowitz
1986-1987	Boyd J. Poulsen	Arthur M. Horowitz

ACADEMY OF PHARMACEUTICAL RESEARCH AND SCIENCES

	Chairman/President	Secretary
1987-1988	Jordan L. Cohen	Arthur H. Kibbe
1988-1989	William F. McGhan	Arthur H. Kibbe
1989-1990	William E. Evans	Arthur H. Kibbe
1990-1991	Anthony Palmieri III	Arthur H. Kibbe
1991-1992	Marvin D. Shephard	Arthur H. Kibbe
1992-1993	Randy P. Juhl	Lucinda L. Maine
1993-1994	Alice Jean Matuszak	Lucinda L. Maine
1994-1995	Francis B. Palumbo	Lucinda L. Maine
1995-1996	Claiborne E. Reeder	Lucinda L. Maine
1996-1997	Betty-ann Hoener	Lucinda L. Maine
1997-1998	Dale B. Christensen	Lucinda L. Maine
1998-1999	Duane M. Kirking	Lucinda L. Maine
1999-2000	Loyd V. Allen, Jr.	Lucinda L. Maine
2000-2001	Rosalie Sagraves	Lucinda L. Maine
2001-2002	Bernard A. Sorofman	Lucinda L. Maine
2002-2003	Arthur H. Kibbe	Lucinda L. Maine

ACADEMY OF PHARMACY PRACTICE AND MANAGEMENT

	Chairman	Secretary
1987-1988	Mark A. Pulido	Maude A. Babington
1988-1990	Eugene M. Lutz	C. Edward Webb
1990-1991	Hazel M. Pipkin	Judy Shinogle
1991-1992	Calvin Knowlton °	Judy Shinogle
1992-1993	Leonard "Red" Camp III	John Hammond
1993-1994	Steve C. Firman	John Hammond
1994-1995	Janet P. Engle °	Susan C. Winckler
1995-1996	Albert F. Lockamy, Jr.	Susan C. Winckler
1996-1997	Benjamin J. Gruda	Susan C. Winckler
1997-1998	Roberta M. Armstrong	Susan C. Winckler
1998-1999	Michael J. Glen	Janet Edward
1999-2000	Anna Charuk Kowblansky	Anne L. Burns
2000-2001	Ed L. Hamilton	Anne L. Burns
2001-2002	Bruce Field	Anne L. Burns
2002-2003	Michael P. Cinque	Anne L. Burns

Sections

(in alphabetical order)

ADMINISTRATIVE PRACTICE SECTION

Chairman

1987-1988	Richard C. Januszewski
1988-1990	W. Ray Burns
1990-1991	Pamela S. Farrior
1991-1992	Kenneth R. Couch
1992-1993	Benjamin J. Gruda
1993-1994	Debra W. Nichol
1994-1995	Anna Charuk Kowblansky
1995-1996	Gary A. Halpern
1996-1997	Michael P. Cinque
1997-1998	Bruce C. Field
1998-1999	Todd A Edgar
1999-2000	James A. Miller
2000-2001	Ann Macro
2001-2002	Deborah Simmrus
2002-2003	Stephen Wickizer

BASIC SCIENCES SECTION

Chairman

1987-1989	Anthony Palmieri III
1989-1990	Stuart Feldman
1990-1991	Alice Jean Matuszak
1991-1992	Betty-ann Hoener
1992-1993	James Blanchard
1993-1994	David W. Newton
1994-1995	Fotios M. Plakogiannis
1995-1996	Anthony Cutie
1996-1997	Ralph Tarantino
1997-1998	Loyd V. Allen, Jr.
1998-1999	Mario Sylvestri
1999-2000	Arthur H. Kibbe
2000-2001	Lawrence H. Block
2001-2002	Shelly Prince
2002-2003	Walter G. Chambliss

BASIC PHARMACEUTICS SECTION

	Chairman	Secretary
1965-1967	Dale E. Wurster	James E. Tingstad
1967-1968	John A. Biles	Stuart P. Eriksen
1968-1969	Alfred N. Martin	William I. Higuchi
1969-1970	James E. Tingstad	George Zografi
1970-1971	David E. Guttman	James Thomas Doluisio °
1971-1972	William I. Higuchi	Arthur R. Mlodozeniec
1972-1973	George Zografi	Emanuel J. Russo
1973-1974	James Thomas Doluisio°	Leslie Z. Benet
1974-1975	John L. Lach	Gordon L. Flynn
1975-1976	Anthony P. Simonelli	Gordon L. Flynn
1976-1977	Leslie Z. Benet	Gordon L. Flynn
1977-1978	Emanuel J. Russo	Arlyn W. Kinkel
1978-1979	Armando J. Agular	Arlyn W. Kinkel
1979-1980	Gordon L. Flynn	Arlyn W. Kinkel
1980-1981	Samuel H. Yalkowsky	James W. McGirity
1981-1982	Kenneth G. Nelson	James W. McGirity
1982-1983	Peter Bernardo	
1983-1984	Theodore J. Roseman	
1984-1985	Gordon L. Amidon	
1985-1986	Thomas F. Patton	
1986-1987	Bradley D. Anderson	

CLINICAL/PHARMACOTHERAPEUTIC PRACTICE SECTION

Chairman

1987-1989	Debra G. Goodman
1989-1990	Janice A. Gaska
1990-1991	Janet P. Engle °
1991-1992	Dominic A. Solimando, Jr.
1992-1993	Bruce Canaday
1993-1994	Donald G. Florridia
1994-1995	Dennis M. Williams
1995-1996	Gary Milavetz
1996-1997	William T. Sawyer
1997-1998	Cathy Worrall
1998-1999	Valerie Prince
1999-2000	Bobby S. Bryant
2000-2001	George Yasutake
2001-2002	Marialice Bennett
2002-2003	Milissa Rock

CLINICAL PRACTICE SECTION

Chairman

1975-1976	Candace B. Bryan (pro tem)
1976-1977	Gary W. Cripps
1977-1978	Thomas J. Mattei
1978-1979	Philip Paul Gerbino °
1979-1980	Thomas P. Reinders
1980-1981	Raymond W. Roberts
1981-1982	Thomas W. Wiser
1982-1983	Robert Earl Davis °
1983-1984	Timothy R. Covington
1984-1985	Philip E. Johnston
1985-1986	Dennis K. Helling
1986-1987	William R. Garnett
1987-1888	Kathleen M. D'Achille
1988-1989	Debra G. Goodman

CLINICAL SCIENCES SECTION

Chairman

1987-1988	Thomas S. Foster
1990-1991	Larry A. Bauer
1991-1992	William R. Garnett
1992-1993	Michael Bottorff
1993-1994	George E. Dukes
1994-1995	James C. Cloyd
1995-1996	Mary E. Teresi
1996-1997	Rosalie Sagraves
1997-1998	Ann B. Amerson
1998-1999	Theodore G. Tong
1999-2000	Mary Lee
2000-2001	Gary C. Yee
2001-2002	Warren Narducci
2002-2003	Mary E. Teresi

COMMERCIAL INTERESTS SECTION

	Chairman	Secretary
1887-1889	Albert H. Hollister	Joseph W. Colcord
1889-1890	Leo Eliel °	Frederick B. Kilmer
1890-1891	Henry Canning	William L. Dewoody
1891-1893	Willard H. Torbert	Arthur Bassett
1893-1894	Wiley Rogers	James O. Burge
1894-1895	George J. Seabury	James O. Burge
1895-1896	George J. Seabury	Clay W. Holmes
1896-1897	Lewis C. Hopp°	John E. D'Avignon

COMMERCIAL INTERESTS SECTION

(continued)

	Chairman	Secretary
1897-1898	Joseph Jacobs	Hendrick G. Webster
1898-1899	Joseph Jacobs	James H.Bobbitt
1899-1900	James M. Good°	Charles A. Rapelye
1900-1901	Charles A. Rapelye	Frederick W. Meissner
1901-1902	Frederick W. Meissner	Eugene G. Eberle°
1902-1903	Thomas V. Wooten	William C. Anderson
1903-1904	William L. Dewoody	Robert C. Reilly
1904-1905	Charles R. Sherman	Robert C.Reilly
1905-1906	Henry P. Hynson	Herman D.Kniseley
1906-1907	Herman D. Kniseley	Charles H.Avery
1907-1908	Jacob Diner	George O. Young
1908-1909	Harry B. Mason	Erich H. Ladish
1909-1910	Waldo M. Bowman	George H.P. Lichthardt
1910-1911	Franklin M. Apple	Benjamin E. Pritchard
1911-1912	Ernest Berger	David W. Ramsaur
1912-1913	Autumn V. Pease	William R.White
1913-1914	Charles G. Lindville & Harry B. Mason	Grant W. Stevens
1914-1915	Edward H. Thiesing	Rudolph R. Kuever
1915-1916	Robert Seel Lehman	James C. McGee
1916-1917	Philip H. Utech	Robert P. Fischelis °
1917-1918	Robert P. Fischelis°	Ferd W.Nitardy
1918-1919	Ernest F. Cook	Henry S. Noel
1919-1920	Henry S. Noel	Charles O. Lee
1920-1921	Adam Wirth	C. W. Holzhauer °
1921-1922	Charles W. Holton°	Bernard H.Eichold
1922-1923	Walter M. Chase	Henry B. Smith
1923-1924	Henry B. Smith	W. Bruce Philip °
1924-1925	W. Bruce Philip°	George Judisch
1925-1926	Ambrose Hunsberger	Bernard M. Keene
1926-1927	Bernard M. Keene	C. Leonard O'Connell
1927-1928	C. Leonard O'Connell	Russell B. Rothrock
1928-1929	Russell B. Rothrock	Joseph G. Noh
1929-1930	Denny Brann	Rowland Jones
1930-1931	Joseph G. Noh	Leon Monell
1931-1932	Rowland Jones	John A. J. Funk
1932-1933	Leon Monell	Henry Brown
1933-1934	John A. J. Funk	Robert W. Rodman
1934-1935	Henry Brown	Roland T. Lakey
1935-1936	Robert W. Rodman	Henry F. Hein
1936-1937	Roland T. Lakey	Joseph H. Goodness

COMMUNITY AND AMBULATORY PRACTICE SECTION

	Chairman
1987-1988	George B. Browning
1988-1990	Calvin Knowlton °
1990-1991	L. N. "Red" Camp, III
1990-1991	Jerry Moore
1991-1992	Albert F. Lockamy, Jr.
1992-1993	J. T. "Tom" Gulick
1993-1994	Roberta M. Armstrong
1994-1995	Michael J. Glen
1995-1996	Bruce C. Field
1996-1997	Charles C. Thomas
1997-1998	Theresa L. Wells Tolle
1998-1999	Mark Hobbs
1999-2000	Karen L. Reed
2000-2001	Richard C. Holm
2001-2002	Daniel Kennedy
2001-2002	Page Dunlop

DRUG STANDARDS, ANALYSIS & CONTROL SECTION

	Chairman	Secretary
1965-1967	Lloyd C. Miller	Dale H. Szulcewski
1967-1968	Klaus Florey	Jack P. Comer
1968-1969	William J. Mader	Jack P. Comer

ECONOMICS AND ADMINISTRATIVE SCIENCE SECTION

	Chairman	Secretary
1966-1967	Joseph D. McEvilla	Robert E. Abrams
1967-1968	Robert V. Evanson	Robert E. Abrams
1968-1969	Richard J. Hampton	Robert E. Abrams
1969-1970	Robert W. Hammel	Michael D. Jacoff
1970-1971	Floyd A. Grolle	Michael D. Jacoff
1971-1972	Albert W. Jowdy	Michael D. Jacoff
1972-1973	M. Keith Weikel	Michael D. Jacoff
1973-1974	Maven J. Myers	Sheldon Siegel
1974-1975	Richard A. Ohvall	Sheldon Siegel
1975-1976	Richard E. Johnson	Sheldon Siegel
1976-1977	G. Joseph Norwood	Charles L. Braucher
1977-1978	Richard E. Faust	Charles L. Braucher
1978-1979	Jean Paul Gagnon	

ECONOMIC, SOCIAL AND ADMINISTRATIVE SCIENCE SECTION

	Chairman
1979-1980	Dewey D. Garner
1980-1981	Dave S. Forbes
1981-1982	Kenneth W. Look
1982-1983	W. Michael Dickson
1983-1984	Patrick L. McKercher
1984-1985	Robert H. Hunter
1985-1986	Paul A. Holberg

ECONOMIC, SOCIAL AND ADMINISTRATIVE SCIENCE SECTION (continued)

	Chairman
1986-1987	Christopher Rodowskas, Jr.
1987-1988	Lee R. Strandberg
1988-1990	Marvin D. Shephard
1990-1991	C. Eugene Reeder
1991-1992	Frank J. Ascione
1992-1993	Francis B. Palumbo
1993-1994	David H. Kreling
1994-1995	Karen L. Rascati
1995-1996	Dale B. Christensen
1996-1997	Duane M. Kirking
1997-1998	Eleanor M. Perfetto
1998-1999	Bernard A. Sorofman
1999-2000	Earlene E. Lipowski
2000-2001	Stephen W. Schondelmeyer
2001-2002	Jon C. Schommer
2002-2003	Joseph Thomas III

FEDERAL PHARMCAY SECTION

	Chairman	Secretary
1973-1974	Ralph C. Boehm	Jordon D. Johnson
1974-1975	A. Gordon Moore	Lawrence D. Smith
1975-1977	Angelo. R. Petoletti	Darrell F. Snook
1977-1978	Jordan D. Johnson	Darrell F. Snook
1978-1979	Angelo. R. Petoletti	Ronald L. Williams
1979-1980	Jordan D. Johnson	
1980-1981	G. Neil Libby	
1982-1983	Richard J. Bertin	
1983-1984	John Ferinde	
1982-1983	William D. Clyde, Jr.	
1985-1986	Vincent J. Fierro	
1986-1987	M. Ray Holt	
1987-1989	Allen D. Whisenant	
1989-1990	R. Duane Tackitt	

GENERAL PRACTICE OF PHARMACY SECTION

	Chairman	Secretary
1961-1963	J. Martin Winton	Benjamin A. Smith
1963-1964	Joseph H. Kern	Benjamin A. Smith
1964-1965	R. Dudley Conness	Thurman H. Miller

HISTORICAL PHARMACY SECTION

	Chairman	Secretary
1902-1903	Edward Kremers	George Mahlon Beringer°
1903-1904	Edward Kremers	Ezra Joseph Kennedy
1904-1905	Albert Ethelbert Ebert°	Caswell Armstrong Mayo°
1905-1906	John Francis Hancock °	Carl S. N. Hallberg
1906-1907	Ewen McIntyre	Eugene Gustave Eberle °

	Chairman	Secretary
1907-1908	Edward Vernon Howell	Eugene Gustave Eberle °
1908-1909	John Catis Bond	Eugene Gustave Eberle °
1909-1910	Eugene Gustave Eberle°	John Augustus Dunn
1910-1911	Joseph Lyon Lemberger°	Otto Raubenheimer
1911-1912	Otto Raubenheimer	Caswell Armstrong Mayo °
1912-1913	John Granville Godding°	Frederick Troup Gordon
1913-1914	William Charles Alpers°	Frederick Troup Gordon
1914-1915	Frederick Troup Gordon	Albert Henry Clark
1915-1916	Charles Holzhauer °	G. G. Marshall
1916-1917	William Laneman DuBois	Lucius Elmer Sayre°
1917-1918	Lucius Elmer Sayre °	Hugo Kantrowitz
1918-1919	Hugo Kantrowitz	William Oscar Richtmann
1919-1920	William Oscar Richtmann	Curt Paul Wimmer
1920-1921	Curt Paul Wimmer	Arthur Wilson Linton
1921-1922	Curt Paul Wimmer	Clyde L. Eddy
1922-1924	Clyde L. Eddy	Robert S. Lehman
1924-1925	Robert S. Lehman	L. K. Darbaker
1925-1926	L. K. Darbaker	William F. Sudro
1926-1927	William F. Sudro	Ezra Joseph Kennedy
1927-1928	William P. Porterfield	Ambrose Mueller
1928-1929	Lyman Frederic Kebler	George Denton Beal °
1929-1930	George Denton Beal °	John Thomas Lloyd
1930-1931	John Thomas Lloyd	Lewis E. Warren
1931-1932	John Thomas Lloyd	Louis Gershenfeld
1933-1934	Louis Gershenfeld	Charles O. Lee
1934-1935	Charles O. Lee	Heber W. Youngken
1935-1936	Heber W. Youngken	Loyd Ervin Harris
1936-1937	Loyd Ervin Harris	Edward J. Ireland
1937-1938	Edward J. Ireland	Willis T. Bradley
1938-1939	Willis T. Bradley	J. Hampton Hoch
1939-1940	J. Hampton Hoch	Learny F. Jones
1940-1941	Ivor Griffith °	F. D. Stoll
1941-1942	Learny F. Jones	Ralph Bienfang
1942-1944	F. D. Stoll	Karl L. Kaufman
1944-1946	F. D. Stoll	Clarence M. Brown
1946-1947	Karl L. Kaufman	Kenneth Redman
1947-1948	Clarence M. Brown	Roland T. Lakey
1948-1949	Kenneth Redman	H. George Wolfe
1949-1950	Roland T. Lakey	Glenn Sonnedecker
1950-1951	H. George Wolfe	Edward S. Brady
1951-1952	Glenn Sonnedecker	George Griffenhagen
1952-1953	Edward S. Brady	Edward J. Rowe
1953-1954	George Griffenhagen	George E. Osborne

	Chairman	Secretary
1954-1955	Edward J. Rowe	George Griffenhagen
1955-1956	George E. Osborne	George Griffenhagen
1956-1957	Eunice R. Bonow	George Griffenhagen
1957-1958	Alex Berman	George Griffenhagen
1958-1959	George A. Bender	George Griffenhagen
1959-1960	Roy Bird Cook °	Donald T. Meredith
1960-1961	Laurence D. Lockie	Donald T. Meredith
1961-1962	Edward J. Ireland	Esther Jane Wood Hall
1962-1963	Donald T. Meredith	Esther Jane Wood Hall
1963-1965	Herbert Raubenheimer	Esther Jane Wood Hall
1965-1966	Norman H. Franke	Esther Jane Wood Hall
1966-1967	Esther Jane Wood Hall	Sami K. Hamarneh

Merged in 1968 with American Institute of the History of Pharmacy.

HOME HEALTH CARE SECTION

	Chairman
1984-1986	J. Thomas Gulick
1986-1987	Madeline Feinberg
1987-1988	Branton G. Lachman
1988-1989	George B. Browning

HOSPITAL AND INSTITUTIONAL PRACTICE SECTION

	Chairman
1987-1988	R. Duane Tackitt
1988-1990	John M. Hammond
1990-1991	Elizabeth A. Simpson
1991-1992	Richard M. Church
1992-1993	Wilson O. Allen
1993-1994	Debra S. Weintraub
1994-1995	Fred C. Hirning
1995-1996	Ronald H. Small
1996-1997	Ed L. Hamilton
1997-1998	Christopher J. Forst
1998-1999	Dominic A. Solimando, Jr.
1999-2000	Fred Schmidt
2000-2001	Valerie Prince
2001-2002	Cathy Worrall
2002-2003	Thomas Worrall

INDUSTRIAL PHARMACEUTICAL TECHNOLOGY SECTION

	Chairman	Secretary
1965-1967	Leon Lachman	Earl A. Kimes
1967-1968	Edward J. Hanus	Earl A. Kimes
1968-1969	Gilbert S. Banker	Earl A. Kimes
1969-1970	Roy Kuramoto	Arge Drubulis
1970-1971	W. Mayo Higgins	Arge Drubulis
1971-1972	Arnold D. Marcus	Arge Drubulis
1972-1973	Ralph S. Levi	Arge Drubulis
1973-1974	James C. Boylan	Arge Drubulis
1974-1975	Hal N. Wolkoff	Arge Drubulis
1975-1976	John C. Griffin	Arge Drubulis
1976-1977	Earl Rosen	Arge Drubulis
1977-1978	Arthur R. Mlodozeniec	Arge Drubulis
1978-1979	James B. Applno	Arge Drubulis
1979-1980	William J. Tillman	Arge Drubulis
1980-1981	Kenneth R. Heimlich	Arge Drubulis
1981-1982	Boyd J. Poulsen	
1982-1983	Paul E. Wray	
1983-1984	Garnet E. Peck	
1984-1985	Joseph B. Schwartz	
1985-1986	Terry L. Benney	
1986-1987	Morgan L. Beatty	
1987-1988	Frank W. Goodhart	

INDUSTRIAL PHARMACY SECTION

	Chairman	Secretary
1959-1960	Jack Cooper	Earl A. Kimes
1960-1961	Paul R. Rasanen	Earl A. Kimes
1961-1962	George F. Hoffnagle	Earl A. Kimes
1062-1963	Richard Zapapas	Earl A. Kimes
1963-1964	Carl J. Lintner	Earl A. Kimes
1964-1965	Walter Charnicki	Earl A. Kimes

LONG TERM CARE SECTION

	Chairman
1975-1976	Monroe D. Lipman (pro tem)
1976-1977	Monroe D. Lipman
1977-1978	Jerry C. Hood
1978-1979	Susan E. Torrico
1979-1980	James W. Cooper
1980-1981	Robert L. Snively
1981-1982	Bruce A. Hufford
1982-1983	Charles H. Brown
1983-1984	Ronald C. Kayne
1984-1985	M. Peter Pevonka
1985-1986	Thomas D. Guidry
1986-1987	Rodney C. Bohn
1987-1988	Eugene M. Lutz
1988-1989	Richard C. Januszewski

MEDICINAL CHEMISTRY SECTION

	Chairman	Secretary
1965-1967	Taito O. Soine	Eugene C. Jorgensen
1967-1968	W. Lewis Nobles	Eugene C. Jorgensen
1968-1969	Howard J. Schaeffer	James C. Kellett, Jr.
1969-1970	Raymond E. Counsell	Blaine M. Sutton
1970-1971	Chester J. Cavallito	Blaine M. Sutton
1971-1972	Eugene C. Jorgensen	Blaine M. Sutton
1972-1973	Lemont B. Kier	George H. Cocolas
1973-1974	James E. Gearien	George H. Cocolas
1974-1975	Monroe E. Wall	George H. Cocolas
1975-1976	Robert E. Willette	George H. Cocolas
1976-1977	Robert A. Wiley	Dwight S. Fullerton
1977-1978	George H. Cocolas	Dwight S. Fullerton
1978-1979	Wendell L. Nelson	

MEDICINAL CHEMISTRY AND PHARMACOGNOSY SECTION

	Chairman
1979-1980	Lee C. Schramm
1980-1981	Leonard R. Worthen
1981-1982	Anthony A. Sinkula
1982-1983	Dwight S. Fullerton
1983-1984	Gary L. Grunewald
1984-1985	Gary W. Elmer
1985-1986	Lindley A. Cates
1986-1987	Paul L. Schiff
1987-1988	William J. Keller

MILITARY PHARMACY SECTION

	Chairman	Secretary-Treasurer
1956-1958	Bernard Aabel	William L. Austin
1958-1959	Kenneth B. Johnson	Solomon C. Pflag
1959-1960	Solomon C. Pflag	Carl Brown
1960-1961	Vernon O. Trygstad	Claude V. Timberlake
1961-1962	Ralph D. Arnold	John M. Gooch
1962-1963	Carl Brown	LeRoy D. Werley, Jr.
1963-1964	Claude V. Timberlake	Melvin W. Crotty
1964-1965	John M. Gooch	Robert Rigg
1965-1966	Leroy D. Werley, Jr.	Arthur W. Dodds
1966-1967	Robert Rigg	Robert Statler
1967-1968	Arthur W. Dodds	Paul E. Hubbard
1968-1969	Jack W. McNamara	Theodore W. Tober
1969-1970	Robert A. Statler	Boris J. Osteroff
1970-1971	Theodore W. Tober	William J. Christopherson
1971-1972	Boris J. Osteroff	Roland F. Harding
1972-1973	Maxine Beatty	Angelo R. Petoletti

Nuclear Pharmacy Practice Section

	Chairman
1975-1977	James F. Cooper
1977-1978	Stanley M. Shaw
1978-1979	David R. Allen
1979-1980	Stanley M. Shaw
1980-1981	Ronald J. Callahan
1981-1982	Kenneth Breslow
1982-1983	Clifford F. Hotte
1983-1984	William J. Baker
1984-1985	Robert W. Beightol
1985-1986	George H. Hinkle
1986-1987	Dennis P. Swanson
1987-1988	Richard J. Kowalsky
1988-1989	William B. Hladik III
1993-1994	David L. Laven
1994-1995	Richard J. Hammes
1995-1996	James A. Ponto
1996-1997	Stanley M. Shaw
1997-1998	Nicki L. Hilliard
1998-1999	Timothy M. Quinton
1999-2000	Kenneth T. Cheng
2000-2001	Neil A. Petry
2001-2002	Duann Vanderslice
2002-2003	Joseph C. Hung

Pharmaceutical Analysis and Control Section

	Chairman	Secretary
1969-1970	William B. Brownell	Carl R. Rehm
1970-1971	John J. Windheuser	Carl R. Rehm
1971-1972	Erik H. Jensen	Lee Timothy Grady
1972-1973	Gerald J. Papariello	Lee Timothy Grady
1973-1974	Jack P. Comer	Charles H. Barnstein
1974-1975	Bernard Z. Senkowski	Charles H. Barnstein
1975-1976	Salvatore A. Fusari	James B. Johnson
1976-1977	Hyman Mitchner	James B. Johnson
1977-1978	Lee Timothy Grady	Leo F. Cullen
1978-1979	Jane C. Sheridan	Nicholas J. DeAngelis
1979-1980	James B. Johnson	Nicholas J. DeAngelis
1980-1981	William F. Beyer	Marilyn Dix Smith
1981-1982	Leo F. Cullen	
1982-1983	James W. Munson	
1983-1984	Nicholas J. DeAngelis	
1984-1985	Robert V. Smith	
1985-1986	Marilyn Dix Smith	
1986-1987	Charles H. Barnstein	
1987-1988	James E. Carter	

Pharmaceutical Economics Section

	Chairman	Secretary
1937-1938	Henry F. Hein	Joseph H. Goodness
1938-1939	Paul C. Olsen	Joseph H. Goodness
1939-1940	Joseph H. Goodness	Clarence M. Brown
1940-1941	Clarence M. Brown	Ira Rothbrock
1941-1942	B. Olive Cole	Henry W. Heine
1942-1944	Bert R. Mull	Stephen Wilson
1944-1946	William F. Sudro	Bernard Bialk
1946-1947	Stephen Wilson	George F. Archambault°
1947-1948	Stephen Wilson	Edward J. Ireland
1948-1949	William L. Califf	Edward J. Ireland
1949-1950	Edward J. Ireland	John A. MacCartney°
1950-1951	John A. MacCartney °	Francis J. O'Brien
1951-1952	Frances J. O'Brien	Alvah G. Hall
1952-1953	Alvah G. Hall	Irving Rubin
1953-1954	Irving Rubin	James Warren Lansdowne °
1954-1955	James Warren Lansdowne°	Noel M. Ferguson
1955-1956	Noel M. Ferguson	Charles C. Rabe
1956-1957	George Scharringhausen	Benjamin A. Smith
1957-1958	Harold W. Pratt	Benjamin A. Smith
1958-1959	Arthur H. Einbeck	Benjamin A. Smith
1959-1960	Harvey J. Norgaard	Benjamin A. Smith
1960-1961	Richard L. Hull	Robert V. Evanson

Pharmaceutical Education & Legislation Section

@ = Section on Pharmaceutical Legislation only
# = Section on Pharmaceutical Education only

	Chairman	Secretary
1887-1888#	John F. Judge	Henry Milton Whelpley °
1887-1888@	Randolph F. Bryant	William Pendleton DeForest
1888-1889#	Peter Wendover Bedford°	Lucius Elmer Sayre°
1888-1889@	Charles W. Day	John Newell Hurty
1889-1890#	Peter Wendover Bedford°	Alviso Burdette Stevens
1889-1890@	Peter Wendover Bedford°	Alviso Burdette Stevens
1890-1891	William Simon	Louis Cass Hogan
1891-1892	Alviso Burdette Stevens	Louis Cass Hogan
1892-1893	Robert Gibson Eccles	Frank Gibbs Ryan
1893-1894	Robert Gibson Eccles	Louis Cass Hogan
1894-1895	James Michener Good°	Carl S. N. Hallberg
1895-1897	Carl S. N. Hallberg	James Hartley Beal°
1897-1898	James Hartley Beal °	Hendrick Gordon Webster
1898-1899	Albert Byron Lyons	James Henry Bobbitt
1899-1901	Clement Belton Lowe	Julius Arnold Koch°
1901-1902	Eugene Gustavus Eberle°	James W. T. Knox
1902-1903	James W. T. Knox	Harry Beckwith Mason

PHARMACEUTICAL EDUCATION & LEGISLATION
SECTION (continued)

	Chairman	Secretary
1903-1905	Harry Beckwith Mason	William Lincoln Cliffe
1905-1907	Oscar Oldberg °	Joseph Winters England
1907-1908	Franklin M. Apple	Joseph Weinstein
1908-1909	Joseph Winters England	Charles Herbert LaWall°
1909-1910	Charles Herbert LaWall°	Charles Willis Johnson°
1910-1911	Charles Wilson Johnson°	Wilber John Teeters
1911-1912	John Crawford Wallace	Wilber John Teeters
1912-1913	Wilber John Teeters	Frank Herman Freericks
1913-1914	Hugh Craig	Frank Herman Freericks
1914-1916	Frank Herman Freericks	Rudolph R. Kuever
1916-1917	Rudolph R. Kuever	Charles Bernard Jordan
1917-1918	Charles Bernard Jordan	Wortley Fuller Rudd
1918-1919	Wortley Fuller Rudd	Clair Albert Dye
1919-1920	Clair Albert Dye	Edward Spease
1920-1921	Edward Spease	Washington Hayne Ziegler
1921-1922	Washington Hayne Ziegler	William Francis Gidley
1922-1923	William Francis Gidley	Gordon Alger Bergy
1923-1924	Gordon Alger Bergy	William Mansfield
1924-1925	William Mansfield	John G. Beard
1925-1926	John G. Beard	Henry M. Faser
1926-1927	Henry M. Faser	Myron Nile Ford
1927-1928	Myron Nile Ford	Arthur L. I. Winne
1928-1929	Arthur L. I. Winne	Glenn Llewellyn Jenkins °
1929-1930	Glenn Llewellyn Jenkins°	Rudolph Henry Raabe
1930-1931	Bernard V. Christensen°	C. M. Anderson
1931-1932	Rudolph Henry Raabe	Charles J. Clayton
1932-1933	W. Henry Rivard	Charles W. Ballard
1933-1934	George Charles Schicks	Charles W. Ballard
1934-1935	Oscar E. Russell	Louis Wait Rising
1935-1936	C. Leonard O'Connell	George Allen Moulton°
1936-1937	George C. Schicks	John F. McCloskey
1937-1938	George Allen Moulton°	A. O. Michelsen
1938-1939	John F. McCloskey	Leslie M. Ohmart
1939-1940	A. O. Michelsen	Roland T. Lakey
1940-1942	Leslie M. Ohmart	Forest J. Goodrich
1942-1944	Edward J. Ireland	P. O. Clark
1944-1946	William F. Sudro	Bernard A. Bialk
1946-1947	Joseph S. Lucas	Bernard A. Bialk
1947-1948	James S. Hill	Ralph W. Clark
1948-1949	Bernard A. Bialk	Ralph W. Clark
1949-1950	Ralph W. Clark	David W. O'Day
1950-1951	David W. O'Day	John L. Voigt

	Chairman	Secretary
1951-1952	C. Lee Huyck	Ralph J. Mill
1952-1953	John L. Voigt	Robert A. Walsh
1953-1954	Ralph J. Mill	Frank L. Mercer
1954-1955	Robert A. Walsh	Hugh C. Ferguson
1955-1956	Frank L. Mercer	Albert L. Picchioni
1956-1957	Hugh C. Ferguson	James R. McCowan
1957-1958	Albert L. Picchioni	Richard K. Mulvey
1958-1959	James R. McCowan	Paul A. Pumpian
1959-1960	Richard K. Mulvey	Cecil P. Headlee
1960-1961	Paul A. Pumpian	Cecil P. Headlee

PHARMACEUTICAL TECHNOLOGY SECTION

	Chairman	Secretary
1961-1962	Lyman Fonda	William J. Sheffield
1962-1963	Jack K. Dale	William J. Sheffield
1963-1964	V. Jean Brown	William J. Sheffield
1964-1965	William J. Sheffield	Ben F. Cooper

PHARMACODYNAMICS AND DRUG DISPOSITION SECTION

	Chairman
1983-1984	Zola P. Horovitz
1984-1985	Herbert Barry III
1985-1986	Avraham Yacobi
1986-1987	William G. Crouthamel
1987-1988	Randall B. Smith

PHARMACOGNOSY AND NATURAL PRODUCTS SECTION

	Chairman	Secretary
1965-1967	Arthur E. Schwarting	Jack L. Beal
1967-1968	Varro E. Tyler, Jr.	Jack L. Beal
1968-1969	Gordon H. Svoboda	Jack L. Beal
1969-1970	Lynn R. Brady	Jack L. Beal
1970-1971	Egil Ramstad	George H. Constantine
1971-1972	David P. Carew	George H. Constantine
1972-1973	Jack L. Beal	George H. Constantine
1973-1974	Elmore H. Taylor	Joseph Schradie
1974-1975	Ralph N. Blomster	Joseph Schradie
1975-1976	James E. Robbers	Joseph Schradie
1976-1977	Heber W. Youngken	Joseph Schradie
1977-1978	E. John Staba	Joseph Schradie
1978-1979	Jerry L. McLaughlin	

PHARMACOLOGY AND BIOCHEMISTRY SECTION

	Chairman	Secretary
1965-1967	Joseph P. Buckley	Allan H. Conney
1967-1968	John William Keating	Tom S. Miya
1968-1969	Ewart A. Swinyard	Tom S. Miya
1969-1970	Allan H. Conney	Kenneth F. Finger
1970-1971	David H. Tedeschi	Kenneth F. Finger
1971-1972	Tom S. Miya	Jane Frances Emele

PHARMACOLOGY AND TOXICOLOGY SECTION

	Chairman	Secretary
1972-1973	Lawrence C. Weaver	Jane Frances Emele
1973-1974	Kenneth F. Finger	John Autian
1974-1975	Harold H. Wolf	John Autian
1975-1976	Raymond P. Ahlquist	Michael C. Gerald
1976-1977	C. Jelleff Carr	Michael C. Gerald
1977-1978	Harvey J. Kupferberg	Michael C. Gerald
1978-1979	Louis Diamond	Alan W. Castellion
1979-1980	Morris D. Faiman	Alan W. Castellion
1980-1981	Albert L. Picchioni	Avraham Yacobi
1981-1982	Morton E. Goldberg	
1982-1983	Lawrence W. Chakrin	

PRACTICAL PHARMACY (AND DISPENSING) SECTION

	Chairman	Secretary
1900-1901	Henry P. Hynson	Laurence S. A. Stedem
1901-1902	Laurence S. A. Stedem	William F. Kaemmerer
1902-1903	George M. Beringer°	William H. Burke
1903-1904	William H. Burke	Edsel A. Ruddiman
1904-1905	Charles A. Rapelye	William C. Kirchgessner
1905-1906	William C. Alpers°	Henry A. B. Dunning°
1906-1907	Henry A. B. Dunning°	Joseph Weinstein
1907-1908	Joseph W. England	Charles H. LaWall °
1908-1909	Leonard A. Seltzer	E. Fullerton Cook
1909-1910	Otto Raubenheimer	Erich H. Ladish
1910-1911	Louis Saalbach	Philip H. Utech
1911-1912	Philip H. Utech	J. Leon Lascoff °
1912-1913	J. Leon Lascoff °	Ferd W. Nitardy
1913-1914	Ferd W. Nitardy	Cornelius Osseward
1914-1915	Cornelius Osseward	Irwin A. Becker
1915-1916	Joseph Weinstein	Hugh B. Secheverell
1916-1917	William H. Glover	David Stoltz

PRACTICAL PHARMACY (AND DISPENSING) SECTION (continued)

	Chairman	Secretary
1917-1918	Josiah C. Peacock	Robert W. Terry
1918-1919	Robert Wood Terry	Edward Davy
1919-1920	Edsel Alexander Ruddiman	Ivor Griffith°
1920-1921	Ivor Griffith°	Henry Minor Faser
1921-1922	Ivor Griffith°	Irwin Atwood Becker
1922-1923	Crosby B. Washburn	Robert J. Ruth
1923-1924	Robert J. Ruth	William H. Ford
1924-1925	John C. Krantz, Jr.	Fred J. Blumenschein
1925-1926	Howard C. Newton °	Gustav Bachman
1926-1927	Adley Bonisteel Nichols	Charles Vail Netz
1927-1928	Adley Bonisteel Nichols	P. H. Dirstine
1928-1929	P. H. Dirstine	Howard C. Newton°
1929-1930	Howard C. Newton °	Eugene O. Leonard
1930-1931	Ralph Eugene Terry	William Paul Briggs
1931-1932	William Goggin Crockett	Ralph Eugene Terry
1932-1933	William Paul Briggs	Ralph Eugene Terry
1933-1934	Marvin Jackson Andrews	Ralph Eugene Terry
1934-1935	Henry Mathew Burlage	Leon W. Richards
1935-1936	Louis Wait Rising	Leon W. Richards
1936-1937	Harvey A. K. Whitney	Leon W. Richards
1937-1938	William J. Husa	Louis C. Zopf
1938-1939	Leon W. Richards	Louis C. Zopf
1939-1940	Ralph William Clark	Louis C. Zopf
1940-1941	Louis C. Zopf	Clark T. Eidsmoe
1941-1942	William Allen Prout	Clark T. Eidsmoe
1942-1944	Earl P. Guth	Ralph William Clark
1944-1946	George E. Crossen	Arthur P. Wyss
1946-1947	Joseph B. Sprowls	Elmer M. Plein
1947-1948	Charles V. Selby	Elmer M. Plein
1948-1949	John Zugich	Elmer M. Plein
1949-1950	Arthur P. Wyss	Elmer M. Plein
1950-1951	Raymond E. Schmitz	Elmer M. Plein
1951-1952	Mary K. Keenan	Elmer M. Plein
1952-1953	Elmer M. Klein	Samuel W. Goldstein
1953-1954	Gordon A. Bergy	Samuel W. Goldstein
1954-1955	H. George DeKay	Samuel W. Goldstein
1955-1956	William R. Lloyd	Samuel W. Goldstein
1956-1957	Leslie M. Ohmart	Samuel W. Goldstein
1957-1958	Samuel W. Goldstein	Glen J. Sperandio
1958-1959	Orville H. Miller	Samuel W. Goldstein
1959-1960	Glen J. Sperandio	Samuel W. Goldstein
1960-1961	Frederick V. Lofgren	Patrick F. Belcastro

PRACTICE MANAGEMENT SECTION

	Chairman
1977-1979	Rinaldo A. Brusadin (pro tem)
1979-1980	Mark J. Sullivan
1980-1981	Roger H. L'Hommedieu
1981-1982	Dennis A. Smith
1982-1983	J. Thomas Gulick
1983-1984	Terry D. Grant
1984-1985	Donald L. Beck
1985-1986	Linda K. Garrelts

SCIENTIFIC SECTION

	Chairman	Secretary
1887-1888	Thomas Roberts Baker	Albert Byron Lyons
1888-1889	Emlen Painter °	Henry Milton Whelpley °
1889-1890	Henry Milton Whelpley *	Charles Ford Darc
1890-1891	Edgar Leonard Patch °	Carl S. N. Hallberg
1891-1892	Carl S. N. Hallberg	Herbert Wesley Snow
1892-1893	Charles T. P. Fennel	Frank Gibbs Ryan
1893-1894	Lucius Elmer Sayre °	Charles Mangan Ford
1894-1895	Alfred R. L. Dohme °	George B. Kauffman
1895-1896	Samuel Philip Sadtler	William Charles Alpers °
1896-1897	William Charles Alpers °	Virgil Coblentz
1897-1898	Edward Kremers	Albert Byron Lyons
1898-1899	Henry Hurd Rusby °	Henry Vincome Arny °
1899-1900	Frank Gibbs Ryan	Caswell Armstrong Mayo °
1900-1901	Oscar Oldberg °	Lyman Frederic Kebler
1901-1902	Lyman Frederic Kebler	Joseph Winters England
1902-1903	Julius O. Schlotterbeck	Joseph Winters England
1903-1904	William August Puckner	Eustace Harold Gane
1904-1905	Eustace Harold Gane	Charles Edward Caspari
1905-1906	Charles Edward Caspari	Daniel Base
1906-1907	Reid Hunt	Virgil Coblentz
1907-1908	Virgil Coblentz	Charles E. Vanderkleed
1908-1909	Charles E. Vanderkleed	Martin Inventius Wilbert
1909-1910	Martin Inventius Wilbert	Albert Henry Clark
1910-1911	Albert Henry Clark	William O. Richtmann
1911-1912	William O. Richtmann	Charles Herbert LaWall °
1912-1913	Frank Randall Eldred	Freeman Preston Stroup

SCIENTIFIC SECTION (continued)

	Chairman	Secretary
1913-1914	Edsel Alexander Ruddiman	Wilbur Lincoln Scoville
1914-1915	Hermann Engelhardt	William Mansfield
1915-1916	Wilbur Lincoln Scoville	Edwin Leigh Newcomb
1916-1917	Joseph L. Turner	Warner W. Stockberger
1917-1918	Warner W. Stockberger	Henry Corbin Fuller
1918-1919	Edmund Norris Gathercoal°	Andrew Grover DuMez °
1919-1920	Jacob Diner	Andrew Grover DuMez °
1920-1921	Andrew Grover DuMez°	Heber W. Youngken
1921-1922	Heber W. Youngken	Arno Vlehoever
1922-1923	Heber W. Youngken	John Paul Snyder
1923-1924	John Paul Snyder	Paul Stewart Pittinger
1924-1925	Paul Stewart Pittinger	Frantz F. Berg
1925-1926	Frantz F. Berg	Paul Stewart Pittinger
1926-1927	John Christian Krantz	Paul Stewart Pittinger
1927-1928	Lewis W. Rowe	Paul Stewart Pittinger
1928-1929	James Clyde Munch	Lewis W. Rowe
1929-1930	Henry August Langehan	Lewis W. Rowe
1930-1931	Edward E. Swanson	Lewis W. Rowe
1931-1932	Lewis E. Warren	Lewis W. Rowe
1932-1933	William John Husa	Lewis W. Rowe
1933-1934	Francis Eugene Bibbins	Lewis W. Rowe
1934-1935	Eldin Verne Lynn	Francis Eugene Bibbins
1935-1936	Henry Mathew Burlage	Francis Eugene Bibbins
1936-1937	Glenn Llewellyn Jenkins°	Francis Eugene Bibbins
1937-1938	Bernard V. Christensen°	Francis Eugene Bibbins
1938-1939	Charles F. Lanwermeyer	Francis Eugene Bibbins
1939-1940	Joseph B. Burt °	Francis Eugene Bibbins
1940-1941	James M. Dille	Francis Eugene Bibbins
1941-1942	Walter H. Hartung	Francis Eugene Bibbins
1942-1944	Charles O. Wilson	Francis Eugene Bibbins
1945-1946	L. W. Hazelton	Ray S. Kelley
1946-1947	Louis C. Zopf	Ray S. Kelley
1947-1948	Ralph E. Anderson	Ray S. Kelley
1948-1949	Paul J. Jannke	Ray S. Kelley
1949-1950	Raymond P. Ahlquist	Ray S. Kelley
1950-1951	Earl P. Guth	Ray S. Kelley

SCIENTIFIC SECTION (continued)

	Chairman	Secretary
1951-1952	Lloyd McClain Parks °	Ray S. Kelley
1952-1953	Ole Gisvold	Ray S. Kelley
1953-1954	Leroy D. Edwards	Arthur J. McBay
1954-1955	Heber W. Youngken, Jr.	Arthur J. McBay
1955-1956	Rudolph H. Blythe	Arthur J. McBay
1956-1957	George P. Hager	Arthur J. McBay
1957-1958	Ewart A. Swinyard	Robert C. Anderson
1958-1959	John E. Christian	Robert C. Anderson
1959-1960	Martin Barr	Robert C. Anderson
1960-1961	Walter. P. Charnicki	Robert C. Anderson
1961-1962	Takeru Higuchi	Robert C. Anderson
1962-1963	Thomas J. Macek	Robert C. Anderson
1963-1964	Eino Nelson	Rudolph H. Blythe
1964-1965	Joseph V. Swintosky	Rudolph H. Blythe
1965-1966	Robert F. Doerge	Rudolph H. Blythe
1966-1967	Dale E. Wurster	

SPECIALIZED PHARMACEUTICAL SERVICES SECTION

	Chairman
1987-1990	David L. Laven
1990-1991	Stephen G. Arter
1991-1992	Martha M. Rumore
1992-1993	Clyde N. Cole
1993-1994	David L. Laven
1993-1994	Stephen G. Arter
1994-1995	Mary Lynn McPherson
1995-1996	R. David Lauper
1996-1997	Paula M. Calvert
1997-1998	William R. Letendre
1998-1999	Michael P. Cinque
1999-2000	Joni I. Berry
2000-2001	Elizabeth A. Gower
2001-2002	Melinda Joyce
2001-2002	Joni I. Berry

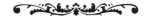

Student Organizations

PHARMACY STUDENT SECTION

	Chairman/President	Secretary-Treasurer
1954-1955	Edward L. Perednia	Harold B. Sparr
1955-1956	Donald J. Vannucci	Edgar P. Filippette
1956-1957	Donald J. Miller	Joann J. Johnson
1957-1958	James G. Dowling	Lucille Trimarco
1958-1959	Carl L. Vitalie	Joann O'Brien
1959-1960	Keith Weikel	Rose Marie Wilkas
1960-1961	Garrett Swenson	Barbara Bell
1961-1962	Dennis J. Hayes	Kathleen Young
1962-1963	Dennis J. Hayes	Bonnie Grundeman
1963-1964	Ramon P. Boswell	Barbara Lowery
1964-1965	Roger Ball	Ruth Millete
1965-1966	Tim Von Dohlen	Diana Haun
1966-1967	Edwin Green	Diane Haun
1967-1968	Dewey A. Gibson, Jr.	Marilyn Bearden
1968-1969	Joseph L. Fink III	Linda A. LaFontaine
1969-1970	Gary R. Lawless	Ann C. Bonham

STUDENT APhA

	President	House Speaker
1969-1970	Gary R. Lawless	Carey V. Post
1970-1971	Raymond L. Sattler	Lawrence J. Frieders
1971-1972	J. Craig Hostetler	Lawrence E. Patterson
1972-1973	Jack V. Nicolais	Harry C. Watters
1973-1974	Stephen W. Schondelmeyer	M. Lynn Crimson
1974-1975	Cedric H. Jones	Michael Ira Smith
1975-1976	John F. Cooper	Keith J. Frederick
1976-1977	Barbara E. Treadwell	Tery Baskin

STUDENT APhA (continued)

	President	House Speaker
1977-1978	Dennis D. Kimmel	James F. Emigh
1978-1979	Nean Molthan	Daryl R. Wesche
1979-1980	Lucinda L. Maine	Brian A. McDonald
1980-1981	Cynthia L. Iannarelli	Michael A. Mone
1981-1982	Pamela J. Koss	Dudley A. Demarest, Jr.
1982-1983	Brian B. Bullock	George E. Jones, Jr.
1983-1984	John M. Coster	Les E. Bennett
1984-1985	Carmela M. Silvestri	Jennifer S. Taylor
1985-1986	Donald D. Cilla, Jr.	Brockman E. Nyberg
1986-1987	Michael L. Manolakis	Daniel C. Malone

ACADEMY OF STUDENTS OF PHARMACY

	Chairman/President	House Speaker
1987-1988	Tracey E. Donahue	Bethany J. Boyd
1988-1989	Carol Leigh Giltner	Lora Hummel Mayer
1989-1990	Kem P. Krueger	Patti L. Gadsek
1990-1991	Marc Watrous	Monique Jackson
1991-1992	Mechelle LeWarre	Jill Bot
1992-1993	Jonathan G. Marquess	Valeria Prince
1993-1994	Tim Watson	Shevan Graham
1994-1995	Gerald B. Trapp	Eric Wolford
1995-1996	Michael D. Hogue	Valerie Schmidt
1996-1997	Joshua S. Benner	Trey Gardner
1997-1998	Jessika C. Stewart-Chinn	Helen Park
1998-1999	Jay R. Phipps	Lawrence Brown
1999-2000	Clarence McMillan, Jr.	Macary Weck
2000-2001	Jean Schreck	Joshua Welborn
2001-2002	John C. Kirtley	

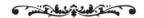

Women's Section

	President	Secretary
1912-1914	Mrs. John G. Godding	Anna Gertrude Bagley
1914-1915	Mrs. John Culley	Anna Gertrude Bagley
1915-1916	Mrs. G. D. Timmons	Anna Gertrude Bagley
1916-1917	Mrs. E. A. Ruddiman	Jean McKee Kenaston
1917-1918	Zada M. Cooper	Jean McKee Kenaston
1918-1919	Anna Gertrude Bagley	Jean McKee Kenaston
1919-1920	Mrs. F. J. Wulling	Jean McKee Kenaston
1920-1922	Mrs. Lewis C. Hopp	Genevieve Simms
1922-1923	Mrs. Lyman F. Kebler	Anna Gertrude Bagley

Section Dissolved

Auxiliary to the APhA

	President	Secretary
1946-1947	Mrs. Charles H. Evans	Mrs. Roy Bird Cook
1947-1948	Mrs. Charles H. Evans	Mrs. Arthur H. Uhl
1950-1952	Mrs. Earl. R. Serles	Mrs. W. Arthur Purdum
1952-1953	Mrs. Ray S. Kelley	Mrs. W. Arthur Purdum
1953-1954	Mrs. Ray S. Kelley	Mrs. Henry M. Burlage
1954-1956	Mrs. Hugo H. Schaefer	Mrs. Henry M. Burlage
1956-1958	Mrs. Leib L. Riggs	Mrs. Elmer M. Plein
1958-1959	Mrs. William P. Cusick	Mrs. Elmer M. Plein
1959-1960	Mrs. William P. Cusick	Mrs. Lee Worell
1960-1961	Miss Thea Gesoalde	Mrs. Lee Worell
1961-1962	Miss Thea Gesoalde	Mrs. George Scharringhausen
1962-1964	Mrs. Clifton E. Miller	Mrs. Reginald W. Lowe
1964-1966	Mrs. Lloyd M. Parks	Mrs. Reginald W. Lowe
1966-1967	Mrs. Wilbur E. Powers	Mrs. Reginald W. Lowe
1967-1968	Mrs. Roy A. Bowers	Mrs. Reginald W. Lowe

	President	Secretary
1968-1969	Mrs. Ivan Rowland	Mrs. Martin Sopocy
1969-1972	Mrs. Reginald W. Lowe	Mrs. Marie B. Kuck
1972-1974	Mrs. William J. Sheffield	Mrs. Joseph A. Oddis
1974-1976	Mrs. John S. Ruggiero	Mrs. Jack S. Heard
1976-1978	Mrs. Harry E. Durham	Mrs. Jack S. Heard
1978-1979	Mrs. Robert G. Gibbs	Mrs. Raymond A. Gosselin
1979-1981	Mrs. Hinton F. Bevis	Mrs. Albert R. Haskell
1981-1982	Mrs. Hinton F. Bevis	Mrs. Roland Leuzinger
1982-1984	Mrs. Raymond A. Gosselin	Mrs. Roland Leuzinger
1984-1986	Mary Ann Parker	Carole Huhn
1986-1988	Sophie Vlassis	Jane Fenno
1988-1990	Carole Huhn	Patricia Cobb
1990-1992	Dorothy B. Kay	Jane Fenno
1992-1994	Anne G. Tyson	Regina Johnson
1994-1996	Peggy Gawronski	Regina Johnson
1996-1998	Nan Tower	Merri Edwards
1998-2000	Blanche Prine	Peggy Gawronski

Auxiliary dissolved in 2001

Honorary Presidents

1907-1908	Philip Charles Candidus	1956-1957	Ferd Wilhelm Nitardy
1908-1909	Samuel A. D. Sheppard	1957-1958	Frank Owen Taylor
1909-1910	Enno Sander °	1958-1959	George O. Young
1910-1911	Ewen McIntyre	1959-1960	Harry Loynd
1911-1912	Henry Biroth	1960-1961	Oscar Rennebohm
1912-1913	Thomas Francis Main	1961-1962	Heber Youngken, Sr.
1913-1914	Albert Brown Lyons	1962-1963	Paul S. Pittinger
1914-1915	George Henry Schafer °	1963-1964	Thomas A. Foster
1915-1916	Fabius Chapman Godbold	1964-1965	Carl T. Durham
1916-1917	James Oscar Burge	1965-1966	Nicholas S. Gesoalde
1917-1918	William Lawrence Dewoody	1966-1967	Henry Mathew Burlage
1918-1919	Oliver Franklin Fuller	1967-1968	Troy C. Daniels
1919-1920	Alviso Burdette Stevens	1968-1969	Hugo Herman Schaefer
1920-1921	John Francis Hancock °	1969-1970	Charles O. Lee
1921-1922	John Crawford Wallace	1970-1971	B. Samuel Rogers
1922-1923	Thomas Dearmond McElhenie	1971-1972	Arthur H. Uhl
1923-1924	William Laneman DuBois	1972-1973	B. B. Brown
1924-1925	Louis Emanuel	1973-1974	Attilio R. Granito
1925-1926	William Arthur Frost	1974-1975	George L. Webster
1926-1927	William Henry Rogers	1975-1976	Justin L. Powers
1927-1928	Edward Mallinckrodt	1976-1977	Nick M. Avellone
1928-1929	Francis Edward Stewart	1977-1978	Fred Meek (posthumously)
1929-1930	Edward Victor Zoeller	1978-1979	Roy A. Bowers
1930-1931	Elie Henry La Pierre	1979-1980	Edward S. Brady
1931-1932	Henry Solomon Wellcome	1980-1981	Marjorie D. Coghill
1932-1933	Charles Frederick Heebner	1981-1982	Conrad A. Blomquist
1933-1934	Edward Kremers	1982-1983	Louise Schmitz Kortz
1934-1935	Josiah Kirby Lilly	1983-1984	Roland T. Lakey
1935-1936	David Marvel R. Culbreth	1984-1985	Allen J. Brands
1936-1937	Willis George Gregory	1985-1986	Glenn Sonnedecker
1937-1938	Henry G. Ruenzel	1986-1987	Gloria Niemeyer Francke
1938-1939	William Christine Anderson	1987-1988	Donald C. Brodie
1939-1940	John William Gayle	1988-1889	Arthur G. Zupko
1940-1941	William Perry Porterfield	1989-1990	Ewart A. Swinyard
1941-1942	Josiah Comegys Peacock	1990-1991	George B. Griffenhagen
1942-1943	James E. Hancock	1991-1992	David Jacob Krigstein
1943-1944	George Judisch	1992-1993	E. Clairborne Robins
1944-1946	Leonard A. Seltzer	1993-1994	Paul F. Parker
1946-1947	A. C. Taylor	1994-1995	Luther R. Parker
1947-1948	Gustavus A. Pfeiffer	1995-1996	Alvin N. Geser
1948-1949	John Culley	1996-1997	August P. Lemberger
1949-1950	Robert Cumming Wilson	1997-1998	Mary Louise Andersen
1950-1951	Ernest Gottlieb Eberhardt	1998-1999	Louis P. Jeffrey
1951-1952	Curt Paul Wimmer	1999-2000	Warren E. Weaver
1952-1953	Rufus A. Lyman	2000-2001	Charles D. Pulido
1953-1954	Eli Lilly	2001-2002	Charles R. Walgreen, Jr.
1954-1955	Ernest Fullerton Cook	2002-2003	Ernest Mario
1955-1956	Max N. Lemberger		

Honorary Members

George D. Armstrong	U.S.A.	(1955)	David Hooper	India	(1899)
John Attfield	Great Britain	(1871)	Hubert H. Humphrey	U.S.A.	(1962)
Franklin Bache	U.S.A.	(1857)	Joseph Ince	Great Britain	(1882)
Madison J. Bailey	U.S.A.	(1856)	Morizo Ishidate	Japan	(1971)
Robert Bentley	Great Britain	(1872)	Edward M. Kennedy	U.S.A.	(2000)
Pierre Boullay	France	(1868)	William Kirby	Great Britain	(1920)
Emile Bourquelot	France	(1919)	I. M. Kolthoff	Netherlands	(1924)
Henry Bowman Brady	Great Britain	(1871)	C. Everett Koop	U.S.A.	(1990)
Christian Brunnengraeber	Germany	(1882)	Dan Kushner	U.S.A.	(1980)
George Arnold Burbidge	Canada	(1931)	Xavier Landerer	Greece	(1877)
John Cameron	Great Britain	(1927)	George P. Larrick	U.S.A.	(1963)
Jose Manuel Cardenas	Mexico	(1999)	Charles A. LeMaistre	U.S.A.	(1985)
Michael Carteighe	Great Britain	(1882)	Desmond Lewis	Great Britain	(1976)
Arthur Casselmann	Russia	(1868)	Hugh N. Linstead	Great Britain	(1962)
Alphonse Chevalier	France	(1871)	Hermann Ludwig	Germany	(1871)
Eugene Collin	France	(1919)	Joseph Henry Maiden	Australia	(1920)
Henry Deane	Great Britain	(1868)	William Mair	Great Britain	(1931)
Augustin A. Delondre	France	(1871)	J. H. M. A. Martens	Netherlands	(1987)
A. T. De Meyer	Belgium	(1868)	J. von Martenson	Russia	(1882)
J. E. De Vrij	Netherlands	(1871)	Stanislas Martin	France	(1872)
Rudolpho Albino Dias S.	Brazil	(1930)	William Martindale	Great Britain	(1898)
Jose Guillermo Diaz	Cuba	(1929)	Charles H. Mayo	U.S.A.	(1929)
G. Dragendorff	Russia	(1868)	Ewen McIntyre	U.S.A.	(1910)
Adolph Duflos	Germany	(1871)	Arthur Meyer	Germany	(1910)
Elias Durand	U.S.A.	(1857)	John P. Miall	U.S.A.	(2000)
Carl T. Durham	U.S.A.	(1943)	Frederick Mohr	Germany	(1868)
Charles C. Edwards	U.S.A.	(1979)	Charles Moore	U.S.A.	(1934)
Thomas Farrington	U.S.A.	(1856)	Mary Kelly Mulane	U.S.A.	(1981)
John Ferguson	Great Britain	(1998)	Juan Manuel Noreiga	Mexico	(1929)
Leroy C. Fevang	Canada	(1996)	Mark Novitch	U.S.A.	(1983)
Frank Field	U.S.A.	(1983)	Paul L. O'Brien	U.S.A.	(1992)
Fredrich Fluckiger	Germany	(1868)	Alberto Garcia Ortiz	Spain	(1967)
Gen-Ichiro Fukuchi	Japan	(1966)	Wolfgang Ostwald	Germany	(1929)
Thomas R. Fulda	U.S.A.	(1995)	Armando Soto Parado	Chile	(1930)
John George Gadamer	Germany	(1923)	Emile Perrot	France	(1923)
Frederick M. Garfield	U.S.A.	(1975)	G. Planchon	France	(1877)
Norbert Gille	Belgium	(1868)	David H. Pryor	U.S.A.	(1991)
William Samuel Glyn-Jones	Great Britain	(1920)	Winton D. Rankin	U.S.A.	(1967)
Albert Goris	France	(1930)	John Redwood	Great Britain	(1871)
Henry George Greenish	Great Britain	(1913)	Richard Reynolds	Great Britain	(1882)
Thomas Greenish	Great Britain	(1882)	Stephane Robinet	France	(1868)
Leon Guignard	France	(1920)	Enno Sander	U.S.A.	(1909)
Hermann Hager	Germany	(1868)	George W. Sanford	Great Britain	(1882)
Daniel Hanbury	Great Britain	(1868)	David Satcher	U.S.A.	(1995)
Arthur Hill Hayes	U.S.A.	(1986)	Karl Schacht	Germany	(1882)
Hans Heger	Austria	(1932)	George F. Schacht	Great Britain	(1882)
F. Gladstone Hines	Great Britain	(1932)	Edward Schaer	Switzerland	(1877)
Frederick Hoffmann	Germany	(1898)	Hermann Schelenz	Germany	(1912)
J. J. Hofman	Netherlands	(1931)	Ernst Schmidt	Germany	(1899)
Edward Morell Holmes	Great Britain	(1899)	Svend A. Schou	Denmark	(1965)

Honorary Members *(continued)*

Marie Schwartz	U.S.A.	(1994)	Max Tishler	U.S.A.	(1972)
Donna E. Shalala	U.S.A.	(2000)	William Alexander Tschirch	Switzerland	(1910)
Samuel Arus D. Sheppard	U.S.A.	(1908)	John C. Turnbull	Canada	(1969)
Shoji Shibata	Japan	(1987)	Arthur Ulene	U.S.A.	(1978)
Stanley Siegelman	U.S.A.	(1989)	George Urdang	Germany/U.S.A.	(1932)
Niccola Sinimberghi	Italy	(1882)	Leopold Van Itallie	Netherlands	(1923)
Knut Magnus Sjoberg	Sweden	(1929)	Anton von Waldheim	Austria	(1871)
Herbert Skinner	Great Britain	(1932)	Anton U. R. Wasicky	Austria	(1937)
Daniel B. Smith	U.S.A.	(1856)	Henry A. Waxman	U.S.A.	(1997)
Jean Leon Soubeiran	France	(1871)	John C. Weaver	U.S.A.	(1973)
James A. Spaulding	U.S.A.	(1928)	Heinrich A. L. Wiggers	Germany	(1868)
Peter Squire	Great Britain	(1882)	Joep H. M. Winters	Netherlands	(1969)
Dieter Steinbach	Germany	(1999)	G. C. Wittstein	Germany	(1868)
C. Joseph Stetler	U.S.A.	(1979)	George B. Wood	U.S.A.	(1857)
Nils-Olaf Strandqvist	Sweden	(1996)	Hector Zayas-Bazan y Perdomo	Cuba/U.S.A.	(1982)
Kozaburo Takeda	Japan	(1971)	Heinrich Zoernig	Switzerland	(1910)
Hermann Thoms	Germany	(1923)			

APPENDIX E

Sources of Information

American Pharmaceutical Association

C[onrad] Lewis Diehl, "The American Pharmaceutical Association," *The Pharmaceutical Era*, vol. 16, pp. 878-886, December 31, 1896.

Frederick Hoffmann, "A Retrospect of the Development of American Pharmacy and the American Pharmaceutical Association," *APhA Proceedings*, vol. 50, pp. 100-145, 1902.

Henry M[ilton] Whelpley, "The American Pharmaceutical Association in 1902," *APhA Proceedings*, vol. 50, pp. 7-24, 1902.

Anonymous, "The American Pharmaceutical Association," *The Druggists Circular*, 50th anniversary issue, pp. 100-103, January 1907.

John F[rancis] Hancock, "The American Pharmaceutical Association: Its Origin, Results, and Possibilities," *Journal of the American Pharmaceutical Association*, vol. 1, pp. 12-17, 1912.

Franklin M. Apple, "Pennsylvania in the American Pharmaceutical Association," *Journal of the American Pharmaceutical Association*, vol. 3, pp. 1135 1138, 1914.

William C[harles] Alpers, "The History of the American Pharmaceutical Association, *Journal of the American Pharmaceutical Association*, vol. 1, pp. 972-992, 1912; vol. 3, pp. 1625-1640, 1914; vol. 4, pp. 3-17, 1915.

Eugene G[ustave] Eberle, "The Original Certificate of Membership of the American Pharmaceutical Association," *Journal of the American Pharmaceutical Association*, vol. 5, pp. 459-461, 1916.

Edgar L[eonard] Patch, "Fifty Years of APhA," *Practical Druggist*, pp. 33-34. January 1922.

William B[aker] Day, "The American Pharmaceutical Association: An Historical Sketch," *Druggist Circular*, July 1924.

James H[artley] Beal, "The Work, Principal Purposes, and Ideals of APhA," *Journal of the American Pharmaceutical Association*, vol. 16, pp. 799-800, 1927.

Eugene G[ustave] Eberle, "Periods in the History of APhA," *Journal of the American Pharmaceutical Association*, vol. 16, pp. 711-712, 1927.

David M. R. Culbreth, "Ex-Presidents of APhA from Baltimore," *Journal of the American Pharmaceutical Association*, vol. 20, pp. 246-252, 1931.

James H[artley] Beal, "Place and Purpose of APhA Among Pharmaceutical Organizations," *Journal of the American Pharmaceutical Association*, vol. 21, pp. 698-703, 1932.

James H[artley] Beal, "APhA as a Factor in American Food and Drug Legislation," *Journal of the American Pharmaceutical Association*, vol. 26, pp. 747-751, 1937.

George Urdang, "The APhA and Her Children," *American Druggist*, August 1946. (Describes APhA's role in the formation of the AACP, ACA, ASHP, NABP, and NARD.)

Charles W. Ballard, "Historical Background on the Founding of the APhA," *Journal of the American Pharmaceutical Association, Practical Pharmacy Edition*, vol. 12, pp. 695-697, 1951

Various Authors, "Founding Members of APhA," *Journal of the American Pharmaceutical Association, Practical Pharmacy Edition*, vol. 13, pp. 704-708, 1952. (Biographies of founding members.)

Bernard Zerbe, "Roster of the Presidents of the American Pharmaceutical Association" (with portraits), *Journal of the American Pharmaceutical Association, Practical Pharmacy Edition*, vol. 12, pp. 493-500, 1952.

Anonymous, "The First Certificate of Membership," *Journal of the American Pharmaceutical Association, Practical Pharmacy Edition*, vol. 12, pp. 490-492, 1952.

American Pharmaceutical Association (continued)

George A. Bender, *Great Moments in Pharmacy*, Northwood Institute Press, Detroit, 1966. (Pages 118-124 describe the founding of APhA, including a reproduction of the Robert Thom painting depicting the founding meeting in Philadelphia, October 6-8, 1852.)

George Urdang, "The Founding Period of the American Pharmaceutical Association 1852-1872," *American Pharmaceutical Association: Tribute in Bronze to the Founding, 1852*, Philadelphia, 1964.

Glenn Sonnedecker, *Kremers and Urdang's History of Pharmacy*, Fourth Edition, J. B. Lippincott Company, Philadelphia, 1976. (Pages 198-205 provide a concise history of the American Pharmaceutical Association.)

George Griffenhagen, "What Is Past Is Prologue," *Journal of the American Pharmaceutical Association*, vol. NS15, p. 375, 1975.

George Griffenhagen, "125th APhA Anniversary," *Journal of the American Pharmaceutical Association*, vol. NS17, pp. 614-616, 1977.

Anonymous, "A New Look Debuts" [History of APhA Logos], *American Pharmacy*, NS25, p. 458, 1985.

APhA Annual Meetings

George Griffenhagen, "The American Pharmaceutical Association in Cincinnati," *Journal of the American Pharmaceutical Association, Practical Pharmacy Edition*, vol. 20, pp. 378-379, 1959.

Anonymous, "APhA in the Nation's Capital: A Look Back," *Journal of the American Pharmaceutical Association, Practical Pharmacy Edition*, vol. 21, pp. 407-409, 1960. See also article with the same title in *Journal of the American Pharmaceutical Association*, vol. NS10, p. 138, 1970.

Anonymous, "APhA Recalls Chicago in Retrospect," *Journal of the American Pharmaceutical Association*, vol. NS1, pp. 214-218, 1961.

George Griffenhagen, "[Meetings in Canada] from 1896 to 1969," *Journal of the American Pharmaceutical Association*, vol. NS9, p. 153, 1969.

Anonymous, "Centenary Travelogue [in San Francisco]," *American Pharmacy*, NS29, pp. 273-275, 1989.

APhA Branches and Chapters

Charles E. Vanderkleed, John E. Kramer, and E. Fullerton Cook, *History of the Philadelphia Branch of APhA 1906-1952*, 94-page manuscript in the APhA Foundation Archives.

APhA Code of Ethics

Robert A. Buerki, *The Challenge of Ethics in Pharmacy Practice*, American Institute of the History of Pharmacy, Madison, Wisconsin, 1985. (Appendix includes evolution of the APhA Code of Ethics.)

Michael L. Manolakis, "Why APhA Should Reject Its Code of Ethics," *American Pharmacy*, NS31, pp. 822-824, 1991.

Robert A. Buerki and Louis D. Vottero, *Ethical Responsibility in Pharmacy Practice*, American Institute of the History of Pharmacy, Madison, Wisconsin, 1994. Appendix A records all APhA Codes of Ethics from 1852 to 1994.

Joseph L. Fink III, "Updating the Code of Ethics," *American Pharmacy*, vol. NS34, p. 80, August 1994.

APhA Headquarters Building

C[arl] S. N. Hallberg, "The Procter Memorial," *APhA Bulletin*, vol. 1, pp. 133-137, May 1906.

Henry S[olomon] Wellcome, "The American Institute of Pharmacy," *Journal of the American Pharmaceutical Association*, vol. 19, pp. 676-679, 1930.

Robert L[ee] Swain, "The American Institute of Pharmacy Dedication Address," *Journal of the American Pharmaceutical Association*, vol. 23, pp. 480-483, 1934.

Anonymous, "APhA Builds Its Annex," *Journal of the American Pharmaceutical Association, Practical Pharmacy Edition*, vol. 21, pp. 426-427, 1960.

George Griffenhagen, *The American Institute of Pharmacy 50th Anniversary*, APhA, Washington, D.C., 1984; reprinted as *The American Institute of Pharmacy*, Washington, D.C., 1989.

Anonymous, "A Restoration Completed: APhA Headquarters," *American Pharmacy*, vol. NS28, pp. 570-572, 1988.

Anonymous, "APhA Building Featured at National Gallery Exhibit," *American Pharmacy*, NS31, p. 171, 1991.

Steven Bedford, "Museums Designed by John Russell Pope," *Antiques Magazine*, pages 750-763, April 1991. [Describes and illustrates Pope's original 1907 design subsequently used for APhA headquarters building.]

Anonymous, *American Pharmaceutical Association Flagpole Memorial*, APhA, Washington, D.C., 1993.

Steven Bedford, *John Russell Pope: Architect of Empire*, pages 140-145, Rizzoli International Publications, New York, 1999.

APhA Sub-Divisions (Foundation)

Anonymous, *American Pharmaceutical Association Foundation*, Washington, D.C., 1990.

APhA Sub-Divisions (Historical Pharmacy)

Anonymous, *Catalogue of the Historical Exhibition: American Pharmaceutical Association 1852-1902*, Philadelphia. September 8-13, 1902.

George Urdang, "The American Pharmaceutical Association's Section on Historical Pharmacy," *American Journal of Pharmaceutical Education*, vol. 17, pp. 389-400, July 1953.

APhA Sub-Divisions (House of Delegates)

Anonymous, "House of Delegates Special Meeting," *Journal of the American Pharmaceutical Association*, vol. NS9, pp. 21-32, 1969. (Includes a history of the APhA House of Delegates.)

David J. Krigstein, "The House of Delegates; A True Representation," *Journal of the American Pharmaceutical Association*, vol. NS15, pp. 310, 320, 1975.

Anonymous, "House of Delegates: the Function and Composition," *Journal of the American Pharmaceutical Association*, vol. NS17, pp. 150-151, 1977.

George Griffenhagen, *APhA House of Delegates: A Review of Policy Development and Implementaton*, June 8, 1992, Manuscript in APhA Foundation Archives.

Hazel M. Pipkin, "APhA's House of Delegates: Overhaul or Tuneup?" *American Pharmacy*, vol. NS32, p. 684, 1992.

APhA Sub-Divisions (Pharmacy Practice)

Alex Berman, "The Section on Practical Pharmacy of the American Pharmaceutical Association," *American Journal of Pharmaceutical Education*, vol. 17, pp. 351-362, July 1953.

Norman H. Franke, "The Section on Pharmaceutical Economics of the American Pharmaceutical Association," *American Journal of Pharmaceutical Education*, vol. 17, pp. 334-341, July 1953.

Glenn Sonnedecker, "The Section on Education and Legislation of the American Pharmaceutical Association," *American Journal of Pharmaceutical Education*, vol. 17, pp. 362-383, July 1953.

William J. Edwards, "Academy of General Practice of Pharmacy: A Decade of Service to the Pharmacy Practitioner," *Journal of the American Pharmaceutical Association*, vol. NS15, pp. 322-324, 1975.

Stanley M. Shaw, "Emergence of the Specialty of Nuclear Pharmacy," *American Pharmacy*, vol. NS19, pp. 304-305, 1979.

James F. Cooper, editor, *Twenty-Five Years APhA Academy of Pharmacy Practice and Management Nuclear Pharmacy Section*, Washington D.C., March 13, 2000.

APhA Sub-Divisions (Scientists)

George Griffenhagen, "The Scientific Section of the American Pharmaceutical Association," *American Journal of Pharmaceutical Education*, vol. 17, pp. 342-350, July 1953.

William L. Blockstein, "Academy of Pharmaceutical Sciences," *Journal of the American Pharmaceutical Association*, vol. NS5, pp. 602-604, 1966.

Louis W. Busse, "The Role of the Academy of Pharmaceutical Sciences," *Journal of the American Pharmaceutical Association*, vol. NS15, pp. 156-158, 1975.

Klaus G. Florey, *The Founding of the APhA Academy of Pharmaceutical Sciences: A History*, APhA, Washington, DC, 1979.

Anthony Palmieri III, *Thirty Years of Scientific Excellence: APhA Academy of Pharmaceutical Research and Science*, APhA, Washington, DC, 1996.

APhA Sub-Divisions (Students)

B[ernard] V. Christensen, "Student Branches of APhA," *Journal of the American Pharmaceutical Association*, vol. 19, pp. 390-393, 1930.

John F. McCloskey, "The Student Branches of APhA," *Journal of the American Pharmaceutical Association, Practical Pharmacy Edition*, vol. 17, pp. 662-663, 1956.

Yvonne Marie Dietrich, *History of the Student Branches of APhA*, Thesis at Loyola University of the South, May 1957 (bound 43-page typescript in APhA Foundation Archives).

Anonymous, "APhA and Its Student Chapters," *The Pharmacy Student*, volume 11, #4, Autumn 1981.

Students (continued)

Various authors, "30th Anniversary of APhA-ASP," *Pharmacy Student*, supplement to the *Journal of the American Pharmaceutical Association*, vol. 39, March-April 1999.

APhA Sub-Divisions (Women)

Eunice R. Bonow, "The Women's Section of the American Pharmaceutical Association," *American Journal of Pharmaceutical Education*, vol. 17, pp. 383-388, July 1953.

Mrs. Reginald Lowe, "Women's Auxiliary: A Bit About the Past," *Journal of the American Pharmaceutical Association*, vol. NS13, p. 164, 1973.

George Griffenhagen, "Woman Power," *Journal of the American Pharmaceutical Association*, vol. NS13, p. 609, 1973.

Marvin D. Shephard and Kenneth W. Kirk, "Women in Pharmacy," *American Pharmacy*, vol. NS21, pp. 237-241, 1981.

Metta Lou Henderson and Tammy Lynn Keeney, "Women in Pharmacy Education: the Pioneers," *American Pharmacy*, vol. NS28, pp. 308-311, 1988.

APhA Sub-Divisions (Publications)

C[onrad] Lewis Diehl, "The Evolution of the *National Formulary*," *APhA Bulletin*, pp. 14-18, 44-47, January 1909.

Samuel L[ouis] Hilton, "The APhA Recipe Book," *Journal of the American Pharmaceutical Association*, vol. 26, pp. 354-355, 1937.

Justin L. Powers, "The Scientific Edition of the Journal of the American Pharmaceutical Association," *Journal of the American Pharmaceutical Association, Scientific Edition*, vol. 33, pp. 520-524, 1944.

Anonymous, "This [APhA] Journal and Its Origins," *Journal of the American Pharmaceutical Association, Practical Pharmacy Edition*, vol. 18, p. 25, 1957.

Anonymous, "Twenty Years of Progress," *Journal of the American Pharmaceutical Association, Practical Pharmacy Edition*, vol. 21, pp. 14-15, 1960.

Glenn Sonnedecker, "The [APhA] Journal is Born," *Journal of the American Pharmaceutical Association*, vol. NS1, pp. 744-745, 776-777, December 1961.

Edward G. Feldmann, "Future of Drug Compendia," *Journal of the American Pharmaceutical Association*, vol. NS15, pp. 198-201, 1975.

Edward G. Feldmann, Gregory J. Higby, William M. Heller, and Glenn Sonnedecker, *One Hundred Years of the National Formulary*, American Institute of the History of Pharmacy, Madison, Wisconsin, 1989.

George Griffenhagen, "Coming Full Circle," *Journal of the American Pharmaceutical Association*, vol. NS56, pp. 5-6, 1996.

APhA Related Activities

Eugene G[ustave] Eberle, "National Pharmaceutical Week," *Journal of the American Pharmaceutical Association*, vol. 14, pp. 369-471, 1925.

Robert J. Ruth, "The History of National Pharmacy Week" *Journal of the American Pharmaceutical Association*, vol. 20, pp. 696-706, 1931.

William John Hajin, "The National Quinine Pool," *The Hospital Corps Quarterly*, vol. 16, pp. 1-46, October 1943.

Hugo H. Schaefer, "Pharmaceutical Education's Great Years 1900 to 1951," *Journal of the American Pharmaceutical Association, Practical Pharmacy Edition*, vol. 12, pp. 280-283, 1951.

Wallace F. Janssen, "Fifty Years of Progress in Food and Drug Protection," *Journal of the American Pharmaceutical Association, Practical Pharmacy Edition*, vol. 17, pp. 339-341, 353, 1956.

Robert Abramson, "National Pharmacy Week: A Brief History," *Journal of the American Pharmaceutical Association, Practical Pharmacy Edition*, vol. 17, pp. 446-449, 473, 1956.

Homer A. George, "Poison Prevention Week," *Journal of the American Pharmaceutical Association, Practical Pharmacy Edition*, vol. 21, pp. 139-140, 1960.

Anonymous, "Birth of Public Relations in the U.S.A.," *Journal of the American Pharmaceutical Association, Practical Pharmacy Edition*, vol. 21, pp. 477-478, 1960.

George Griffenhagen, "Participation of U.S. Pharmacists in International Congresses," *American Journal of Hospital Pharmacy*, vol. 20, pp. 121-131, March 1963.

Aaron J. Spector, *The Pharmacy as a Health Education Center: An Experimental Study Conducted by National Analysts, Inc. for the American Pharmaceutical Association*, Washington, DC, 1964.

APhA Related Activities (continued)

Chet Huntly, "National Survey Evaluates Community Pharmacy as Health Education Center," *Journal of the American Pharmaceutical Association*, vol. NS4, pp. 475-481, 1964.

Anonymous, "World Fairing with APhA Through the Ages," *Journal of the American Pharmaceutical Association*, vol. NS4, pp. 264-267, 1964.

K. M. Reese, "Drug Standards Laboratory Enters Second Decade," *Journal of the American Pharmaceutical Association*, vol. NS12, pp. 16-20, 1972.

George Griffenhagen, William L. Blockstein, and David J. Krigstein, *The Remington Lectures: A Century in American Pharmacy*, American Pharmaceutical Association, 1994.

Maurice Q[uinn] Bectel, "Employer-Employee Relations in Historical Perspective," *Journal of the American Pharmaceutical Association*, vol. NS10, pp. 91-92, 1970.

Virginia Bates Johnson, "Drug Product Selection Through the Decades," *American Pharmacy*, vol. NS20, pp. 572-576, 1980.

Wallace F. Janssen, "Milestones in U.S. Drug Law History," *American Pharmacy*, vol. NS21, pp. 212-221, 1981.

Anonymous, "APhA's Major Antitrust [Mail Order] Victory," *American Pharmacy*, vol. NS21, pp. 606-609, 1981.

Roger E. Parker, Domingo R. Martinez, and Timothy R. Covington, "Drug Product Selection: History and Legal Overview," *American Pharmacy*, vol. NS31, pp. 524-531, 655-664, 1991.

Gregory J. Higby, *In Service to American Pharmacy; The Professional Life of William Procter, Jr.*, University of Alabama Press, Tuscaloosa, c. 1992. 269 pp.

Board of Pharmaceutical Specialties

Vicki Meade, "Specialization in Pharmacy," *American Pharmacy*, vol. NS31, pp. 24-29, 1991.

Anonymous, "Board of Pharmaceutical Specialties Going Strong After 25 Years," Offset report issued in 2001.

Related Organizations

American Association of Colleges of Pharmacy

Anonymous, "The Organization of the Drug Trade," *American Druggist*, pp. 68-70, 1931.

Harry L. Kendall and C[harles] O. Lee, "College of Pharmacy Associations," *American Journal of Pharmaceutical Education*, vol. 8, pp. 195-230, 1944.

George Urdang, "College of Pharmacy Associations," *American Journal of Pharmaceutical Education*, vol. 8, pp. 333-339, 1944.

Robert A. Buerki, "The First Century of the American Association of Colleges of Pharmacy," *American Journal of Pharmaceutical Education*, vol. 63, 210 pages, Fall Supplement 1999.

American Association of Consultant Pharmacists

Becky Comer and Michael Posey, *Twenty-Five Years of Caring*, American Association of Consultant Pharmacists, 1994.

American College of Apothecaries

Henry V[income] Arny, "The American Institute of Prescriptionists," *Journal of the American Pharmaceutical Association*, vol. 3, pp. 1542-1547, 1914.

Leonard J. Piccoli, "A Proposed American College of Pharmacists," *Journal of the American Pharmaceutical Association, Practical Pharmacy Edition*, vol. 1, pp. 174-175, 1940.

Ernst W. Stieb, *First Quarter Century of the American College of Apothecaries*, ACA, 1970.

American Council on Pharmaceutical Education

Anonymous, "American Council on Pharmaceutical Education," *Journal of the American Pharmaceutical Association*, vol. 27, pp. 64-65, 1938.

Robert L[ee] Swain, "A.C.P.E. Conceived," *Journal of the American Pharmaceutical Association, Practical Pharmacy Edition*, vol. 15, pp. 484-485, 1954.

American Foundation for Pharmaceutical Education

Edward S. Rogers, "The Objectives of the American Foundation for Pharmaceutical Education," *American Journal of Pharmaceutical Education*, vol. 8, pp. 316-327, 1944.

W. Paul Briggs, *American Foundation for Pharmaceutical Education 25th Anniversary Year*, Washington, DC, 1967.

Albert B. Fischer. Jr., *A Half Century of Service to Pharmacy 1942-1992*, American Foundation for Pharmaceutical Education, June 1992.

American Institute of the History of Pharmacy

George Urdang, "Why the AIHP Was Organized at Madison, Wisconsin," *Badger Pharmacist*, March 1941.

American Institute of the History of Pharmacy
(continued)

George Urdang, *The First Five Years of the American Institute of the History of Pharmacy*, AIHP, Madison, Wisconsin, 1946.

Anonymous, "AIHP 10th Anniversary," *Wisconsin Druggist*, pp. 11-12, June 1951.

Ernst W. Stieb, *American Institute of the History of Pharmacy Through Two Decades*, Madison, Wisconsin. 25 pp.

American Society of Health-System Pharmacists
John F. Miller and Russell H. Stimson, "Our Hospital Pharmacists' Association," *Journal of the American Pharmaceutical Association*, vol. 28, pp. 606-609, 1939.

Blossom L. Lehrke, "A Survey of Hospital Pharmacy Associations in the U.S.," *Journal of the American Pharmaceutical Association*, vol. 28, pp. 680-683, 1939.

Don E[ugene] Francke, "The Hospital Pharmacist," *Journal of the American Pharmaceutical Association, Practical Pharmacy Edition*, vol. 6, pp. 77-78, 1945.

Anonymous, "Hospital Pharmacy Division Established," *Journal of the American Pharmaceutical Association, Practical Pharmacy Edition*, vol. 8, p. 76, 1947.

Gloria Niemeyer, Alex Berman, and Don E[ugene] Francke, "Ten Years of the American Society of Hospital Pharmacists 1942-1952," *Bulletin of the American Society of Hospital Pharmacists*, vol. 9, pp. 277-421, 1952.

Alex Berman, *The American Society of Hospital Pharmacists: A Bicentennial Perspective*, ASHP, 1975, 16 pp.

Ruth Roy Harris and Warren E. McConnell, "The American Society of Hospital Pharmacists: A History," *American Journal of Hospital Pharmacy* Supplement, 1993.

American Society for Pharmacy Law
Joseph L. Fink III, "Pharmacist-Lawyers," *Journal of the American Pharmaceutical Association*, vol. NS14, pp. 565-569, 1974.

American Society of Pharmacognosy
Anna Koffler Wannamaker, *The History of the Plant Science Seminar*, American Society of Pharmacognosy, 1973.

Consumer Healthcare Products Association
Frederick Humphreys and Ray Vaughn Pierce, "Association of Manufacturers and Dealers in Proprietary Articles in the U.S.," *The Pharmaceutical Era*, vol. 16, pp. 901-905, December 31, 1896.

Anonymous, "The Proprietary Association of America," *The Druggists Circular*, 50th anniversary issue, pp. 112-114, January 1907.

Ervin F. Kemp, "Some Notes on the History of the Proprietary Association," *Journal of the American Pharmaceutical Association*, vol. 15, pp. 973-979, November 1926.

Healthcare Distribution Management Association
Anonymous, "The National Wholesale Druggists Association," *Western Druggist*, vol. 19, pp. 32-34, 1893.

M[ahlon] N. Kline, "The National Wholesale Druggists Association," *The Pharmaceutical Era*, vol. 16, pp. 896-900, December 31, 1896.

Anonymous, "The National Wholesale Druggists Association," *The Druggists Circular*, 50th anniversary issue, pp. 110-112, January 1907.

Charles H. Waterbury, *A History of the National Wholesale Druggists Association*, NWDA, New York, 1924.

Lyman F. Kebler, "The Western Wholesale Drug Association (1876-1882)," *Journal of the American Pharmaceutical Association*, vol. 15, pp. 293-297, 1926.

Anonymous, "The Organization of the Drug Trade," *American Druggist*, pp. 33-50, 1931.

John T. Fay, Jr., *NWDA First One Hundred Years 1876-1976*, Wholesale Drugs Centennial Issue, Indianapolis, Indiana, 1976.

National Association of Boards of Pharmacy
H[enry] C. Christensen, "The Influence of Henry Milton Whelpley in the Formation of the National Association of Boards of Pharmacy," *Journal of the American Pharmaceutical Association*, vol. 17, pp. 782-784, 1928.

Robert L[ee] Swain, "National Association of Boards of Pharmacy in Appreciation of its 50 Years of Achievement," *Journal of the American Pharmaceutical Association, Practical Pharmacy Edition*, vol. 15, pp. 482-485, 1954.

Roy Bird Cook, Patrick H[enry] Costello, Glenn Sonnedecker, Robert L[ee] Swain, and George Urdang, *National Association of Boards of Pharmacy 1904-1954*, American Institute of the History of Pharmacy in cooperation with NABP, Madison, Wisconsin, 1955.

Melvin W. Green, *The First 75 Years of the National Association of Boards of Pharmacy*, NABP, Chicago, Illinois, 1979.

National Association of Chain Drug Stores

Frank H. Freericks, "The Chain Store," *Journal of the American Pharmaceutical Association*, vol. 16, pp. 1175-1179, 1927.

Anonymous, *NACDS: The First 50 Years*, National Association of Chain Drug Stores, 1983.

Jane Mobley, *Prescription for Success: The Chain Drug Story*, Hallmark Cards, Lowell Press, Kansas City, Missouri, 1990.

National Community Pharmacists Association

Anonymous, "The National Association of Retail Druggists," *The Druggists Circular*, 50th anniversary issue, pp. 104-109, January 1907.

Samuel C. Henry, "Concerning the N.A.R.D.," *The Druggists Circular*, vol. 68, pp. 299-302, August 1924.

George Urdang, "The Precedents of the NARD and Its Founding 50 Years Ago," *American Journal of Pharmaceutical Education*, vol. 13, pp. 358-375, 1949.

C. Fred Williams, *A Century of Service and Beyond: 1898 NARD / 1998 NCPA: A History of One Hundred Years of Leadership for Independent Pharmacy*, National Community Pharmacists Association, Alexandria, Virginia, 1998.

National Conference of Pharmaceutical Organizations

James D. Cope, *The Story of the National Drug Trade Conference*, Washington, DC, 1989.

James D. Cope, *The Story of the National Conference of Pharmaceutical Organizations*, Washington, DC, 1996.

Pharmaceutical Research and Manufacturers of America

Birdsey L. Maltbie, "High Points in the History of American Pharmaceutical Manufacturers' Association," *Journal of the American Pharmaceutical Association*, vol. 16, pp. 1192-1194, 1927.

Anonymous, "The Organization of the Drug Trade," *American Druggist*, pp. 3-20, 1931.

Birdsey L. Maltbie, *A Quarter Century of Progress in Manufacturing Pharmacy*, American Pharmaceutical Manufacturers Association, New York, New York, 1937.

Herbert S. Wilkinson, "History and Evolution of the Pharmaceutical Industry," *Journal of the American Pharmaceutical Association, Practical Pharmacy Edition*, vol. 20, pp. 592-593, 1959.

William C. Cray, *The First 25 Years of the Pharmaceutical Manufacturers Association Foundation*, Pharmaceutical Manufacturers Association Foundation, Washington, DC, 1984.

William C. Cray, *The First 30 Years [of] the Pharmaceutical Manufacturers Association*, Pharmaceutical Manufacturers Association, Washington, DC, 1989.

United States Pharmacopeial Convention

Glenn Sonnedecker, "The Founding Period of the U.S. Pharmacopeia," *Pharmacy in History*, vol. 35, pp 151-162, 1993; vol. 36, pp 3-25, 103-122, 1994.

Lee Anderson and Gregory J. Higby, *The Spirit of Volunterism: The United States Pharmacopeia 1820-1995*, The United States Pharmacopeial Convention, Rockville, Maryland, 1995.

Lee Anderson and Kathy Penningroth, *Good Work & True: The United States Pharmacopeial Convention Board of Trustees 1900-2000*, The United States Pharmacopeial Convention, Rockville, Maryland, 2000.

Fraternities and Sororities

Jerome Boonshoft and Robert Kirschner, *Forty Years of AZO*, Alpha Zeta Omega, 1960.

A. Richard Bliss, "A Brief History of Kappa Psi Fraternity," *Journal of the American Pharmaceutical Association*, vol. 11, pp. 352-356, 1922.

Frank H. Eby, *The History of Kappa Psi Pharmaceutical Fraternity 1879-1966*, Kappa Psi Fraternity, 1967.

Dewey D. Garner, *The History of Kappa Psi Pharmaceutical Fraternity 1879-1993*, Kappa Psi Fraternity, 1993.

Lewis N. Brown, "A Brief History of Phi Delta Chi Fraternity," *Journal of the American Pharmaceutical Association*, vol. 11, pp. 351-352, 1922.

John D. Grabenstein, *Phi Delta Chi: A Tradition of Leaders in Pharmacy*, Phi Delta Chi, Athens, Georgia, 1995.

Zada M. Cooper, "Rho Chi Honorary Pharmaceutical Society," *Journal of the American Pharmaceutical Association*, vol. 14, pp. 734-736, 1925.

Glenn L[lewellyn] Jenkins, "The Rho Chi Society — 1922-1932," *Journal of the American Pharmaceutical Association*, vol. 21, pp. 1033-1037, 1932.

Roy A. Bowers and David L. Cowen, *The Rho Chi Society: The Development of the Honor Society of American Pharmacy*, 3rd edition, Rho Chi Society, Madison, 1966.

Index of Persons

This index includes every person mentioned in the text and/or appendices, with the page number(s) on which the person is referenced one or more times. A "p" following the page number indicates that this page includes a portrait photograph of the person; a "b" following the page number indicates that this page includes a biographical sketch of the person.

P

Packard, Charles H...55, 76, 242pb, 254, 256, 257, 259

Painter, Emlen...216, 243pb, 253, 255, 257, 275

Palmieri III, Anthony...266, 267, 283

Palumbo, Francis B...264, 266, 269

Papariello, Gerald J...272

Parado, Armando Soto...279

Parascandola, John...3

Parisen, George W...257, 264

Park, Helen...276

Parks, Lloyd M...242pb, 254, 256, 262, 276

Parks, Mrs. Lloyd M,,,142, 277

Parker, Luther R...278

Parker, Mrs. Luther R...277

Parker, Paul F...278

Parker, Roger E...285

Parran, Thomas...181

Parrish, Edward...Frontispiece, 7, 17, 18, 19, 113, 154, 173, 216, 242pb, 253, 255, 258

Patch, Edgar L...123, 218, 243pb, 253, 275, 281

Patterson, Lawrence E...153, 276

Patton, John F...33, 217, 243pb, 253

Patton, Thomas F...267

Pauley, Alfred W...255

Payne, George F...19, 61, 62, 66, 222, 243pb, 254, 255, 256

Peacock, Josiah C...274, 278

Pease, Autumn V...268

Peck, Garnet E...271

Peck, Samuel P...256

Penna, Richard P...107, 266

Penningroth, Kathy...287

Perednia, Edward L...150, 276

Perfetto, Eleanor M...269

Perrot, Emile...279

Perruso, Judith F...107

Perry, Frederick W. R...259

Petoletti, Angelo R...269, 271

Petry, Neil A...272

Pevonka, M. Peter...271

Pfeiffer, Gustavus A...278

Pflag, Solomon C...271

Philbrick, Samuel...Frontispiece

Philip, W. Bruce...83, 90, 179, 243pb, 254, 258, 260, 268

Phipps, Jay R...276

Picchioni, Albert L...273, 274

Piccoli, Leonard J...285

Pierce, Ray Vaughn...286

Pipkin, Hazel M...87, 142, 223, 261, 264, 266, 283

Pittinger, Paul S...255, 264, 275, 278

Plakogiannis, Fotios M...267

Planchon, G...279

Plein, Elmer M...274

Plein, Mrs. Elmer M...277

Ponto, James A...272

Pope, John H...256

Pope, John Russell...Preface, 88, 91

Porterfield, William P...258, 264, 270, 278

Posey, L. Michael...106, 107, 285

Post, Carey V...276

Poulson, Boyd J...60, 200, 271

Power, Frederick B...191

Powers, Justin L...104, 114, 278, 284

Powers, Thomas H...159, 167

Powers, Wilbur E...260

Powers, Mrs. Wilbur E...277

Pratt, Harold W...272

Prescott, Albert B...9, 47, 121, 122, 123, 222, 243pb, 253, 256

Prescott, Donald E...107

Preston, Andrew P...255, 264

Price, Constance...140

Prince, Shelly...267

Prince, Valerie...267, 270, 276

Prine, Blanche...277

Pritchard, Benjamin E...268

Pritchard, Mearl D...36, 219, 255, 260, 264

Pritchard, M. Donald...256, 264

Procter, Jr., William...Frontispiece, 6, 10, 17, 63, 101, 108, 160, 177, 190, 191, 192, 193, 197, 199, 243pb, 253, 255, 258

Prout, William A...274

Provost, George P...105

Pryor, David H...279

Puckner, William A...275

Pulido, Charles D...264, 278

Pulido, Mark A...266

Pumpian, Paul A...273

Purdum, W. Arthur...264

Purdum, Mrs. W. Arthur...277

Putnam, Mary Corinna...137

Q

Quinton, Timothy M...272

R

Raabe, Rudolph H...273

Rabe, Charles C...220, 256, 264, 272

Ragland, Jr., Fred...264

Ramsaur, David W...268

Ramseth, James R...46, 266

Ramsperger, Gustavus...264

Ramstad, Egil...273

Rankin, Jesse W...258

Rankin, Winton D...279

Rapelye, Charles A...256, 264, 268, 274

Rasanen, Paul R...271

Rascati, Karen L...269

Raubenheimer, Herbert...270

Raubenheimer, Otto...115, 270, 274

Reagan, Ronald...11

Reamer, Thomas...56, 57

Redman, Kenneth...270

Redsecker, Jacob H...264

Redwood, John...279

Reed, Karen L...269

Reeder, C. Eugene...264, 266, 269

Reese, J. A...124

Reese, K.M...285

Rehm, Carl R...272

Reilly, Robert C...268

Remington, Joseph P...28, 75, 110, 123, 163, 193, 200, 217, 223, 244pb, 250p, 253, 258

Rennebohm, Oscar...257, 264, 278

Rennick, Dan...106, 200

Reynolds, Richard...279

Rhudy, Marily H...142, 205, 222, 223, 244pb, 254, 259

Rice, Charles...110, 111, 112, 255, 259, 264

Richards, A. E...257

Richards, Leon W...274

Richards, Richard Q...244pb, 254, 260

Richardson, James...166

Richardson, Willard S...260

Richardson, William S...258, 264

Richtmann, William O...270, 275

Rico, Ulysses...93

Ridway, Ethel...90

Reinders, Thomas P...268

Rigg, Robert...271

Riggs, Leib L...257, 260, 264

Riggs, Mrs. Leib L...277

Rising, Louis Wait...51, 273, 274

Rittenhouse, Henry N...258

Rivard, W. Henry...273

Y

Yacobi, Avraham...273, 274
Yalkowsky, Samuel H...267
Yasutake, George...267
Yeager, Alvin A...257, 265
Yee, Chester D...221, 265
Yee, Gary C...268
Young, George O...268, 278
Young, Kathleen...276

Youngken, Jr., Heber W...204, 205, 273, 276
Youngken, Sr., Heber W...200, 270, 275, 278

Z

Zapapas, Richard...271
Zayas-Bazan, Hector...280
Zellmer, William...53

Zerbe, Bernard...104, 281
Ziegler, Ronald...47
Ziegler, Washington H...256, 265, 273
Zoeller, Edward V...278
Zoernig, Heinrich...280
Zografi, George...266, 267
Zopf, Louis C...56, 124, 260, 274, 275
Zugich, John...274
Zupko, Arthur G...278

Illustration Credits

Photographs and illustrations employed in this book have been obtained from the following sources. The photographer is identified when known.

Adams & Frank Co. Photography, 64 (now in APhA Foundation Archives)

American Institute of the History of Pharmacy, 10, 35, 60 (top), 68, 172, 204, 207-208

American Pharmaceutical Association Foundation Archives, Frontispiece, 2, 4-6, 12-13, 15-16, 18-19, 20 (top), 21-26, 29-31, 34, 36-38, 41-42, 44, 46-47, 52, 56-57, 60 (bottom), 65-66, 69-70, 72-73, 75-77, 79-81, 84, 86, 89 (bottom), 90, 92-97, 102, 105-106, 109-110, 112-114, 116, 118-119, 121-122, 125-127, 130, 132, 139 (top), 139, 141, 143, 145, 149, 153 (bottom), 158, 161-162, 164, 167, 170, 174, 176, 178-180, 182 184, 186, 188, 190, 192, 194-195, 199-200, 202-203, 209-215, 217-219, 221-223, 225-249, 251.

Aron, Don, Photography, 153 (top), 169 (top), 220 (now in APhA Foundation Archives)

Babst, Ed, Photography, 198 (now in APhA Foundation Archives)

Broadway Photo Shop, 104 (now in APhA Foundation Archives)

Caspari, C. S., Collection, 158 (now in APhA Foundation Archives)

Chase Photo, Ltd., 42 (now in APhA Foundation Archives)

Culver Pictures Inc., 61 (now in APhA Foundation Archives)

Davis, Freemont, Photography, 99 (now in APhA Foundation Archives)

deTurro, L. V., Photography, 134 (now in APhA Foundation Archives)

Dohme City Photographers, 82 (now in APhA Foundation Archives)

Dupuy, Eugene, Collection, 17 (now in APhA Foundation Archives)

Finnigan & Associates Photography, 146 (now in APhA Foundation Archives)

Giorno, Chuck, Photography, 87, 224 (now in APhA Foundation Archives)

Glatt, Larry, Photography, 49 (now in APhA Foundation Archives)

Griffenhagen, George, Collection, 131, 165, 196-197

Hathcox, David, Photography, 53, 140 (bottom), (now in APhA Foundation Archives)

Helfand, William H., Collection, 28, 55, 155, 160, 163, 165

Kaufmann-Fabry Photographers, 168 (now in APhA Foundation Archives)

Library of Congress, 129

McLuaghlin Brothers Photography, 181 (now in APhA Foundation Archives)

McNulty & Graham Photography, 71, 150 (now in APhA Foundation Archives)

Munson of Long Beach Photography, 63 (now in APhA Foundation Archives)

Neary, Lowell, Photography, 136 (now in APhA Foundation Archives)

Oscar & Associates Photography, 169 (bottom) (now in APhA Foundation Archives)

Philadelphia College of Pharmacy and Science, 14 (photograph by Dennis Worthen)

Runge, Mary Munson, Collection, 138 (bottom)

Reni Newsphoto Service, 31, 95 (bottom), (now in APhA Foundation Archives)

Reedy, Bruce, Photography, 205 (now in APhA Foundation Archives)

Schick, Jules, Photography, 140 (top), (now in APhA Foundation Archives)

Smithsonian Institution, 2, 68, 89 (top)

Spencer Photographers, 152 (now in APhA Foundation Archives)

U. S. Army, 201

U. S. Goverment Printing Office, 8

U. S. National Archives, 11, 108

U. S. Pharmacopeial Convention, 115

Whelpley, Henry M., Collection, 20 (bottom), 33, 58 (bottom), 100, 102 (now in APhA Foundation Archives)

Author and Collaborating Editors

George B. Griffenhagen (author) is a 1949 graduate in pharmacy from the University of Southern California, with a 1950 M.S. in pharmaceutical chemistry. He served as 1952-1959 curator of the Smithsonian Institution Division of Medical Sciences; 1959-1989 senior staff member of the American Pharmaceutical Association; 1962-1976 editor of the *Journal of the American Pharmaceutical Association*; and 1990-1991 APhA honorary president. Author of 15 books and more than 100 articles on the history of pharmacy and pharmaceutical philately; his first book, *The Story of California Pharmacy* (1950), and his most recent book, *History of Drug Containers and Their Labels* (1999), were published by the American Institute of the History of Pharmacy of which he is a past president and current secretary.

Gregory J. Higby (collaborating editor) is a 1977 graduate in pharmacy from the University of Michigan, and 1984 recipient of a Ph.D. in the history of pharmacy from the University of Wisconsin-Madison. He has served as the director of the American Institute of the History of Pharmacy since 1988; editor of *Pharmacy in History* since 1987; and adjunct professor at the University of Wisconsin School of Pharmacy. A third generation pharmacist, he has written extensively on the history of American pharmacy. His first book, *In Service to American Pharmacy*, published in 1992 by the University of Alabama Press, discusses the career of William Procter, Jr., a primary founder of APhA.

Glenn Sonnedecker (collaborating editor) is a 1942 graduate in pharmacy from Ohio State University, and became the first American to earn a Ph.D. degree in the history of pharmacy and science, granted in 1952 by the University of Wisconsin-Madison. He was a member of the editorial staff of Science Service 1942-1943, and editor of the *Journal of the American Pharmaceutical Association* 1943-1948. He served on the faculty of the University of Wisconsin (history of pharmacy) 1952-1986; and director of the American Institute of the History of Pharmacy 1957-1973 and 1981-1985. He was also 1983-1991 president of the International Academy of the History of Pharmacy, and is author or co-author of more than one hundred articles and books.

John P. Swann (collaborating editor) is a 1979 graduate in chemistry and history from the University of Kansas, and 1985 recipient of a Ph.D. in pharmacy and the history of science from the University of Wisconsin-Madison. He served as senior research associate at the University of Texas Medical Branch 1986-1989, and since 1989 he has served as historian at the U.S. Food and Drug Administration in Rockville, Maryland. His publications have focused on the history of drugs, biomedical research, the pharmaceutical industry, and regulatory history. His book, *Academic Scientists and the Pharmaceutical Industry*, was published by Johns Hopkins University Press in 1988, and translated and published in Japanese in 1992.

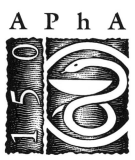

APhA

1852–2002